Field's

Anatomy, Palpation
and Surface Markings

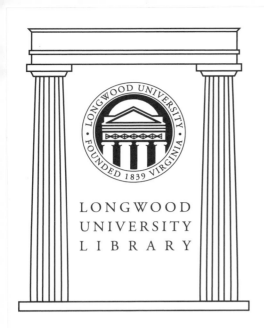
For Elsevier Ltd:

Publisher: Heidi Harrison
Associate Editor: Siobhan Campbell
Production Manager: David Fleming
Design: Andrew Chapman
Illustrator: Derek Field

Field's

Anatomy, Palpation and Surface Markings

Fourth edition

Derek Field Grad Dip Phys, FCSP, Dip TP
Former Vice Principal , North London School of Physiotherapy, City University, London

Jane Owen Hutchinson MA(ED), MCSP, SRP, Dip TP
Manager, Physiotherapy Support Service, Royal National Institute of the Blind, London

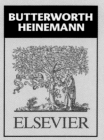

EDINBURGH LONDON NEW YORK OXFORD PHILADELPHIA ST LOUIS SYDNEY TORONTO 2006

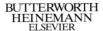

BUTTERWORTH
HEINEMANN
ELSEVIER

An imprint of Elsevier Limited

First published 1994
Second edition 1997
Third edition 2001
Fourth edition 2006

© 2006, Elsevier Ltd

The right of Derek Field and Jane Owen Hutchinson to be identified as authors of this work has been asserted by them in accordance with the Copyright, Designs and Patents Act 1988.

ISBN 10: 0 7506 8848 3
ISBN 13: 978 0 7506 8848 2

British Library Cataloguing in Publication Data
A catalogue record for this book is available from the British Library.

Library of Congress Cataloging in Publication Data
A catalog record for this book is available from the Library of Congress.

Note
Neither the Publisher nor the Authors assume any responsibility for any loss or injury and/or damage to persons or property arising out of or related to any use of the material contained in this book. It is the responsibility of the treating practitioner, relying on independent expertise and knowledge of the patient, to determine the best treatment and method of application for the patient.

Printed in China

The Publisher's Policy is to use Paper manufactured from sustainable forests.

ELSEVIER
your source for books,
journals and multimedia
in the health sciences
www.elsevierhealth.com

Working together to grow
libraries in developing countries

www.elsevier.com | www.bookaid.org | www.sabre.org

ELSEVIER   BOOK AID International   Sabre Foundation

The
Publisher's
policy is to use
**paper manufactured
from sustainable forests**

Contents

Introduction to prefaces

It was again decided, that in this Fourth Edition of Field's Anatomy, Palpation and Surface Markings, (formerly, Anatomy, Palpation and Surface Markings), it would be of some interest to the student of anatomy to include the preface to the First, Second and Third Editions. This would explain how the book was conceived and some of the reasoning and developments which have taken place in the production of this Fourth Edition. The basic plan has always been the same; to produce a book which is easy to read with clear photographs and drawings facilitating the accumulation of knowledge of the human body and endeavouring to make the study of anatomy a pleasant and enjoyable assignment.

In this Fourth Edition we have introduced a new self assessment section at the end of each main area of study. This will give the student a more active role in the learning process and add a sense of participation in their accumulation of anatomical knowledge. To make full use of this additional facility it is recommended that the preface to the Fourth Edition is studied with care.

Preface to the first edition

The aim of this book is to familiarize the student of anatomy with a basic plan of the human body, combining this knowledge with the art of palpation. This is a vital discipline for a true understanding of the relationship of structures with the surface, and provides both students and practitioners with an ability to visualize these structures through the skin.

The book is designed to be an adjunct to the study of anatomy; therefore, only details of bone, joint structure, muscle attachments, nerve origins and distributions which can be palpated or determined from the surface will be included. Nevertheless, the text, with its illustrations on facing pages, where possible, provide the student and practitioner with a source of information which is designed to be clear and easy to understand. It should also stimulate the anatomist to develop the ability to palpate all types of structure below the skin, as well as the quality of movement in joints, and tension and texture in tissues. Finally, with practice, it is hoped that the palpator will develop the ability to identify fine movements, tissue and joint damage and other anomalies which will facilitate patient assessment.

There are five main sections of the book: the upper limb, the lower limb, the head and neck, the thorax and the abdomen. Each is divided into the following subsections: bones, joints, muscles, nerves, arteries and veins. The lymphatic system has been excluded as it is normally impossible to palpate, although the drainage routes can be seen from time to time, particularly when there is an infection in the region drained. The lymph nodes are also difficult to palpate unless they are enlarged as a consequence of pathological reaction.

Wherever possible, the left-hand page of text contains information on palpation, with an outline of the surface markings. The facing page consists of photographs of the region taken from different angles, beside which is a line drawing indicating the underlying structures, together with measurements, where possible, showing the relationship between the structures. Between the photographs and the line drawings is a list of structures of importance, identified by arrows where appropriate.

Much of the information in the following pages has been acquired from the study of the living body, dissections and numerous standard anatomical textbooks. The reader is recommended to refer to as many authors as possible to ensure a broad knowledge and understanding of anatomy.

Preface to the second edition

Due to the popularity and success of the first edition of this book it has been decided to cease reprints and move immediately into the production of a second edition.

The aims and layout of this second edition are very similar to those in the first, with improvements being made to the index and text. Drawings and photographs are, where possible, facing relevant text with the labelling shared between photographs and drawings. Full colour has now been used to give greater clarification to the photographs and in addition the headings of each section have been highlighted. The cover illustration has been altered to portray the palpating hands on the surface of the shoulder.

To improve the accuracy of the identification of structures below the surface and for the benefit of those searching for the structure, small black dots were applied to the surface marking of the structures before the photographs were taken. This, combined with accurate photography, has ensured the portrayal of the exact location of structures not seen below the surface.

These improvements have been incorporated to enhance the clarity and appearance of the book. It is hoped that the reader, whether studying anatomy for medicine, sport or purely for pleasure will derive as much information and interest from this second edition as from the first.

Preface to the third edition

With the continuing popularity and success of the second edition of Anatomy, Palpation and Surface Markings there was a great deal of discussion as to whether it was going to be necessary or even helpful to produce a third edition. The second edition has become a 'best seller' in the Butterworth-Heinemann medical books section and appeared to give the reader the information and stimulus that was needed for the application of the art of palpation to the study of living anatomy. The author, however, being presented with the opportunity to develop some of the ideas which had been impossible to use in the first and second editions, due to cost and space, felt that vast improvements could be made.

Much of the text assumed that the student had a basic knowledge of anatomy and that the shape and construction of underlying structures would be known. With the additional space for text it meant that a short description could precede the area to be examined, thus avoiding the necessity of checking in other books. It must be pointed out, however, that only a basic outline of description is given. This extra space for text also allowed the introduction of additional sections on:

Outline descriptions of bones and muscles
Palpation on movement
Functional anatomy
General location and description of organs
Outline of joint structure, etc.

All of these, it is hoped, will increase the quest for further knowledge in the student.

Having the photograph and drawing opposite the relevant text in the first and second editions was a feature which was praised by many readers. It was therefore decided to improve this facility by, where possible, placing the photograph opposite the drawing and labelling them both so that they line up on each page. This allows more labels to be added to the drawings to help with the location of more bony features. It was also felt that being able to locate the labelled point in the text would save time. The relevant word in the text has therefore been highlighted in blue.

The photographs and drawings have been enlarged to improve their clarity and the text has been divided into four separate blocks below, while still maintaining the clear print. The page headers are again highlighted in a blue strip but the sections have been re-ordered to improve their location.

The enlargement of photographs and drawings, the positioning of the text below with highlighted labels, the additional sections and the improved general layout of this third edition should ease the burden of study for the student of anatomy and help to develop an enjoyment in the investigation of anatomical structures which are palpable deep to the skin.

Preface to the fourth edition

Whilst the success of the three previous editions of this book has been considerable, it was deemed appropriate, when preparing this 4th edition, to undertake a complete re-evaluation of the text in the light of current professional educational philosophy and clinical practice.

As a consequence, Chapter 1 has been re-written with a view to reflecting current trends in relation to the underpinning principles of medical practice; further, it attempts to provide a more detailed analysis of the nature of touch and its significance in relation to the practice of the art of palpation. Throughout the remainder of the book, a different approach to the study of anatomy and palpation skills has been adopted which more accurately reflects the study methods undertaken by students on many professionally validated programmes throughout the UK. Because this approach is based on the principle that individuals learn best when they play an active part in the learning process, students are required to become more self-directed than before, to take a greater responsibility for their own learning and to engage in exploring the practical significance of their theoretical knowledge. To date, our experience indicates that whilst learners often find these methods more challenging initially, they eventually regard them as extremely rewarding and more enjoyable than the more traditional approaches to teaching which might have been encountered during secondary education.

It is worth emphasising that the student cannot practice the art of palpation successfully without having gained a sound knowledge base in anatomy and physiology. Our text is designed to encourage and enable the student to undertake a regular evaluation of theoretical knowledge and its practical application. To be a skilled palpator requires the practitioner to be able to identify and locate the various anatomical structures of the body which requires regular practice, evaluation and modification of techniques.

For these reasons, we have introduced a self-assessment section which follows each separate anatomical area of the body. This consists of a series of questions, diagrams and photographs relating to the text of the particular section. The questions are set out in sections, with page numbers and with each question having a space below for the answer. The number indicates the page on which the answer to the question can be found. This system will enable the reader to return to the appropriate page, should a gap in knowledge have been identified following review. Some of the questions are based on knowledge and understanding which should have been gained from the study of that particular section although the specific answers may not be found in the text itself. In such cases, the question will be followed by a sign (fr) which will indicate to the student that further reading from other texts will/may be required.

The diagrams and/or photographs will be found on the right hand page facing the appropriate set of questions. Each diagram and/or photograph will be furnished with a set of leader lines and a space for the reader to insert the name of the part indicated. Once again, after completing the task of inserting text into all of the spaces provided, the student should refer back to the original diagram/photograph If any omissions or mistakes are identified, the student should return to the diagram/photograph for further study and then enter or/alter any text in the spaces provided.

If, on review of each of the sections, the student discovers several omissions and/or mistakes, a return to each relevant section in order to undertake further study is strongly recommended. If, on the other hand, the student discovers the presence of omissions and/or mistakes in several sections, it is recommended that an in-depth study of the entire chapter should be undertaken before proceeding further.

Derek Field
Jane Owen Hutchinson
June 2005

Acknowledgements

I would like to welcome Jane Owen Hutchinson M.A.(Ed.). MCSP SRP. Dip.TP., to the writing team of this book. I have known and worked with Jane for many years and have always admired her ability to express in text her knowledge and original ideas. With her input we intend this book to become an even more popular addition to the student's bookshelf and with the changes we are making it should become an essential part of the modern student's self assessment programme.

I would also like to take this opportunity to thank my colleagues, friends and readers from all over the world who have assisted me in the production of this 4th edition of Field's Anatomy, formerly just Anatomy, Palpation and Surface Markings.

My thanks go to Anthony B. Ward LBIPP, of Churchill Ward Associates, Long Hanborough, for shooting the many photographs used in the 3rd and 4th editions. My thanks also go to Tim Brown and Sally Ede for posing for the many photographs.

I must express a special thank you to Heidi Allen and Siobhan Campbell, who, together with their colleagues at Reed Elsevier, Oxford, made our task more enjoyable by easing our workload wherever possible.

Finally, I would like to express a very special thank you to Yvonne, my wife, who has spent many hours of organizing schedules and work sessions, reading and editing all manners of information and research, helping to collate the dots on the photographs with the labels and most importantly for her encouragement.

Derek Field

Palpation: definition, application and practice

Contents

SOME DEFINITIONS AND CONCEPTS

Palpation: some definitions

The Oxford Dictionary of English defines the verb to palpate as: 'to examine (a part of the body) by touch, especially for medical purposes'. Its derivative noun is 'palpation' (from the Latin verb 'palpare': to 'feel or touch gently'.) According to *The Chambers Dictionary*, the term 'palp' means 'to feel, examine or explore by touch'; 'palpare' is defined as 'to touch softly, stroke, caress or flatter'. *Churchill's Medical Dictionary* defines palpation as 'to stroke, caress; to explore or examine by touching and probing with the hands and fingers'.

Whilst 'stroking', 'caressing' or (tactile) 'flattering' represent practices (through 'gentle touch') that are essentially designed to give physiological and psychological 'healing' to the recipient, palpation, for the purposes of this text, is primarily a purposeful activity requiring considerable skill. It is associated with methodical exploration and detailed manual examination, the aim of which is to acquire objective information that will eventually lead to a reasoned medical diagnosis upon which a subsequent treatment regimen can be based. *Gould's Medical Dictionary* makes the direct link between the activity of palpation and diagnosis by gentle touch which involves the detection of the 'characteristics and condition of local tissues of the underlying organs or tumors'.

In *The Oxford Dictionary of English,* to examine is defined as 'to test; to inquire into; to question; to look closely at or into; to inspect'. According to *The Chambers Dictionary*, to examine is to 'inspect (someone or something) thoroughly in order to determine the nature of a condition'. The activity involves critical, reflective thinking: the systematic weighing up of evidence in an attempt to arrive at a balanced conclusion.

General characteristics of palpation

Palpation is a highly complex and sophisticated manual skill. Citing Frymann, Chaitow (2003) draws attention to the potential which palpation offers members of the healing professions:

> The human hand is equipped with instruments to perceive changes in texture, surface texture, surface humidity, to penetrate and detect successively deeper tissue textures, turgescence, elasticity and irritability. The human hand, furthermore, is designed to detect minute motion, motion which can only be detected by the most sensitive electronic pick-up devices available. This carries the art of palpation beyond the various modalities of touch into the realm of proprioception, of

changes in position and tension within our own muscular system.

> (Chaitow 2003)

As Frymann emphasizes, the hand is particularly well equipped to play the key role in this activity. With reference to palpation of the human body, Chaitow reminds us that different parts of the hand possess the ability to discriminate between variations in tissue features: '… relative tension, texture, degree of moisture, temperature and so on.' He then makes the important point that 'This highlights the fact that an individual's overall palpatory sensitivity depends on a combination of different perceptive (and proprioceptive) qualities and abilities' (Chaitow 2003).

TOUCH

Some general characteristics

Palpation involves the use of one of the primary senses, that of touch, in order to investigate and obtain information or to supplement that already gained by other means, such as by visual and auditory input. As Poon (1995) points out:

> The act of touching and the feeling of being touched are very powerful experiences … (and touch) is the earliest and most primitive form of communication.

> (Poon 1995)

Montague (1978) reminds us that:

> Touch is the first of the senses to develop in the embryo and it plays a very important role in the birth process itself and in the early life of the individual.

> (Montague 1978)

Not only is it the earliest system to become functional in the human being but touch is also thought to be the last of the senses to be lost immediately prior to death.

Touch plays a very significant part in our everyday experience:

> When the other senses are not wholly effective, we return to the sense of touch to rediscover reality. Clothing is *felt* to determine its quality, fruit is *squeezed* to determine its ripeness and paint is *touched* to test for dryness.

> (Mason 1985)

Experience suggests, however, that there are instances when touch is often subjugated in favour of reliance upon other sensory modalities. Only when an awareness of an alteration in incoming stimuli occurs do we become conscious of the sense of touch. An example of this phenomenon might be when picking up a garment, we recognize its unfamiliarity through its texture or 'feel'; another example might be an awareness of the material of trousers touching the legs immediately after a long period of wearing shorts.

Touch may be divided into two distinct categories: instrumental and expressive. Touch is described as instrumental when it is associated with a deliberate action: locating an anatomical structure for the purposes of examination during a clinical assessment, for example. Touch is identified as expressive when it is associated with spontaneous, affective actions: touching a distressed person's arm in order to convey sympathy and offer comfort (MacWhannell 1992, Poon 1995).

Touch can be experienced as safe or unsafe; physically comfortable or uncomfortable. It can be used to establish rapport: hand-shaking as a formal greeting at the beginning of a clinical interview or as a means of ending a treatment session. Communication by touch is specifically permitted within particular interpersonal relationships (see later). In certain contexts, however, permission to touch may be required, for example, at the commencement, and during the various stages of a clinical examination and treatment session. Touch is associated with psychological reactions: it is difficult to touch or be touched by those who elicit negative responses. The anticipation of touching or being touched can increase stress levels and these reactions may be influenced by personality, cultural and social factors: some female patients may deliberately avoid consulting a male therapist; some patients may be reluctant to remove clothing. It is important to remember that professional personnel are placed in an extremely powerful and privileged position in relation to others: they are given a license to touch and this power and privilege should never be abused.

The physiology of touch

All areas of the skin supplied with appropriate receptors are normally able to perceive a variety of sensations (pain, degrees of pressure, temperature changes, etc.) to a greater or lesser degree. Some areas, however, are more sensitive to stimuli than others because:

> The degree of tactile sensitivity in any area is in direct proportion to the number of sensory units present and active in that area, as well as to the degree of overlap of their receptive fields, which vary in size. Small receptive fields with many sensory units therefore have the highest degree of discriminatory sensitivity.
>
> (Chaitow 2003)

Sensitivity to spatial discrimination is poor in the lumbar region, the legs and the back of the hands. In the back of the hands, for example, two points can only be perceived separately if they are more than 50–100 mm apart. The lips, tongue and fingertips, however, rate high (1–3 mm). Thus individuals with normal sensation in the fingertips should be able to distinguish between two points even when they are less than six mm apart. This is referred to as the 'Two Point Discrimination Test' (see Chaitow 2003, Evans 2000, Magee 1997). The significance of this is that only relatively large objects can be recognized by the receptors in the lumbar region whereas fine point discrimination can be achieved when employing the fingertips.

Chaitow makes the further point that:

> Not only is there a difference of perception relating to spatial accuracy, but also one relating to intensity. An indentation of 6 micrometers is capable of being registered on the finger pads, while 24 micrometers is needed before the sensors in the palm of the hand reach their threshold and perceive the stimulus.
>
> (Chaitow 2003)

Additionally, Evans (2000) contends that:

> Under normal conditions, touch is an exploratory sense rather than purely receptive, and it is becoming increasingly evident that tactile acuity is enhanced in active exploration when compared with passive reception.
>
> (Evans 2000)

Citing Meyers, Etherington and Ashcroft (1958) Evans suggests that:

> An early indication of the phenomenon may be seen in an examination of the parameters of perception required to read Braille. The dots are separated by 2.3 mm, which is close to the threshold value for two-point discrimination at the pad of the index finger. Reduction of the inter-dot space to 1.9 mm only moderately reduces the legibility of the Braille text.
>
> (Evans 2000)

While sighted Braille transcribers, relying solely on visual input, have been known to become proficient at reading Braille by the end of only three weeks, experience confirms that individuals attempting to conquer the system by touch are estimated to take an average of 1½–2 years to reach a speed suitable for serious study, even with regular practice. This is not due to lack of knowledge of the system; rather it is because the palpation and recognition of the signs using tactile input requires a considerable amount of dedicated time and practice in which to develop. As with all skills, the speed and quality of reading depends upon the frequency and amount of use. The ability to palpate with any finger or fingers can usually be developed, the use of the index finger being the most popular. Reading speed is further enhanced by using the fingers of both hands. In some cases, this skill never develops if the individual has not learnt to employ touch from an early age. In rare instances, people who have been unable to use their fingers have developed the same ability to read Braille by using their toes or even their lips! (see above). This means that regardless of the method by which this skill is acquired, the ability to increase the information received through sensory input can be improved, given time and serious dedication to regular practice. This can be of great benefit to the clinical practitioner who wishes to 'read' information that lies deep to the skin. The controlled use of pressure and movement, coupled with feedback and experience, unlocks a vast quantity of information that is often unavailable to the eye.

Obtaining information through touch is a skill, the practical significance of which is often not fully appreciated or valued until it is needed, perhaps to compensate for the impairment or loss of one of the other senses: sight or hearing, for example. Because of this, considerable practice is often required before the skill of palpation becomes developed to the point where it is of practical use to the individual concerned (see above). Initially, new techniques have to be devised and then undertaken slowly and carefully, with regular practice and evaluation, often involving feedback from other observers with consequent modification of behaviour. Efforts to recognize and accurately interpret tactile sensory input demand high levels of concentration which necessarily cause anxiety and additional stress to an individual who is unaccustomed to placing such reliance on this variety of incoming stimuli. These reactions are likely to be experienced by the novice clinical practitioner as well as by the recently disabled person and should be regarded as normal responses to the process of acquiring a new range of sophisticated psychomotor skills and personal strategies (Owen Hutchinson, Atkinson and Orpwood 1998).

In other non-medical contexts, touch-related skills are used to acquire general information about the environment such as establishing the temperature of water. A thermometer could be employed for this purpose, but it is often easier (and quicker) to test water temperature by utilizing the input from the sensory endings in the skin. While the results of this method of temperature testing are likely to be far less accurate than if a thermometer were to be used, they provide a range of potentially significant information upon which subsequent action could be based. The water temperature, for example, might be experienced as burning, scorching, boiling, extremely hot, very hot, fairly hot, hot, quite hot, very warm, blood heat, warm, fairly warm, slightly warm, cool, cold, quite cold, very cold, bitterly cold, freezing and icy cold. A temperature of 42°C read from a thermometer has little practical meaning as to whether something is too hot or too cold to touch.

The social significance of touch

The concept of the novice engaged in learning to interpret incoming stimuli received through touch extends, of course, into the realm of social interaction. As suggested above, touch can represent a powerful means of expressive communication (Nathan 1999). The way in which this communication is interpreted will be contingent upon such variables as personality, upbringing, culture and social situation and, in these contexts, it seems unhelpful to separate touch into mechanical and psychosocial categories. Referring to a medical intervention, Nathan contends that:

> Touching a person's body in a non therapeutic context is not normally considered an act of merely mechanical significance. Nor is it a procedure of a technique – rather it is an act of self-expression, or occasionally self-assertion, or preservation.
>
> (Nathan 1999)

The degree to which people will engage in touching will be dictated by the nature of the interpersonal relationship in which they are involved at the time. Nathan continues:

> In the main, frequent touching is reserved for parent–child relationships, lovers and close friends. In these contexts it both signifies emotional intimacy and is emotionally significant.
>
> (Nathan 1999)

Touch can be employed to communicate a variety of emotions. For example, affection may be conveyed by a gentle squeeze of the hand whereas a loose handshake may imply indifference or even dislike. Touching and being touched can be extremely therapeutic. Montague summarizes the observations of many researchers who conclude that:

> Cutaneous stimulation in the various forms in which the newborn and young receive it is of prime importance for their healthy physical and behavioural development … It appears probable that for human beings, tactile stimulation is of fundamental significance for development of healthy, emotional and affectional relationships.
>
> (Montague 1978)

Montague quotes examples of cases that were studied by Lorna Marshall, a researcher who spent much time between 1950 and 1961 living among the Bushmen of the Kalahari Desert in Botswana, South West Africa. He observed that, within this society, the development of the newborn, infant, adolescent and adult appeared to be influenced by the way in which the child was handled in early life. Montague also refers to accounts by Margaret Mead, who studied the Arapesh and Mundugumor societies in New Guinea during the 1930s and documented the characteristics of their respective social practices. In the former tribe, the child was in contact with the mother for most of the day. The adults of this tribe were observed to be kind, happy and peace-loving people. In the latter tribe, the child had little human contact, being kept in a rough plaited basket which was usually suspended from the mother's forehead. The adults of this tribe were observed to become unattractive, aggressive and cannibalistic.

The tendency to avoid close physical contact can be demonstrated in adults from certain cultures and within some social backgrounds of particular nationalities. Montague comments that 'There exists not only cultural and national differences in tactile behaviour but also class differences.' He cites the English upper class as a an example of a social group that is characterized by non-tactile social behaviour when compared with social groups of other nationalities: French and Italian people display more demonstrative behaviour when greeting one another and are observed to engage in more physical interpersonal contact.

When considering the practice of palpation skills, the significance of Montague's observations cannot be underestimated. Not only is it crucial for us to recognize the relevance of culture, nationality and social class on the degree to which people communicate by touch, but also the impact of living in a multicultural society in which we are likely to encounter unfamiliar and potentially disconcerting practices. Additionally the effect of globalization on our patterns of non-verbal communication has been considerable.

In contrast to the somewhat reserved behaviour of English people in the 19th and early 20th centuries, we now regularly witness overt instances of emotion (love and friendship, happiness and sadness) through physical contact. Behaviour such as mutual embracing, hand-holding and kissing is frequently to be observed in public places. Sportspeople will leap in the air and hug each other following a winning achievement such as the scoring of a goal in football; equally, it is not uncommon for athletes to display tears of misery and frustration and to engage in mutually sympathetic embraces after a failure to attain high standards of performance.

Touch and clinical practice

Palpation, then, would seem to be a practice which involves a combination of many other skilled activities: the appropriate use of touch, the application of methodical investigatory techniques, accurate interpretation of sensory feedback (based upon sound general knowledge), the ability to draw on previous experience, to reflect, critically, upon findings and arrive at a reasoned conclusion.

Palpation is the art of feeling tissues with your hands in such a manner that changes in tension and position within these tissues can be readily noticed, diagnosed and treated.

(Mitchell, Moran and Pruzzo (1979) cited in Chaitow 2003)

A skill is attained and retained by its continual use, evaluation and modification of practice (Phillips 2004). The study and practice of manual contact techniques over a long period of time enables the practitioner to become highly skilled in the art of palpation. The development of this skill provides valuable supplementary information to that which can be obtained through observation and verbal questioning and is crucial to arriving at a meaningful clinical diagnosis. After many years experience of practising palpation skills, the moving, stretching and compression of tissues will be undertaken with precise control. This will enable the therapist to receive and interpret vital information from the patient and to apply and modify techniques as appropriate. Small changes in tension, temperature, dampness, movement and swelling will be identified by the sense of touch; these will then be noted and the appropriate course of action taken. Grieve states:

Of the entire objective examination of the vertebral column, the palpation examination of accessible tissues is probably the most informative and therefore the most valuable.

(Grieve 1986)

As has been noted above, however, learning to palpate is also associated with acquiring the skills to 'read', accurately, the patient's problem. Citing Ford (1989) Chaitow reminds us that:

In days gone by, when a physician had to diagnose by touch a good practitioner did not feel a tumour at his fingertips but he projected his vibratory and pressure sensations into the patient. So we regularly project our sense of touch beyond our physical being and … merely make the ordinarily unconscious process available to our conscious mind. In so doing, we cross the delicate boundary between self and other, to explore, to learn, and ultimately to help.

(Chaitow 2003)

Personal experience confirms that patients can easily distinguish between a novice and an expert practitioner. During the initial examination, both the practitioner and the person being palpated progress through a learning process in which each is engaged in assessing the other by the giving and receiving of information. Relatively little significant information can be obtained if one of the participants in this relationship is reluctant to communicate. This learning process takes time and it is often the case that an accurate picture of the underlying issues does not appear until much later in the treatment session. The reason for this is partly due to the need for each participant to become comfortable with the other, so permitting mutual reduction in anxiety and the relaxation of tension. It is also due to the need for both parties to become familiar with the learning process itself, so that each can benefit from the knowledge gained as a result of their participation in this two-way event. The skill of palpation, therefore, should not be regarded merely as an arbitrary form of physical intervention; rather it must be respected as a highly skilled investigative process which elicits specialized information to both participants. In our experience, the skill of palpation is estimated to be only 10% innate: the other 90% is acquired through dedicated practice.

EFFECTS OF PALPATION ON THE PATIENT

Patient and person

It is far beyond the scope of this book to enter into the complexities of the mind–body debate, but its significance in relation to clinical diagnosis and management cannot be ignored. Traditionally, medical practice has been characterized by the biomedical model of health. This model is underpinned by the philosophical principles of dualism: the mind and body are regarded as separate and distinct entities that do not interact and, essentially, the practitioner is engaged in treating one or the other. The manual therapist would, in this context therefore, be regarded as being concerned only with the treatment of the patient's body. Indeed, it is not uncommon to hear therapists refer to a patient as 'a neck' or 'a back'. The body is considered to resemble a sophisticated machine; if part of that machine is malfunctioning, physical intervention is required in order to rectify the fault (Chaitow in Nathan 1999, Christensen, Jones and Edwards 2004, Owen Hutchinson 2004).

The 1990s, however, have witnessed significant changes in the approach towards illness and disability with the consequent development of the biopsychosocial model of disability which 'is a way of conceptualizing the multifactorial and complex system that shapes a person's experiences of pain and disability' (Christensen, Jones and Edwards 2004.) Citing various sources, Christensen, Jones and Edwards explain the biopsychosocial theory:

> … the degree of disability a person develops will be based upon the reactions of that person to the pain experienced far more than on the physical experience of the pain itself. The biopsychosocial model places a complaint of pain into a more holistic context, and views the pain as important not in isolation, but in relation to any disability the person with pain is experiencing as a result of that pain.
>
> (Christensen, Jones and Edwards 2004)

(See also Ramsden 1999, Stevenson, Grieves and Stein-Parbury 2004).

The last decade has also witnessed a growth in the popularity of complementary medicine, whose underlying holistic principles stand in direct contrast to those of orthodox medical practice. This trend would suggest that patients prefer to be treated as whole persons rather than as bodies requiring cures. When they seek consultation with a therapist, patients are asking for help with more than just a painful neck or back: they want far more than to be the passive recipient of skillfully performed physical techniques. Indeed, patients regard a satisfactory healing experience as one that acknowledges the inextricable links between mind and body and which therefore treats the whole person who is more than just the sum of a collection of constituent parts. Recognizing this, the therapist must adopt an empathic and sensitive approach to all input from the patient, both in terms of verbal and non-verbal communication. Social and cultural factors must also be taken into account.

The quality of all clinical interventions will improve dramatically if the person-centered approach to patient management is adopted. The therapist, however, should not underestimate the degree to which patients have learned the conventions associated with society in general and medicine in particular. During the session, patients will often choose to use language to conceal as well as to reveal emotional states: 'That movement does not hurt any more'; 'I feel much freer now'. It must always be remembered that the patient has this choice. It must also be borne in mind that some patients may not have recognized the link between physical and psychological states and may need to be encouraged to reflect upon their choice of language in order to gain insight into certain aspects of their emotional lives.

As has been suggested above, the act of touching and the feeling of being touched are very powerful experiences and the degree to which people engage in touching is largely contingent upon personality, cultural and social factors. Both patient and therapist may experience an increase in stress levels due to unfamiliarity within particular therapeutic contexts. The practitioner must demonstrate a respect for the patient as a person. Permission to touch should be obtained at the commencement, and during the various stages of a clinical intervention. Abuse of power and the privilege of being licensed to touch must be avoided.

The consultation process

For a variety of physical and psychosocial reasons, many patients remain reluctant to consult professional personnel on matters associated with their personal issues, especially those problems relating to their own bodies. Barriers may be erected by one or both participants in the therapist–patient relationship, although both must contribute to the dismantling of these barriers if effective communication and co-operation are to be achieved. Experience suggests that each patient usually presents with a combination of issues which are revealed by the identification of problems, the giving of information and the posing of a number of questions during the consultation process. Typically, no particular order of priority emerges except perhaps that associated with the overriding presence of pain. Some of the information provided by the patient may appear to be somewhat peripheral in relation to the practitioner's objective of establishing a clinical diagnosis, but it nevertheless represents a vital component of the overall clinical picture and must be thoroughly evaluated before it can be discounted.

The practitioner must be sympathetically receptive to all forms of information offered by the patient. Standards governing all areas of professional practice demand that the clinician must objectively evaluate all clinical evidence and attempt to produce a comprehensive analysis of the presenting situation. On some occasions, a prescribed plan will be used to facilitate the compilation and evaluation of data; at other times, the practitioner will be expected to tailor the procedure according to the patient's individual circumstances. The use of such strategies will enable the practitioner to arrive at a reasoned clinical diagnosis. Care must be taken, however, that any prescribed plan does not preclude the practitioner from obtaining relevant information from the patient; adherence to such standard proforma can sometimes adversely affect the practitioner's judgement and thus lead to an incorrect clinical assessment of the patient's current problem.

It is crucial that the practitioner should manage the initial investigation with great care and sensitivity as this process is likely to have a significant influence on both parties during the subsequent clinical examination. The practitioner should exercise the same degree of tact and diplomacy when conducting the subsequent physical examination, which should be undertaken with equal care, precision and gentleness. Physical or verbal clumsiness at this stage of the proceedings could lead to a complete breakdown of the interpersonal relationship between the therapist and patient, who may become reluctant to communicate vital information. The therapist employs palpation techniques during the first contact with the patient and it is vital that efficient methods of obtaining information are employed at this time. Experience suggests that most patients have an expectation that a clinical examination involving the use of palpation techniques will take place; indeed, they

would consider it to be unprofessional practice if such a procedure were not undertaken. Inevitably, each person will exhibit different reactions to being touched and it is important that the practitioner should establish and evaluate the patient's unique reaction to such interventions at the earliest opportunity. An initial indication of the patient's reaction to physical contact can be obtained by the act of hand-shaking at the commencement of the session. Additionally, information gained by the act of assisting the patient to and from a chair can provide the practitioner with valuable feedback relating to the patient's degree of willingness or reluctance to accept help. Of course, such strategies represent only part of the range of techniques being employed during this initial session. The use of visual, auditory and olfactory input can also provide useful sources of relevant clinical information.

During the period of questioning, the practitioner is recommended to make sensitive and careful physical contact with the area of the patient's pain. When these techniques are performed successfully, this encourages both parties to focus attention on the patient's motivation in seeking the consultation. All movements should be tested carefully, palpation skills being employed simultaneously with continual observation of the ongoing situation, the therapist monitoring any reluctance on the part of the patient to perform movements due to tension, muscle spasm, joint anomalies and pain. Inadvertently eliciting symptoms of acute pain will inevitably destroy the patient's confidence resulting in an unwillingness to offer potentially significant information.

In most cases, the patient will gradually gain confidence and learn to trust the practitioner. Much of the apprehension of meeting will have passed during the initial contact. When the time comes for the therapist to undertake an objective physical examination of the patient's movements, rapport should have been well established which overcomes that initial reluctance to seeking of medical advice.

Palpation continues throughout the examination and subsequent treatment. If it is carried out carefully and sympathetically, it reveals valuable information concerning the patient's physical and psychological condition. Indeed, palpation has the potential to 'unlock' psychological issues which had hitherto been deliberately ignored or unrecognized by the patient as having any relevance to the presenting physical problem. Many practitioners will have experience of patients who seek medical consultation for a relatively minor physical ailment which, during the examination or treatment, will be found to be masking much deeper and more complex issues. All practitioners should be sensitive to this possibility and should note any incongruous sentiments that the patient may express during the session. Experience suggests that it is the physical contact with the patient which appears to facilitate the unveiling of these underlying issues but the importance of recognizing this phenomenon is contingent upon the quality of the practitioner's professional training.

That the patient must have confidence in the practitioner cannot be over-emphasized. This will promote the offering of information through both verbal and non-verbal communication methods. Throughout the consultation, the practitioner should be receptive to the patient; as the session progresses, continual evaluation of the patient's verbal and non-verbal reactions to events should take place. Whether complex or simple, all treatment sessions should promote mutual trust and understanding. Experience indicates that the degree to which a patient contributes to the treatment session is directly proportional to the practitioner's input; this reciprocal relationship is, however, contingent on the practitioner's willingness to impart information and the patient's genuine interest in receiving it.

TECHNIQUES OF PALPATION

It is not enough merely to place the hands on the patient's body and hope to receive the information required. Positive steps must be taken to search for the data. As has been noted above, palpation is associated with the seeking of information and all techniques must be approached in a rational and logical manner. The practitioner can gain very little by contacting a surface with the hands and remaining stationary. Movement of the hands is required so that structures can pass under the fingers in a controlled manner so that any alterations in skin temperature, surface tension, and bone structure can be evaluated and recorded. The practitioner's speed of movement can be adjusted to facilitate the full interpretation of information. The importance of regularly modifying the speed of movement can be demonstrated by the following example. If the fingers are run over Braille script too quickly, dots can be felt but no information is obtained; if the individual adapts the speed accordingly, however, what initially appeared to be an incomprehensible mass of dots now becomes an intelligible text.

Sometimes palpation techniques need to be performed slowly and at considerable depth; at other times they should be carried out quickly and at a superficial level. For example, palpation of the transverse processes of the spines of the lumbar region or the hook of the hamate needs careful application of deep pressure, combined with slow movement and sensitivity to the patient's reactions. Palpation of the spines of the thoracic vertebrae – particularly when counting downwards – is much easier if the fingertips are gently moved up and down three or four centimetres at a time, marking each spine with the finger of the other hand and holding it until the position of the next spine is confirmed. This type of palpation works in a similar way to a scanner using a beam to build up a clearer picture. The technique can be used to obtain a clearer picture of the rib cage, particularly from the posterior aspect.

In our experience, using one or even two complete palms and fingertips conveys more information regarding movement below the skin surface and about the patient's general reaction to physical contact than if the fingertips alone were used. The application of the fingertips alone, for example, would be used for palpating a pulse. Generally, if the structures below the surface are stationary, the hands will have to be used in a controlled movement, whereas if the structures are mobile, the hands should remain stationary. The finer the movement below the surface, the more delicate the palpation technique must be: this is clearly demonstrated when searching for a faint pulse.

If joints are being manipulated to examine the quality of movement and to assess limiting factors, the hands should be moved as little as possible so as to avoid any feedback from the palpator's own tissues which would obscure information from those of the patient. In fact, with this kind of palpation, a minimum of all other movements – with the exception of the joint being examined – is required. This involves adopting a stance which will avoid movement of the feet, applying a hold that will allow the full range of movement without change and also reducing all skin sliding by firm contact. Finally, the palpator must be absolutely sure that the patient's position is stable and that the movement being tested is localized to the joint being examined and is in the plane around the axis required. It is not uncommon, when testing the movements of the upper or lower limb, for a 'clicking' or crepitus to occur and neither the patient nor the examiner are able to locate its source. Conversely, if the examiner's thumb nails touch when pressure is being applied to the posterior aspect of the lateral mass of the atlas (C1), the patient may, erroneously, report a grinding sound located in the atlanto-occipital joint.

When examining the end-range of a joint, all variations must be known in advance so that movement, physiological and accessory, is tested accurately, noting the range available and the limiting factors. This is a highly skilled form of palpation, requiring a great deal of practice on normal joints in order to perfect the technique, considerable experience with abnormal joints to be able to recognize the variations and an expert knowledge of the various conditions to assess how much or how little testing should be undertaken. It is not suggested that this form of palpation should be employed by an expert only; on the contrary, the technique should be practised at the earliest opportunity and based on palpation of normal anatomy. Gradually, if care is taken and limits set, considerable skill can be gained.

Experience suggests that some palpators either under-employ the use of touch and try to compensate by observation, or they tend to palpate over-enthusiastically but fail to interpret the significance of what they feel. Some may also feel what they believe they are meant to feel. It is easy to be persuaded by an eager patient, by prior knowledge or by a more experienced observer that one can feel changes that are not actually present. An open and honest interpretation of what is beneath the fingertips is essential: remember Hans Andersen's story of the Emperor's new clothes!

IMPROVING THE ART OF PALPATION

Returning to the example of the Braille reader, improvement in palpation techniques can only be achieved with practice. As with all areas of knowledge, the motivation to learn is crucial. In relation to clinical practice, the learning of good palpation skills is contingent upon the need to know what lies beneath the surface of the body and the desire to find some means of offering help to patients. Practitioners frequently express the wish to be able to 'see what is happening beneath the surface'. These sentiments confirm the importance of developing appropriate palpation techniques which can then be employed as a means of providing assistance. Inextricably linked with this process is the development of manual dexterity and sensitivity.

It is worth noting that, when practising any technique that necessarily involves the use of the hands, the quality of the information that is received through the sense of touch can often be enhanced by reducing the input from the other senses. Closing the eyes and using the hands to recognize different textures, weights, surfaces, liquids, coins, etc. often reveals hitherto unrecognized characteristics of what are regarded as familiar objects. The palpator must endeavour to obtain as much information from the sense of touch as possible. In order to develop this skill, different objects can be placed in a bag and identified only by using the hands. As the skill improves, less familiar objects can be chosen so that they are less recognizable: their shape might be more unusual and/or they may be smaller. All of these objects should be handled sensitively by the palpator who should attempt to identify their distinctive features (such as blemishes). Progression of this exercise would be to require the palpation and identification of the same objects through the material of the bag. The material of the bag could be chosen so that the exercise becomes progressively more difficult: beginning with a relatively thin surface such as fine plastic and gradually changing to a thicker material. Practise should be undertaken regularly during the course of everyday activities, the practitioner always noting the technique which is most suitable for the identification of each object. One suggestion would be habitually to identify the loose change in a pocket or purse before removing the correct amount to make a purchase. Recognition of coins is a relatively easy task and it should be unnecessary to use vision in order to verify the amount tendered. Take care: this could prove to be an expensive way to learn the art of palpation if adequate practice is not undertaken! Another exercise might be to select clothing on a daily basis using tactile and not visual input. It is a salutary point that all visually impaired people necessarily employ these tactual skills every day.

The development of the sense of touch needs to be nurtured. It is recommended that each contact with an object should be treated as if no visual or auditory input is available whilst attempting to obtain the maximum amount of information. Those who have the privilege of handling patients professionally possess a constant source of practice in their study of structure and function and examination of normal and abnormal phenomena. Those professionals are even more fortunate if they specialize in the use of massage, movement, mobilization and manipulation techniques as part of clinical practice. Individuals who have undertaken formal study and practice of the art of massage are indeed already well versed in the appropriate knowledge and skills relating to palpation. Their contribution to the increased public recognition of palpation as a crucial element in the diagnosis and treatment of clinical conditions cannot be underestimated. Indeed it is gratifying to note the increased status of all the manual therapies during the past decade: people are deliberately selecting practitioners who possess skills that rely on touch for their efficacy. It should never be forgotten, however, that all such therapists are required to demonstrate a serious commitment to Continuing Professional Development (CPD): they are required to revise and update their anatomical and physiological knowledge on a regular basis in order to maintain the high standards of professional practice demanded by their respective professional organizations.

CARE OF THE HANDS

All skills in which complex manual techniques are employed in the performance of precise movements, necessarily rely on the regular care and maintenance of the hands: their mobility, sensitivity and dexterity. Prior to engaging in any form of manual contact, however, the practitioner should ensure that the temperature of the skin is warm; patients do not appreciate being touched by therapists whose hands are cold!

Cleanliness is essential and its positive contribution to the quality of tactile input cannot be underestimated. Traces of grease, cream, dirt, dust, etc.

effectively create an additional intervening layer between the sensory receptor organs and nerve endings in the hand and the object or subject to be palpated. It is significant that most Braille readers will make every effort to keep their hands clean while reading Braille; many tend to avoid eating anything sticky in order to prevent their fingers from losing sensitivity. A routine of washing the hands in warm water using a mild soap and drying them thoroughly after washing should be adopted, The use of additional creams or ointments is not recommended unless this is absolutely necessary. A good, oil-based hand cream can be used at night in order to maintain a smooth, soft condition of the skin; some authorities also recommend the regular use of Vaseline and sugar. Whichever maintenance routine is adopted, the hands must always be washed thoroughly prior to attempting palpation techniques. In addition, the nails should be kept clean and short so that the risks of injury or infection are avoided. No wrist or hand jewellery should be worn. The quality of the palpation depends, to a great extent, upon the texture and suppleness of the hands. They should look and feel good, thus promoting the patient's confidence in the palpator. Poorly maintained hands which are dirty, stiff and with hard skin will be off-putting to patients: a reluctance to be touched will act as a barrier to the passage of information from the body of the patient to the receptors of the palpator.

The joints of the hands must be maintained in a supple condition with the musculature being firm and strong. Regular exercises should be practised in order to maintain joint mobility and increase muscle strength. Contact with all abrasive surfaces and detergents should be avoided as far as possible and gloves should be worn at all times when manual work is performed, particularly during activities such as washing-up, cleaning, gardening, car maintenance and building work. Many liquids, certain soaps and detergents, tend to remove the natural greases from the skin and the use of these should, therefore, be minimal. Any activity that is likely to lead to the production of blisters, finger calluses or general hard skin should also be minimized: examples might include such pastimes as rowing, playing a stringed musical instrument, rope-climbing and woodwork. Additionally, great care must be taken when using sharp instruments or engaging in any activity that is likely to cause trauma and/or skin infection. Lack of vigilance whilst performing any of these activities may prejudice the ability to perform high-quality palpation techniques.

PALPATION OF DIFFERENT TISSUES

Experience suggests that normal palpation when performed by the lay person – and even when undertaken by some professionals – is sometimes ineffective. It may enable the operator to differentiate between such tissues as bone, muscle or tendon etc. but often does little more. By contrast, the skilled student practitioner will be able to distinguish different parts of bones, contrasting shapes and texture of muscles, identify their connections to tendons and trace them to their attachments. Such students will also be able to count vertebrae, palpate lumbar transverse processes and other deep bony structures, locate certain ligaments, palpate elusive pulses and determine abnormalities such as different types of swelling, misalignment and rupture. The expert clinician must progress far beyond this concept in order to complete the picture that lies hidden within the body. Bony landmarks should be studied, linking them together and obtaining a clear mental image of the skeletal layout. This programme should include studying rib angles, transverse processes and spines of all vertebrae including their differing features. For example, the bifid spinous processes of the cervical region contrast with the pointed spines in the thoracic and the rectangular-shaped spines of T12 and in the lumbar region. Alignment of one bone to another is relatively easily examined in the upper and lower limbs whereas this is much more difficult to examine in the vertebral column. Defects in the contour of a bone can also be located and possible avulsions recognized.

Variations in muscle texture should be identifiable and note taken of differences occurring in normal muscle, enabling the examiner to recognize any abnormal variations. Some muscles, such as gluteus maximus and the middle fibres of deltoid, have a coarse structure due to the type of muscle fibres involved, whereas muscles such as the oblique abdominals and quadratus lumborum have a smoother texture. Fibrous tissue between the muscle fibres may give a stringy feel, while local areas of spasm are hard but regular in shape. The former tend to remain in the same position irrespective of what technique is performed on them; the latter will often disappear on applying either heat or massage. Both types of muscle spasm can be found in the rhomboid muscles between the scapula and spinous processes of the vertebral column.

Careful palpation will reveal where each muscle joins its tendon and where and how the tendon is attached. Palpation can also determine how tightly the muscle is bound down by fascia and whether the tendon is maintained in its position by a retinaculum. The extent of the retinacula can be examined and a study made of those structures which pass under or over them.

Swellings in muscle are often caused by bruising (contusion) and bleeding (haematoma) between the muscle fibres. These are normally contained within a localized area and become hard and painful, often warm to the touch and sometimes produce redness over the area. There is nearly always a history of trauma to the region. Care should be taken, however, when palpating any area of swelling as this symptom could be caused by other more serious conditions. It is important to be sensitive to local changes in temperature, noting whether these are higher or lower than expected. The condition of the underlying structures must be recorded and a knowledge of the possible causes of such variations will contribute to the establishment of a clinical diagnosis and subsequent treatment of the condition.

When palpating joints, other considerations must be taken into account. The precise location of the joint line is essential, the quality of this technique being based on the accurate identification of bony landmarks and measurements, taking into account the general size and shape of other bones and the patient's posture at the time. A detailed knowledge of the structure and extent of the adjacent joint surfaces, as well as where ligaments may obscure the joint space, is essential. The presentation of tissue-filled joint spaces under differing circumstances – for example, whether fluid is contained within the joint capsule or within a bursa – together with a detailed knowledge of the surrounding tendons is also a necessary pre-requisite when examining joints. As Chaitow points out:

> There are many important features to note during the examination of joints: the range and smoothness of movement, whether the axis varies according to the position of the joint and to what degree movement may be limited. Employing great care and skill, movement of joints can be examined indirectly through the bones of either side of that joint. The movement between the joint surfaces may be experienced as smooth or grinding; the restriction felt at 'the end of a joint's range of motion may be described as having a certain feel and this is called (the) 'end-feel'.
>
> (Chaitow 2003)

In his discussion of barriers to joint movement Chaitow continues:

> If there is, for any reason, a restriction in the range of motion then a pathological barrier would be apparent on active or passive movement in that direction. If the reason for the restriction involved interosseous changes (arthritis, for example) the end-feel would be sudden or hard. However, if the restriction involved soft tissue dysfunction the end-feel would have a softer nature.
>
> (Chaitow 2003)

Most joints possess additional movements which are of small range and not under voluntary control: these are essential for the efficient functioning of the joint. These are known as 'accessory' movements.

Accessory or joint play movements are those movements of a joint that cannot be performed actively by the individual. Such accessory movements include the roll, spin and slide which accompany a joint's physiological movements.

> (Hengeveld and Banks 2005)

A simple example of this type of movement would be found in the axle of a bicycle wheel. On each side, the axle is surrounded by a ring of ball-bearings maintained in position by a cone which screws on to the axle. When the cones are loose, they allow the wheel to be moved slightly from side to side; when the cones are tight, there is no side-to-side or accessory movement. When there is side-to-side movement, the wheel is free to turn; as the cones are tightened, the ball-bearings become 'close packed' and more difficult to turn so finally locking the wheel. The side-to-side (or accessory) movement is thus essential for the free turning of the wheel, since its elimination results in no movement.

Accessory movements are most demonstrable in human joints within a certain range of the joint movement: when the ligaments allow joint surfaces to be parted or when the surfaces are not congruent. This is termed the 'loose packed' position. When the ligaments of a joint become taut and its surfaces are congruent, no further movement is possible, either physiological or accessory. The joint is now said to be in a 'close packed' position (Standing 2004). If the accessory movements of a joint are lost, the joint becomes extremely difficult to move, similar to the cones of the bicycle wheel being tightened (see above). If, however, accessory movement is restored, as in loosening the cones in the bicycle wheel, normal movement is also restored. The restoration of accessory movements is an important principle underlying the practice of mobilization and manipulation techniques to restore normal movement in joints. With care and expertise, by using a combination of accessory and *normal* movements, joint function can be assessed and the treatment varied accordingly. The use of 'quadrant' techniques (combined movements at the end of range) is a good example of this testing. (For further information on the application of these types of examination and techniques, see Grieve 1986, Hengeveld and Banks 2005.)

Chaitow's definition of 'joint play' is also useful:

> Joint play refers to the particular movements between bones associated with either separation of the surfaces (as in traction) or parallel movement of joint surfaces (also known as translation or translatoric gliding).
>
> (Chaitow 2003)

This information is important in establishing the joints' condition.

Swelling around a joint deforms its shape and contour, the extent of the deformity being dependent upon the degree of swelling involved. The bony features can usually be identified between the areas of swelling. In some instances, the swelling is so profuse that it is difficult to locate bony landmarks; on other occasions, the amount of fluid is so small that precise techniques have to be employed to palpate the swelling which is interfering with normal joint function. Most joint swelling is contained within the capsule, causing a build-up of pressure which results in increasing pain. The swelling may have to be removed surgically, although this is usually deferred until absolutely necessary because of the risk of infection into the joint. Blood can also escape into a joint space (haemarthrosis), resulting in a similar appearance, but this is usually accompanied by some discoloration and an increased local temperature. Any swelling can lead to severe damage to the mechanics of the joint; this damage may vary according to the type of fluid involved.

Careful palpation of the swelling can produce more information than at first thought. The swelling may appear soft and movable with the application of pressure; this often gives a fluid feel as it passes from one part of the joint cavity to another. Alternatively it may appear thick and pliable although difficult to move unless sustained pressure is applied. Swelling may appear to be a solid mass, pitting under pressure from the fingers but taking a considerable time before signs of movement are evident.

SUMMARY

Palpation is a detailed examination using the hands as tools to enable the palpator to elicit information about structures beneath the skin and fascia. It is, in our opinion, still under-used and undervalued, mainly because of lack of practise and appreciation of its intrinsic value. In addition, its teaching and practice are time-consuming, requiring expert instruction from experienced practitioners, genuine interest, patience and commitment from students. While its techniques can be practised and developed, however, expertise, takes time and dedication to acquire.

Palpation is more than just a desire to 'see' through the skin and interpret the underlying anatomy. It can be developed in such a way that information can be imparted to the patient through the practitioner's hands. It is not difficult to appreciate the ways in which the expert palpator can employ the art of instrumental and expressive touching in combination to obtain clinical diagnosis and establish sympathetic communication. Indeed, the philosophy that underpins the practice of many therapists emphasizes the intrinsic therapeutic qualities of touch per se. (See for example Dennis, Jones and Holey 1995, Everett 1997, Nathan 1999, Charman 2000). Healers who practise the 'laying on of hands' and Therapeutic Touch also share this belief. (See Krieger 1986, 1993, 1997, 2002, Macrae 1987, Sayre-Adams and Wright 2001.) The increasing popularity of complementary therapies amongst the general public further confirms the general tendency to place considerable value in an holistic approach to patient care. Rather than relying solely on orthodox medical practice, patients and therapists alike are now recognizing the importance of healing in the management of chronic physical and psychological problems (Nathan 1999, Charman 2000).

Palpation must be learned, practised and developed before it can be applied professionally. The study of anatomy, physiology and the human sciences, together with the additional information obtained through the appropriate use of touch are excellent ways of learning the art of palpation. Anatomy will become clearer and more understandable as the hands become more sensitive to what lies below the skin, leading to an enhancement of knowledge and improvement in assessment: an asset in therapeutic application. Finally, and perhaps most importantly, the skilled palpator should be aware of the patient's reaction to movement. By observing the patient's face, listening to the patient's comments and being sensitive to all reactions in muscle and joint movement, a total picture of the patient's condition becomes available. With care and sensitivity, a great deal of information can easily be obtained.

The following pages contain a detailed study of the surface markings of many of the body's structures, including a guide to the palpation of particular areas. It must be remembered, however, that the development of effective palpation skills for the purposes of clinical intervention requires more than the acquisition of sound theoretical knowledge upon which to base practice. As Chaitow emphasizes, expertise in palpation techniques is achieved '... by application (and repetition) of hundreds of carefully designed exercises that are capable of refining palpation skills to an astonishing degree of sensitivity' (Chaitow 2003).

Citing Frymann (1963) he adds:

> ... palpation cannot be learned by reading or listening; it can only be learned by palpation. This learning process is not just about hard dedicated labour; it should be fun and it should be exciting. The thrills to be experienced when taking this journey of exploration of the tissues of the human body is hopefully contagious ...
>
> (Chaitow 2003)

We hope that readers will take inspiration from this and other related texts and strive to attain expertise in palpation skills in the interests of improving the quality of their clinical practice.

Contents

At the end of this chapter you should be able to:

A. Find and recognize the shape and position of the clavicle, scapula, humerus, radius, ulna, carpal, metacarpal bones and the phalanges.

B. Recognize and palpate many of the bony features.

C. Name all the joints of the upper limb and understand their formation.

D. Trace the lines of the joints, and where possible indicate their bony landmarks and surface markings.

E. Describe or carry out any accessory movements possible noting the ranges in which they are most obvious.

F. Note the ranges of each of the joints and indicate the factors limiting the movement.

G. Give the class and type of each joint noting the axes of movement where possible.

H. Name and demonstrate the action of all the muscles palpable in the upper limb.

I. Draw the shape of the muscle on the surface and palpate its contraction.

J. Palpate tendons and attachments where possible.

K. Name all the main nerves supplying the upper limb.

L. Demonstrate the course and distribution of each of the main nerves of the upper limb.

M. Name the main arteries of the upper limb showing their course and giving their distribution.

N. Name the main veins of the upper limb noting their drainage areas and course.

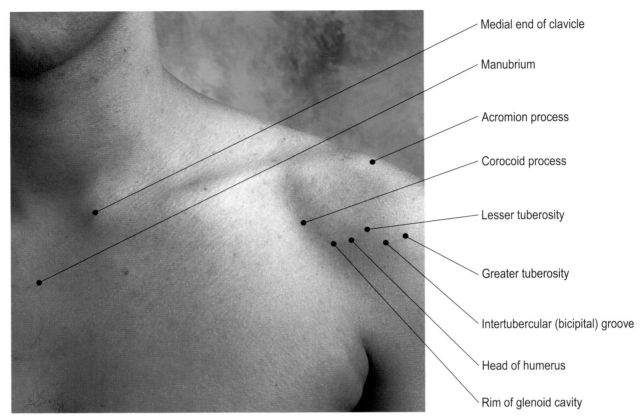

Medial end of clavicle

Manubrium

Acromion process

Corocoid process

Lesser tuberosity

Greater tuberosity

Intertubercular (bicipital) groove

Head of humerus

Rim of glenoid cavity

Fig. 2.1 (a)
The left shoulder (anterior view)

BONES

The pectoral region

The bones in this region are the clavicle and scapula, forming the pectoral girdle, with the upper end of the humerus situated vertically under its lateral margin. The clavicle is situated on the upper part of the anterolateral aspect, and the scapula on the upper part of the posterolateral aspect of the chest wall. The humerus is the upper bone of the arm articulating with the glenoid [*glene* (Gk) = a socket] cavity of the scapula at the shoulder (glenohumeral) joint.

The clavicle [Fig. 2.1]

The clavicle [*clavis* (L) or *kleis* (Gk) = key; also, *clavis* (L) was an S-shaped bar for striking a gong) is about 10 cm long and situated between the manubrium sterni medially and the acromion process of the scapula laterally (Fig. 2.1). It is a long bone and has a shallow S-shape when viewed from above. It ossifies in membrane, which means that its articular surfaces are covered with fibrocartilage and it has no medullary cavity.

Palpation

At the lower boundary of the front of the neck, locate the sternal (jugular) notch centrally. This is formed by the superior border of the manubrium sterni inferiorly, and the medial end of each clavicle on either side. Articular cartilage together with an interarticular disc and interclavicular ligament are interposed between the medial ends of the clavicles and the skin.

Moving laterally, the medial third of the bone is convex forward with a superior and anterior surface, both of which are easily palpable despite giving attachment to the sternocleidomastoid superiorly and pectoralis major anteriorly. Below, the anterior end of the first rib is palpable, particularly where it articulates with the lateral border of the manubrium sterni. Further laterally, the middle third of the clavicle begins to curve backwards, being a little more rounded in cross-section. Posterior to the superior surface a depression, the supraclavicular fossa, can be palpated containing the cord-like structures of the trunks of the brachial plexus running downwards and laterally towards

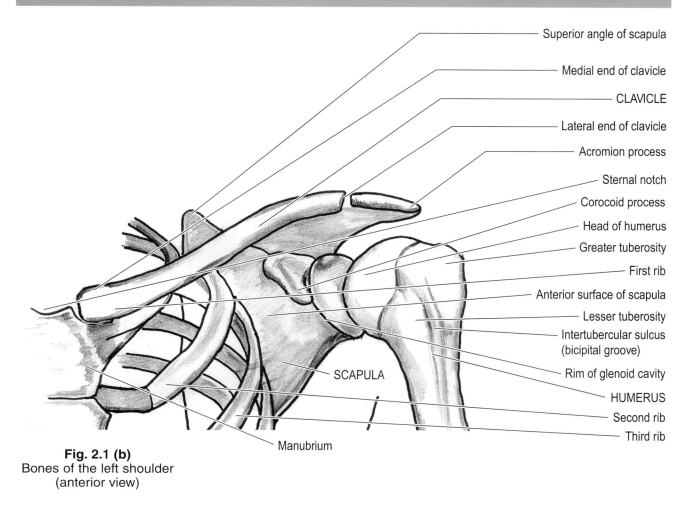

Superior angle of scapula

Medial end of clavicle

CLAVICLE

Lateral end of clavicle

Acromion process

Sternal notch

Corocoid process

Head of humerus

Greater tuberosity

First rib

Anterior surface of scapula

Lesser tuberosity

Intertubercular sulcus
(bicipital groove)

Rim of glenoid cavity

HUMERUS

Second rib

Third rib

SCAPULA

Manubrium

Fig. 2.1 (b)
Bones of the left shoulder
(anterior view)

the upper limb. If deep, but careful, pressure is applied in this notch in an inferomedial direction, the upper surface of the first rib, over which the trunks of the brachial plexus pass, can be recognized. The lateral third of the clavicle becomes flattened from above down and its sharper anterior border is concave forward. Its subcutaneous superior surface can readily be palpated through the skin, becoming thicker at the lateral end toward the acromioclavicular joint. Below the anterior border is a depression, the infraclavicular fossa, situated between deltoid laterally and pectoralis major inferomedially. Here the tip of the coracoid [*korax* (Gk) = a crow and *oeides* (Gk) = shape] process can readily be palpated lying approximately 3 cm below the junction of the middle and lateral thirds of the anterior border and just medial to the anterior fibres of the deltoid. Both anterior and posterior borders of the clavicle give attachment to muscles, deltoid anteriorly and trapezius posteriorly. The lateral end of the clavicle can be identified by a small tubercle on its superior surface which lies just medial to the acromioclavicular joint (see joints of upper limb).

The upper end of the humerus

This comprises the head, the greater tuberosity and the lesser tuberosity. The head is slightly more than half a sphere, smooth and being directed medially, slightly backwards and upwards. The greater tuberosity lies laterally and the lesser tuberosity projects forwards with the intertubercular groove running vertically between the two tuberosities.

Moving lateral to the coracoid process, a slightly pointed projection, the lesser tuberosity of the humerus [*humerus* (L) = the shoulder] can be palpated. This forms the medial border of the intertubercular groove, through which passes the tendon of the long head of biceps. The groove can easily be palpated at this point as it runs vertically downwards (Fig. 2.1). Lateral to the tendon of biceps, the anterior surface of the greater tuberosity may be difficult to palpate as it is covered by the deltoid muscle. However, with your fingers on the anterior aspect, bring the thumb in just below and lateral to the angle of the acromion, and the greater tuberosity can be grasped between the thumb and fingers between the separate fibres of deltoid. The greater tuberosity accounts, in part, for the rounded bulge of the shoulder region.

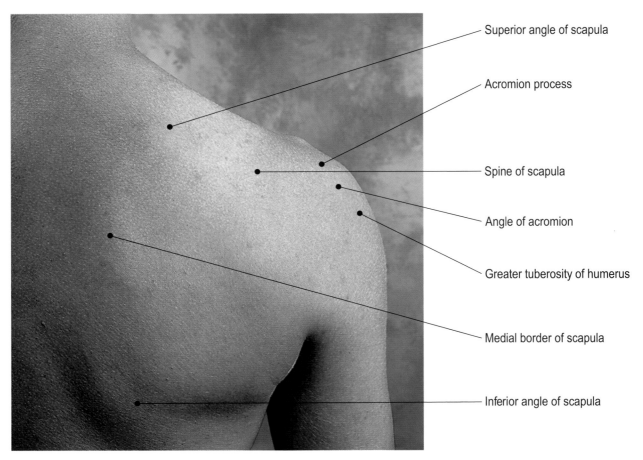

- Superior angle of scapula
- Acromion process
- Spine of scapula
- Angle of acromion
- Greater tuberosity of humerus
- Medial border of scapula
- Inferior angle of scapula

Fig. 2.2 (a)
The right shoulder (posterior view)

The scapula [Fig. 2.2]

The scapula [*scapulae* (L) = shoulder blades], (Fig. 2.2) is a flat triangular bone situated on the posterolateral aspect of the upper chest wall. It has three angles, three borders and costal and dorsal surfaces, the latter being marked by a ledge-shaped spine running almost horizontally.

The spine is wider laterally where it joins the acromion process, but narrows as it passes medially. Its upper and lower borders diverge as it meets the medial border forming a small smooth triangular area. Above the spine there is a deep hollow called the supraspinous fossa and below a larger but shallower depression called the infraspinous fossa.

The lateral angle is expanded and forms the glenoid cavity for articulation with the head of the humerus at the shoulder joint. It also has a sharp bony projection passing forward just below the lateral end of the clavicle called the coracoid process, which is roughened for the attachment of muscle.

Palpation

The whole length of the spine can be palpated between the acromion process laterally and the medial border of the scapula medially. Its upper and lower lips can be recognized easily, even though they give attachment to the trapezius and deltoid muscles, respectively. The posterior surface is clearly palpable and visible, being narrow medially but gradually broadening as it passes laterally to become the superior surface of the acromion. At this point it is covered by a bursa (the supra-acromial bursa), enabling the skin to move easily over this bone. The bone then appears to form a large quadrilateral surface, which is directed upwards and slightly backwards having a posterior, lateral and short anterior border. On its medial side can be palpated the lateral end of the clavicle and the small gap produced by the acromioclavicular joint. The smooth triangular area at the medial end of the spine is also covered by a bursa and can be palpated through the tendinous lower fibres of the trapezius.

The medial border of the scapula is approximately 5 cm lateral to the spines of the second to eighth thoracic vertebrae. Its full length can only be palpated with difficulty, except in lean subjects, as it gives attachment to levator scapulae above and rhomboid major and minor below, as well as being mostly covered by the trapezius muscle. The superior angle is buried in muscle and is tender on deep palpation, but the inferior angle can be identified lying on the posterolateral parts of the seventh and eighth ribs. When the upper limb is

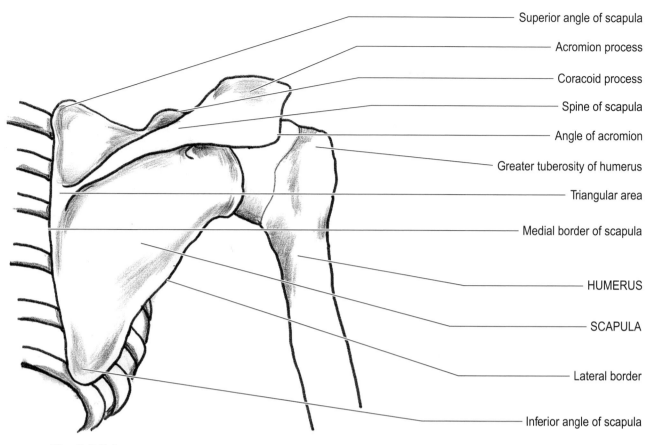

- Superior angle of scapula
- Acromion process
- Coracoid process
- Spine of scapula
- Angle of acromion
- Greater tuberosity of humerus
- Triangular area
- Medial border of scapula
- HUMERUS
- SCAPULA
- Lateral border
- Inferior angle of scapula

Fig. 2.2 (b)
Bones of the right shoulder
(posterior view)

raised above the head, the inferior angle can be seen and felt moving laterally around the chest wall as far as the mid-axillary line. The **lateral border** is very difficult to palpate as it is embedded in thick muscle (teres major and minor). It is by far the thickest of the borders and acts as a lever for its strong muscles to pull it laterally in rotation of the scapula.

Anteriorly, in the infraclavicular fossa, 3 cm below the junction of the lateral and middle thirds of the clavicle, the coracoid process can be palpated despite it giving attachment to three muscles, the short head of the biceps, coracobrachialis and pectoralis minor. Just lateral to the coracoid process running downwards and laterally for approximately 3 cm, the concave anterior rim of the glenoid cavity can be palpated with the head of the humerus lying on its lateral side.

Palpation on movement

Once the boundaries of the scapula have been recognized by palpation, it is important to be able to follow its movements around the chest wall during activities of the shoulder girdle and upper limb.

Place your right hand on the point of the model's right shoulder and place your left hand on the

inferior angle and the lower part of the medial border. Get the model to pull the shoulder girdles forward as in hunching the shoulders (protrusion). The scapula is observed moving forwards around the chest wall but staying in its vertical position. Now get the model to brace back the shoulder girdles. The scapula is observed moving backwards and again not changing its vertical position.

Keeping your hands in the same positions, ask the model now to raise (elevation) and lower the shoulder girdles as in shrugging. The scapula will be observed rising and lowering (depression), but still holding its vertical position.

Now ask the model to raise the right arm above the head. When the upper limb reaches 20 degrees the scapula will be observed rotating around an axis just below the spine nearer to its medial end. The superior angle will rise moving medially and the inferior angle will be observed moving laterally and slightly upwards around the chest wall (lateral rotation). In fact, the inferior angle will reach as far as the mid-axillary line on full elevation of the humerus.

When the arm is lowered the scapula will be seen to return to its original position (medial rotation). If, however, the arm is taken behind the chest, medial rotation continues and the inferior angle will come close to the spines of the vertebrae.

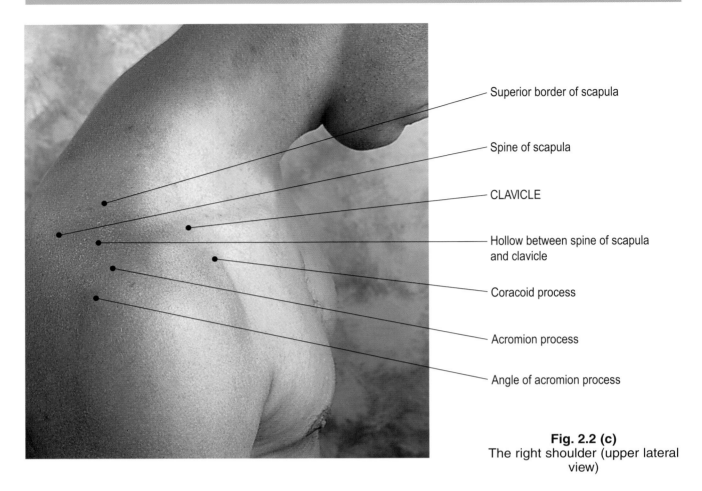

Superior border of scapula

Spine of scapula

CLAVICLE

Hollow between spine of scapula
and clavicle

Coracoid process

Acromion process

Angle of acromion process

Fig. 2.2 (c)
The right shoulder (upper lateral
view)

Anatomy

Viewed from above and slightly laterally with the upper limb in about 45 degrees of abduction, the shoulder girdle forms a 'V' shape with the clavicle being the anterior and the spine of the scapula the posterior stem. They form an angle with each other of approximately 70 degrees and are joined at the acromioclavicular joint. The greater tuberosity of the humerus is now tucked underneath the arch of the acromion. Below the junction of the middle with the lateral third of the clavicle lies the coracoid process and below the lateral third of the clavicle lies the head of the humerus. The acromion appears quadrilateral from above and continues medially and backwards as the spine of the scapula. The upper third of the scapula lies above and anterior to the spine with the superior angle being most medial and the superior border passing laterally, presenting the suprascapular notch and continuing to the base of the coracoid process.

The anterior border of the lateral third of the clavicle continues laterally with the short anterior border of the acromion process, which is again continuous with the lateral border and its posterior border. This continues as the inferior border of the spine.

The posterior border of the lateral third of the clavicle is in the same line as the superior border of the spine of the scapula but acutely angled.

Palpation

Run your fingers from the anterior border of the clavicle across the acromioclavicular joint where the anterior border of the acromion process of the scapula continues in line for approximately 1.5 cm. It then passes backwards as the lateral border of the acromion [akros (Gk) = summit and omos = shoulders] for a further 5 cm before turning medially (acromial angle) to become the inferior lip of the spine of the scapula, all of which is palpable and gives attachment to the deltoid muscle.

Palpation on movement

Place the fingers and thumb of your right hand on the medial end and the fingers and thumb of the left hand on the lateral end of the right clavicle.

As the model draws the shoulder girdle forward (protraction), the lateral end will move forward accompanying the sliding of the scapula around the chest wall. The medial end, however, will be felt gliding backwards in the clavicular notch of the sternum. The axis around which this occurs is approximately 3 cm from its medial end, where the costoclavicular ligament attaches to the under surface of the clavicle. If the shoulder is now drawn backwards (retraction), the lateral end of the clavicle will move backwards, but the medial end will move forwards and become proud of the sternum.

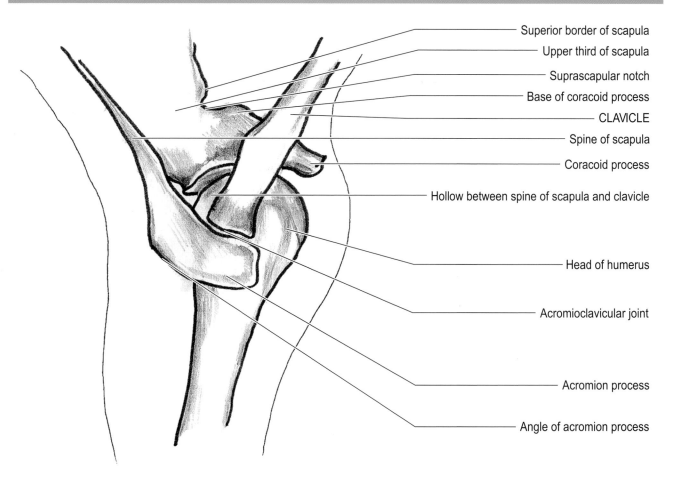

Superior border of scapula
Upper third of scapula
Suprascapular notch
Base of coracoid process
CLAVICLE
Spine of scapula
Coracoid process
Hollow between spine of scapula and clavicle
Head of humerus
Acromioclavicular joint
Acromion process
Angle of acromion process

Fig. 2.2 (d)
Bones of the right shoulder (upper
lateral view)

If the model now raises the shoulder girdle (elevation), the lateral end will rise and the medial end will move down, rolling into the clavicular notch of the sternum using the same fulcrum as above. When the shoulder girdle is lowered the lateral end will drop, and the medial end will rise to its original position or even protrude upwards if the girdle is further depressed.

If the arm is now raised above the head the clavicle will first of all move as in elevation but will, in the final stage, rotate as a whole with the anterior surface moving upwards. This movement accompanies lateral rotation of the scapula. Lowering the arm will return the shoulder girdle to its original position.

Movements of the clavicle, scapula and humerus and the joints between them are highly complex and should be studied in *Anatomy and Human Movement* (Palastanga, Field and Soames 1998).

Functional anatomy

The clavicle acts as a rigid lever bracing the shoulder girdle backwards, allowing the upper limb to move freely away from the chest wall.

With the powerful upper fibres of the trapezius muscle raising or supporting its lateral end and the adjoining acromion process, it helps to transmit weight from the upper limb to the vertebral column via the manubrium sterni and the upper ribs. The clavicle moves around an axis close to its medial end at the attachment of the costoclavicular ligament and is tightly bound to the coracoid laterally by the coracoclavicular ligament. Fractures of the bone may occur due to a fall on the shoulder, as in horse riding, motorcycling and rugby. Normally the fracture will take place where the medial two-thirds joins the lateral third, medial to the coracoclavicular ligament. The shoulder girdle may protrude forwards and a large hard swelling can be palpated and seen at the site of the fracture. Complications can occur from fractures of this bone if it is more central and the sharp bone ends are forced backwards, thus damaging the brachial plexus and/or the subclavian artery. Provided there are no serious complications the fracture will unite readily in approximately six weeks, although movements of the upper limb and shoulder girdle can begin in two weeks or when the sharp pain has subsided.

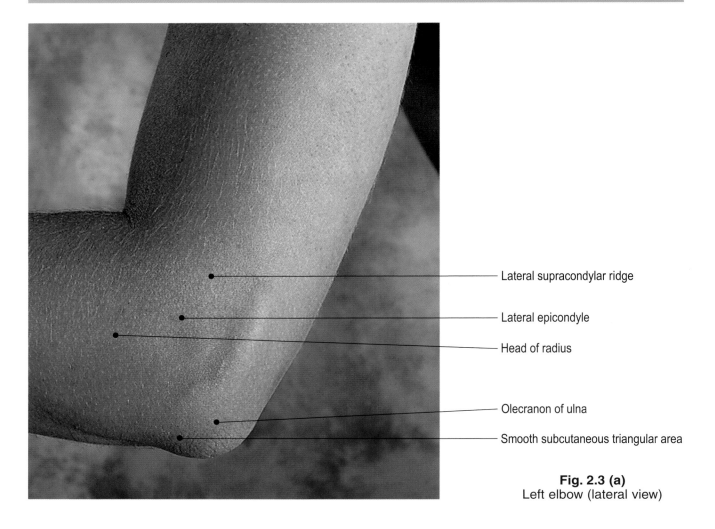

Lateral supracondylar ridge

Lateral epicondyle

Head of radius

Olecranon of ulna

Smooth subcutaneous triangular area

Fig. 2.3 (a)
Left elbow (lateral view)

The elbow region [Fig. 2.3]

This region is made up of the lower end of the humerus, and the upper ends of the radius and ulna.

The lower end of the humerus is composed of a medial and lateral condyle, having two articular surfaces, the trochlea and the capitulum respectively. Above these surfaces anteriorly are two fossae, the coronoid medially and radial laterally. Posteriorly there is a larger depression called the olecranon fossa. On the lateral side of the lateral condyle is a prominence called the lateral epicondyle, which lies at the lower end of the lateral supracondylar ridge.

The upper end of the radius is composed of a head, button-shaped and articular on its upper surface and on the medial third of its rim, a neck, which is cylindrical, joining the head to the upper end of the shaft, and a large tuberosity (bicipital tuberosity), which projects from its medial side at the base of the neck and is roughened on its posterior aspect for the attachment of the tendon of the biceps brachii.

Palpation

Just below the lower attachment of deltoid, halfway down the lateral side of the arm, the humerus can be palpated. It is crossed laterally by the radial nerve running downwards and forwards. Trauma in this area can cause pain, tingling and, sometimes, numbness of the posterolateral aspect of the hand. Inferiorly, the bone can be palpated as a sharp border, the lateral supracondylar ridge, terminating at the large lateral epicondyle. The posterior surface of this epicondyle is subcutaneous and with the elbow flexed can be traced medially across the back of the humerus to the commencement of the olecranon [*olekranon* (Gk) = the point of the elbow] fossa. With the elbow extended, the lateral side of the button-shaped head of the radius [*radius* (L) = spoke of a wheel] can be felt immediately below the epicondyle. The narrow groove running horizontally between the two is the radiohumeral part of the elbow joint. Palpate around the lateral half of the radial head, posteriorly as far as the posterior aspect of the superior radioulnar joint. Just below the head, laterally, the narrowed neck can be identified, being hidden by muscles anteriorly and posteriorly.

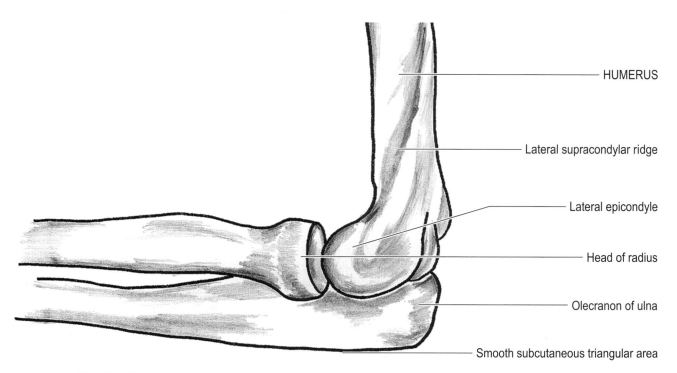

HUMERUS

Lateral supracondylar ridge

Lateral epicondyle

Head of radius

Olecranon of ulna

Smooth subcutaneous triangular area

Fig. 2.3 (b)
Bones of the left elbow (lateral view)

The large bony formation of the olecranon (Fig. 2.3a,b) can be palpated, particularly when the elbow is flexed. Its superior surface is more difficult to feel as it is covered by the tendon of triceps, as it inserts into its posterior aspect. With your fingers now placed on the posterior triangular surface of the olecranon, the skin and superficial fascia can easily be moved owing to the presence of the subcutaneous olecranon bursa. If pressure is applied for some time to this area, as in leaning on the elbows, the bursa can become inflamed and swollen (bursitis). The narrow triangular surface has its apex downwards and is continuous with the posterior border of the ulna, which is subcutaneous as far as its head. The medial and lateral surfaces of the olecranon can readily be palpated; however, lower down they become covered by muscle.

The olecranon is much more difficult to palpate when the elbow is extended, as it moves into the olecranon fossa of the posterior surface of the distal end of the humerus.

Palpation on movement

With the right elbow flexed to 90 degrees, place the fingers of your left hand on the superior surface of the olecranon, which will be at the back of the elbow. Now, with your right hand place the fingers on the medial epicondyle and the thumb on the lateral epicondyle of the humerus. When the model extends the elbow you will observe that the olecranon will virtually disappear into the olecranon fossa on the posterior aspect of the humerus.

With the right elbow again in flexion, find the lateral epicondyle of the humerus. At its lower end there is a small space and then the outer edge of the disc-like head of the radius. If the model now pronates and supinates the forearm you will feel the head of the radius rotating below your fingers.

Finally, stand in front of the fully flexed elbow. Take the arm in your left hand and the forearm in your right. If the model now extends the elbow joint you will observe that the forearm, which was slightly medial to the line of the humerus, now moves more to the lateral side forming an angle with the upper part of the arm. This is termed 'the carrying angle'.

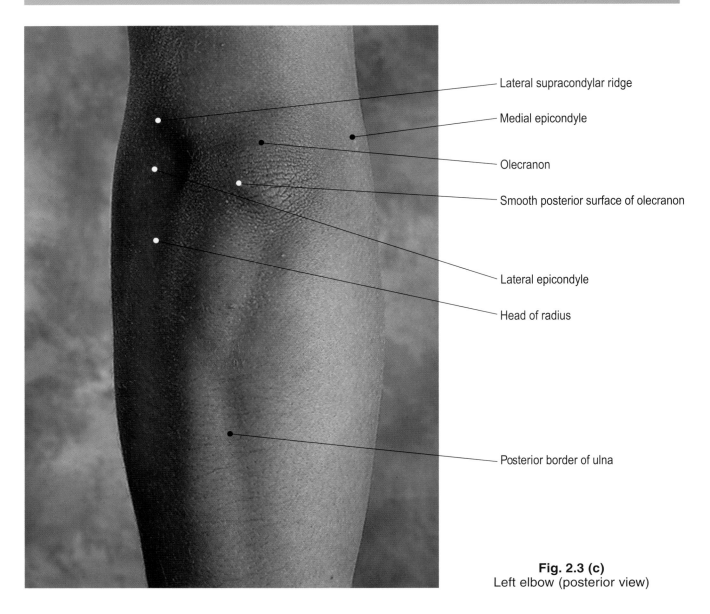

Lateral supracondylar ridge

Medial epicondyle

Olecranon

Smooth posterior surface of olecranon

Lateral epicondyle

Head of radius

Posterior border of ulna

Fig. 2.3 (c)
Left elbow (posterior view)

Bones

On the medial surface of the medial condyle of the humerus there is a large projection called the medial epicondyle, being slightly hollowed posteriorly. Above this is the medial supracondylar ridge which passes up to the medial side of the shaft.

The pulley-shaped trochlea is articular and covers the anterior, inferior and posterior aspect of the bone. Its medial flange is lower than the lateral and accounts for the angle at the elbow joint.

The upper end of the ulna, lying below the trochlea of the humerus, is composed mainly of a hook-shaped process called the olecranon and a shelf-like process projecting forwards from the upper end of the shaft called the coronoid process. The two form a socket shape facing forwards and is called the trochlear notch. This articulates with the trochlea of the humerus in the elbow joint.

Palpation

On the medial side of the elbow, the sharp medial supracondylar ridge can be palpated and traced upwards for approximately the lower quarter of the humerus. At its lower end a large, bony prominence can be palpated 2 cm above the elbow joint and approximately 1 cm below the level of the lateral epicondyle. This is the medial epicondyle behind which there is a deep groove for the ulnar nerve. Palpation of this area may be quite tender and could cause tingling or even numbness on the medial side of the hand due to pressure on the ulnar nerve. This is often referred to as the 'funny bone', owing to the strange sensation when it is compressed.

With the elbow fully flexed, it is just possible to feel the depression of the olecranon fossa through the tendon of the triceps. From the posterior, locate the medial and lateral epicondyles. At a point midway between the two, press your thumb onto the back of the triceps tendon – it will sink

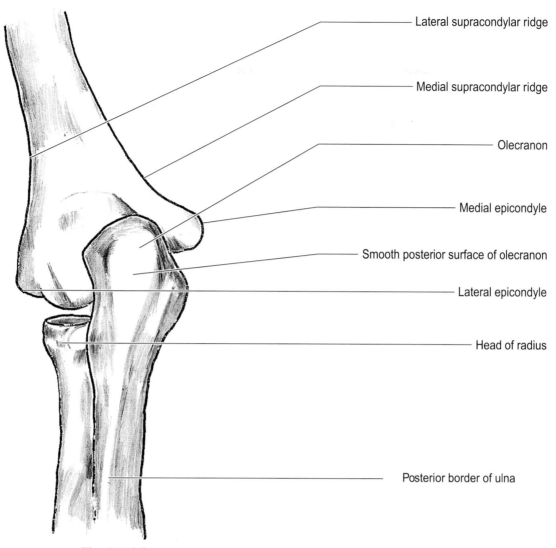

Lateral supracondylar ridge

Medial supracondylar ridge

Olecranon

Medial epicondyle

Smooth posterior surface of olecranon

Lateral epicondyle

Head of radius

Posterior border of ulna

Fig. 2.3 (d)
Bones of the left elbow (posterior view)

slightly into the olecranon fossa. Just below your thumb you will palpate the bony olecranon.

With the right elbow fully extended and the forearm fully supinated, examine the anterior of this region. Place the flat surface of your right hand 2.5 cm below and 2.5 cm lateral to the medial epicondyle. You will feel a hard bony projection deep to the mass of flexor muscles. This is the coronoid [*corone* (Gk) = crown; also the name given to the pointed front of a ship or plough] process. The contrast can be observed by placing your left thumb in a similar position laterally.

Functional anatomy

The title 'carrying angle' at the elbow joint must have been given when the carrying of pails of water was common. In fact most objects carried in the hand with the elbow extended are normally accompanied by the forearm being held in the mid prone position. This eliminates the angle at the elbow. You will also observe that when the elbow is fully flexed the hand does not oppose the shoulder joint but locates itself to mid clavicle position.

If the shoulder is now flexed you will observe that the hand is taken first to the chin and then to the mouth, thus facilitating feeding. Keeping the arm in this position, if the forearm is now fully pronated and the fingers extended, the hand now becomes a protection to the face.

Injuries and degeneration of the elbow and superior radioulnar joint often lead to loss of flexion or extension or both. This results in serious dysfunction of the upper limb, with its ability to shorten and position the hand impeded. In one elbow this is perhaps acceptable, but if this dysfunction is present in both elbow complexes it may be devastating to a person's quality of life. Not only is dressing and eating affected, but the use of the hands when visiting the toilet may be impossible.

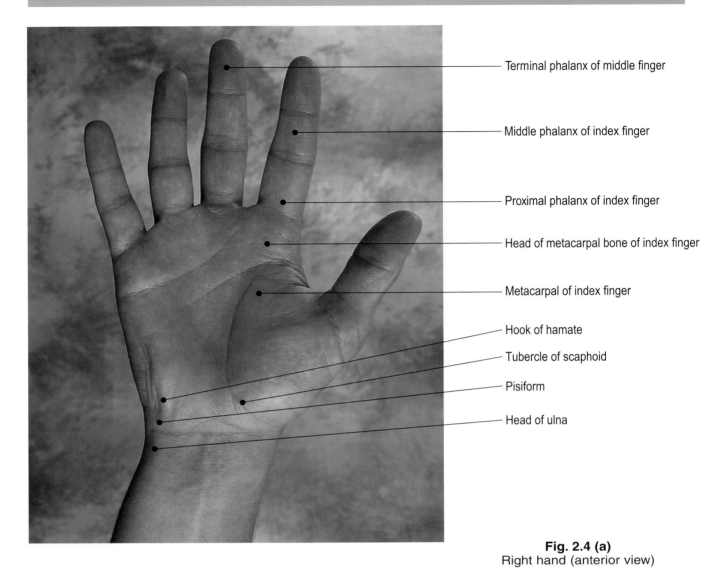

Terminal phalanx of middle finger

Middle phalanx of index finger

Proximal phalanx of index finger

Head of metacarpal bone of index finger

Metacarpal of index finger

Hook of hamate

Tubercle of scaphoid

Pisiform

Head of ulna

Fig. 2.4 (a)
Right hand (anterior view)

The wrist and hand

The lower ends of the radius and ulna form a shallow mortice into which three of the four bones of the proximal row of carpals – scaphoid, lunate and triquetral – fit. The fourth bone in the proximal row, the pisiform, lies anterior to the triquetral. Distally, the proximal row of carpal bones forms another concavity for the reception of the second row of carpal bones – the trapezium, trapezoid, capitate [*capitate* (L) = head-shaped] and hamate. The capitate is the largest of the four and fits snugly into the deepest part of the concavity, being in contact with all the carpal bones except the pisiform, triquetral and trapezium (Fig. 2.4b).

The metacarpals are miniature long bones lying distal to the carpals: that for the thumb articulating with the trapezium; the second mainly articulating with the trapezoid; that for the middle finger mainly articulating with the capitate; and the fourth and fifth articulating with the hamate.

Each metacarpal head articulates with a proximal phalanx.

Each finger has a middle and a distal phalanx, the thumb just a distal phalanx.

Anterior, medial and lateral aspects

Palpation

The bones of the wrist and hand are more difficult to locate on the anterior surface as they tend to be hidden by the muscles which arise and insert in the hand.

Return to the wrist joint and locate the head of the ulna on its medial side (Fig. 2.4). Immediately distal to this, the medial and posterior surfaces of the triquetral [*triquetrus* (L) = having three corners] can be palpated with the pea-shaped pisiform [*pisum* (L) = a pea] lying on its anterior surface, being easily recognizable owing to its prominence, and by the attachment of the tendon of flexor carpi ulnaris to its proximal side.

Deep pressure applied with the tip of the thumb 1 cm distal and slightly lateral to the pisiform reveals a small but distinct bony prominence. This is the hook of the hamate [*hamatus* (L) = hooked]. If the thumb is moved from side to side, two small nerves, the superficial terminal branches of the ulnar nerve, can be compressed against this prominence.

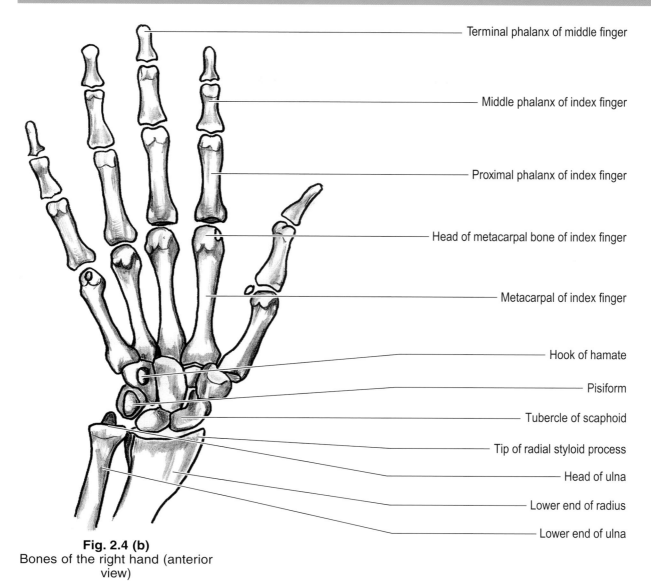

Terminal phalanx of middle finger

Middle phalanx of index finger

Proximal phalanx of index finger

Head of metacarpal bone of index finger

Metacarpal of index finger

Hook of hamate

Pisiform

Tubercle of scaphoid

Tip of radial styloid process

Head of ulna

Lower end of radius

Lower end of ulna

Fig. 2.4 (b)
Bones of the right hand (anterior
view)

On the lateral side of the wrist, locate the **tip of the radial styloid process**. It lies within a space termed the 'anatomical snuff box'. The styloid process can be traced upwards for a short distance, its anterior border continuing as the sharp anterior border of the shaft. Just medial to this crest lies the radial artery. Distal to the styloid process are the lateral surface of the scaphoid [*skaphe* (Gk) = a skiff], the trapezium [*trapezion* (Gk) = an irregular four-sided figure] and the base of the first meta-carpal, marked by a small tubercle. Its shaft leads distally to its head. The base, shaft and the head of the proximal phalanx are clearly palpable, as also are the base and shaft as far as the nail of the distal phalanx [*phalanx* (Gk) = a band of soldiers]. You should note that the posterior surface of the bones of the thumb face laterally due to the thumb lying at right angles to the palm. Medially, the anterior surfaces are difficult to determine due to the presence of muscle and tendon.

The **tubercle of the scaphoid** can be found at the proximal end of the thenar eminence, on the front of the carpal region, 1 cm medial to the tip of the radial styloid process. It is often quite difficult to palpate, although this is made easier if the wrist is extended. The vertical ridge of the trapezium is just palpable with deep pressure 1 cm distal to the scaphoid tubercle. This can often be a painful area for deep palpation, which is best done sparingly. The tubercle is prominent enough to be damaged by falls on the outstretched hand and a fracture may cause pain and dysfunction of the hand for many months due to its poor blood supply leading to a long healing time (see next page).

The anterior surfaces of the remaining carpal, metacarpal and phalangeal bones are difficult to palpate as they lie deep to the muscle and fascia. Only if the fingers are fully extended can the ante-rior surfaces of the heads of the metacarpals be felt in line with each finger, 2 cm proximal to the web between the fingers. The heads of each phalanx are also palpable in full or hyperextension, being just proximal to the creases of the interphalangeal joints. They normally present a small tubercle on either side, palpable if the lateral sides of the head are gripped between finger and thumb.

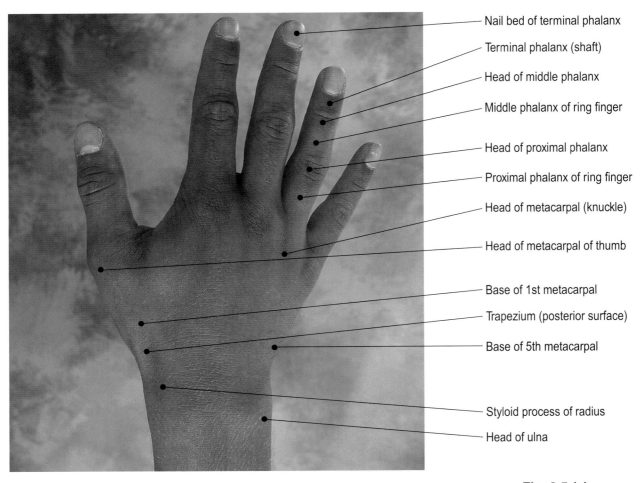

Nail bed of terminal phalanx

Terminal phalanx (shaft)

Head of middle phalanx

Middle phalanx of ring finger

Head of proximal phalanx

Proximal phalanx of ring finger

Head of metacarpal (knuckle)

Head of metacarpal of thumb

Base of 1st metacarpal

Trapezium (posterior surface)

Base of 5th metacarpal

Styloid process of radius

Head of ulna

Fig. 2.5 (a)
Right hand (posterior view)

Posterior aspect [Fig. 2.5]

Palpation

Place your finger on the button-shaped head of the ulna, clearly palpable posteromedially, but hidden by the tendon of flexor carpi ulnaris anteriorly. On its posteromedial aspect, a small projection, the ulnar styloid process, can be palpated, although it is partially hidden by the tendon of the extensor carpi ulnaris. If the wrist is radially deviated, the head of the ulna and its styloid process become much easier to identify.

On the lateral side of the wrist, the radial styloid process can be identified, having tendons running in front and behind. If traced upwards, the lower half of the lateral side of the radius can be palpated before being covered by the bulk of the brachioradialis muscle. This region may be quite tender to palpate as it is often crossed by the superficial terminal branch(es) of the radial nerve.

On the posterior aspect of the distal end of the radius, just above the level of the styloid process, the dorsal tubercle of the radius can be palpated, with the tendon of the extensor pollicis longus grooving its medial side and using it as a pulley. Below the level of the dorsal tubercle and the head of the ulna is a hollow, limited 2 cm below by the bases of the metacarpal bones. With the subject's wrist flexed, the posterior surfaces of the scaphoid, lunate [luna (L) = the moon] and triquetral can be identified in a line distal to the tips of the radial and ulnar styloid processes. Just beyond these the trapezoid, at the base of the second metacarpal, the capitate, at the base of the third, and the hamate, at the base of the fourth and fifth metacarpals, can all be identified if the bones are gripped between the fingers posteriorly, and the thumb anteriorly. The lower limit of this area is marked by the bases of the metacarpal bones with their shafts running distally to end in rounded heads, all of which are easily palpable. The base, shaft and head of each phalanx are again readily palpable posteriorly, particularly when the subject's fingers are flexed. Anteriorly, they are hidden by tendons and the pulp of the fingers.

Palpation on movement

With the wrist in extension, locate the tubercle of the scaphoid and the pisiform bone. As the wrist is taken into flexion they appear to move backwards and become indistinct. Keeping the wrist in flexion, the posterior aspect of the carpal bones can be palpated just below the ulna and

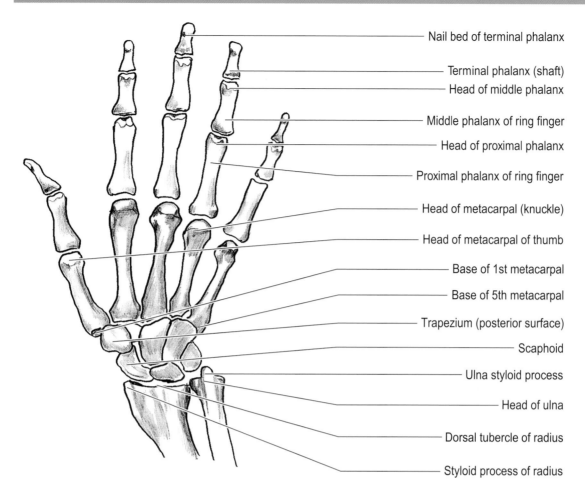

Nail bed of terminal phalanx

Terminal phalanx (shaft)

Head of middle phalanx

Middle phalanx of ring finger

Head of proximal phalanx

Proximal phalanx of ring finger

Head of metacarpal (knuckle)

Head of metacarpal of thumb

Base of 1st metacarpal

Base of 5th metacarpal

Trapezium (posterior surface)

Scaphoid

Ulna styloid process

Head of ulna

Dorsal tubercle of radius

Styloid process of radius

Fig. 2.5 (b)
Bones of the right hand (posterior
view)

radius. If the wrist is taken back into extension, they appear to move forwards and become indistinct.

With the model's index finger in extension, grip the base of the proximal phalanx with your thumb anteriorly and the fingers posteriorly. When the model now flexes the finger you will note that the phalanx moves round to the front of the head of the metacarpal leaving the head prominent (the knuckle). This is common to all the fingers, but more obvious in the index finger. Apply the same procedure to the base of the proximal phalanx of the thumb and you will note that only half the movement is available and the head of the metacarpal is only partially exposed.

If the same procedure is carried out on the inter-phalangeal joints, the head of the most proximal of the two bones becomes palpable as a small 'knuckle' shape.

Functional anatomy

Fractures of the carpal bones are rare except in the case of the scaphoid, which is sometimes damaged by a fall on the outstretched hand. Palpation of the area will normally identify swelling and a rise in temperature around the area, but may elicit acute pain. It is more common in young adults and may need 2–3 months in plaster before healing occurs. As the blood supply to the tubercle of the scaphoid passes through its neck, if the fracture occurs at this point there may be delayed or even non union and a prolonged period in plaster or even an operation may have to be performed. (See orthopaedic literature for further information.)

Fractures of the metacarpal bones is fairly common at all ages and is often due again to a fall on the outstretched hand or a longitudinal force along the metacarpal, as in punching. Displacements are easily palpable combined with the swelling and increase in temperature. Only if there is displacement is there a need for intervention.

Injuries to the phalanges are usually due to direct violence such as trapping the fingers in a door. Displacement is easily palpable, along with the swelling, increase in temperature and acute pain. Alignment must be restored and minimal splinting should be used, perhaps just to the adjoining finger.

All splinting of the hand should be kept to a minimum due to the serious complication of stiffness.

SELF ASSESSMENT

Page 14

1. Identify and name the two bones which comprise the shoulder girdle.

2. Which of these bones lies anteriorly?

3. What is the alternative name for the shoulder joint?

4. With which two bones does the clavicle articulate?

5. Describe the ways in which the clavicle differs from other long bones.

6. Which bones form the sternal notch?

7. Name two muscles which attach to the medial end of the clavicle.

8. Name and palpate the structure below the middle third of the clavicle.

9. Name and palpate the structures in the supraclavicular and infraclavicular fossae.

Page 15

10. Which two muscles are attached to the anterior and posterior borders of the lateral end of the clavicle?

11. Name and palpate the three bony processes which form the upper end of the humerus.

12. What structure lies between the two tuberosities of the humerus?

13. Name the muscle whose tendon passes between these two tuberosities.

Page 16

14. Describe the general location of the scapula.

15. Name the fossa lying above the spine of the scapula.

16. List the three features which form the lateral angle of the scapula.

17. How much of the spine can be palpated?

18. What structure attaches to the lower lip of the spine of the scapula?

19. Name and palpate the structure which lies immediately on top of the acromion process.

21. In the anatomical position, locate and name the rib on which the superior angle of the scapula lies.

22. In the same position, on which ribs is the inferior angle located?

Please complete the labels below.

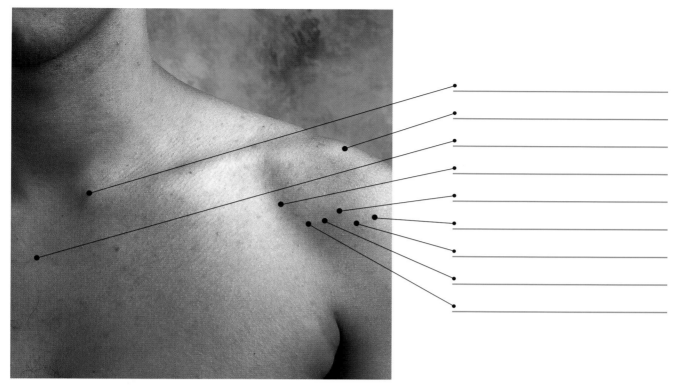

Fig. 2.1 (a) The left shoulder (anterior view)

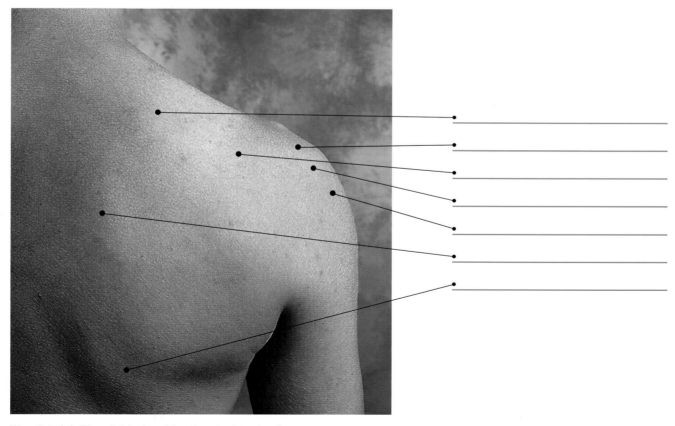

Fig. 2.2 (a) The right shoulder (posterior view)

Page 17

23. From above downwards name the three muscles which attach to the medial border of the scapula.

24. Name the muscles which attach to the lateral border of the scapula.

25. Describe the surface markings for locating the coracoid process.

26. Name the muscles which attach to the coracoid process.

27. Demonstrate and describe protrusion of the scapula.

28. Describe scapula movement in elevation of the shoulder girdle.

29. Demonstrate shoulder abduction and identify the point at which the scapula begins to move.

30. In which direction does the inferior angle of the scapula move when the arm is elevated?

31. In the same movement, in which direction does the superior angle of the scapula travel?

Page 18

32. Approximately what angle does the clavicle form with the spine of the scapula when viewed from above?

33. Name and palpate the two borders which form the acromial angle.

34. In which direction does the medial end of the clavicle move on protrusion of the shoulder girdle?

35. Which ligament acts as the axis around which the clavicle moves?

Page 19

36. In which direction does the medial end of the clavicle move when the shoulder girdle is elevated?

37. Describe the final movement of the clavicle in full elevation of the upper limb.

38. What functions does the clavicle perform?

39. Which ligament attaches the coracoid process to the clavicle?

40. In which region do clavicular fractures usually occur?

41. Describe and explain the serious complications which can occur with this fracture (fr).

42. Under normal circumstances, how long does it take for the clavicle to unite?

Please complete the labels below.

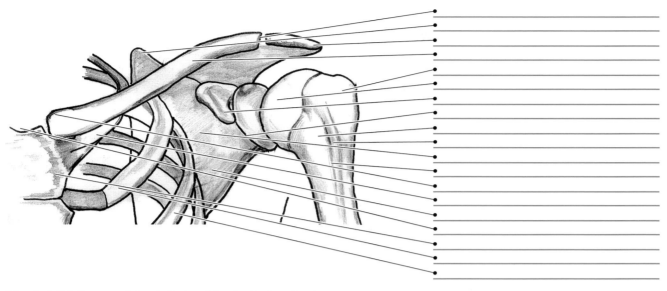

Fig. 2.1 (b) Bones of the left shoulder (anterior view)

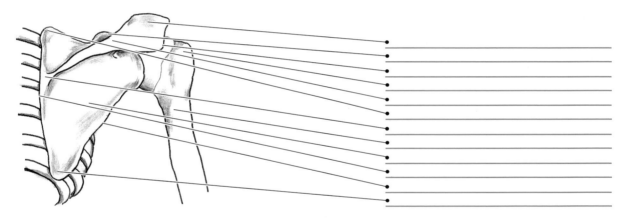

Fig. 2.2 (b) Bones of the right shoulder (posterior view)

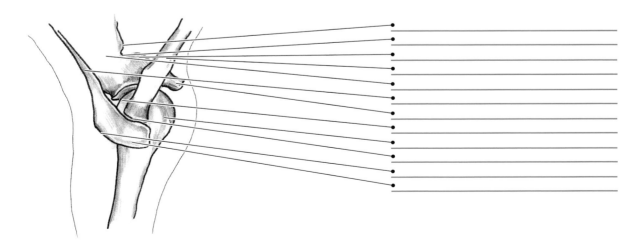

Fig. 2.2 (d) Bones of the right shoulder (upper lateral view)

Page 20

43. Name the lateral articular condyle of the humerus.

44. Name the medial articular condyle of the humerus.

45. Identify the two fossae above the anterior surfaces of the condyles.

46. Name the fossa above the articular condyles posteriorly.

47. The lateral epicondyle lies at the lower end of which ridge?

48. Name and palpate the bony processes which form the upper end of the radius.

49. Describe the lower attachments of the tendon of biceps brachii.

50. Which nerve crosses the middle of the lateral border of the humerus?

51. Name and palpate the structure below the lateral epicondyle of the humerus.

Page 21

52. Name and palpate the bony processes which comprise the upper end of the ulna.

53. What lies on the posterior surface of the olecranon?

54. Which feature of what bone is subcutaneous on the posterior surface of the forearm?

55. Explain why the olecranon is more difficult to palpate when the elbow is extended.

56. Which muscle attaches to the superior surface of the olecranon?

57. Describe what happens to the radial head when the forearm is pro and supinated.

58. Name the angle formed between the humerus and the forearm when the arm is extended.

Page 22

59. Name and indicate the prominence which lies at the lower end of the medial supracondylar ridge.

60. Which is the lowest flange of the trochlea?

61. What process projects forward from the trochlear notch?

62. How far below the medial epicondyle is the line of the elbow joint?

63. Explain why palpation posterior to this area is tender.

64. In 90 degees of elbow flexion state the structures which can be palpated posteriorly between the medial and lateral condyles of the humerus.

Please complete the labels below.

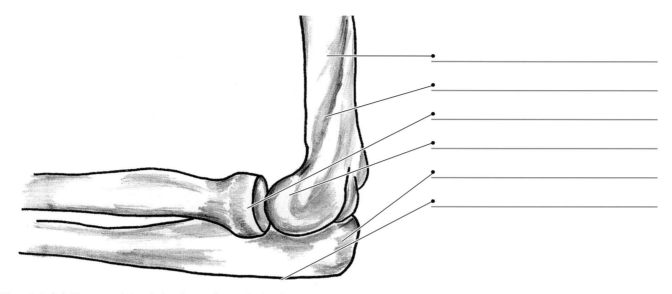

Fig. 2.3 (b) Bones of the left elbow (lateral view)

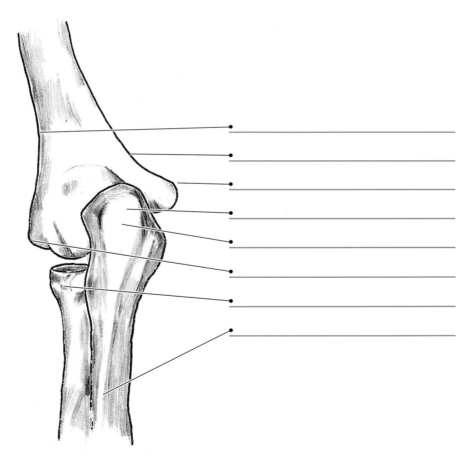

Fig. 2.3 (d) Bones of the left elbow (posterior view)

Page 23

65. Below and lateral to the medial epicondyle, at what distance can the tip of the coranoid process be identified?

Page 24

66. Name the proximal row of carpal bones from lateral to medial.

_____

67. Name the distal row of carpal bones from lateral to medial.

_____

68. Name and palpate the largest carpal bone.

_____

69. Which bone lies on the anterior surface of the triquetral?

_____

70. Which muscle tendon attaches to this bone?

_____

71. What structure can be palpated 1 cm distal to the pisiform bone?

_____

72. Name and palpate the two nerves which can be rolled against this bony prominence.

_____

Page 25

73. Name and indicate the space in which the radial styloid process is found.

_____

74. Identify the structure which lies just medial to the anterior crest of the radial styloid.

_____

75. Describe how the position of the first metacarpal bone differs from the other bones.

_____

76. What distance medial to the styloid process of the radius is the scaphoid tubercle?

_____

77. Name and palpate the structure which can be felt just distal to the scaphoid tubercle.

_____

Page 26

78. Identify the process which lies on the posteromedial side of the head of the ulna.

_____

79. Name the structure which often crosses the lower end of the lateral surface of the radius.

_____

80. Which metacarpal articulates with the capitate bone?

_____

81. The trapezoid articulates with which metacarpal?

_____

Page 27

82. Name the bony features which form the knuckles in the clenched fist.

_____

83. How much less movement occurs in the first metacarpophalangeal joint compared with the movements of the fingers?

_____

84. Explain the reasons for delayed union of the scaphoid with its tubercle (fr).

_____

85. Explain the reasons for restricted splinting of the hand (fr).

_____

Please complete the labels below.

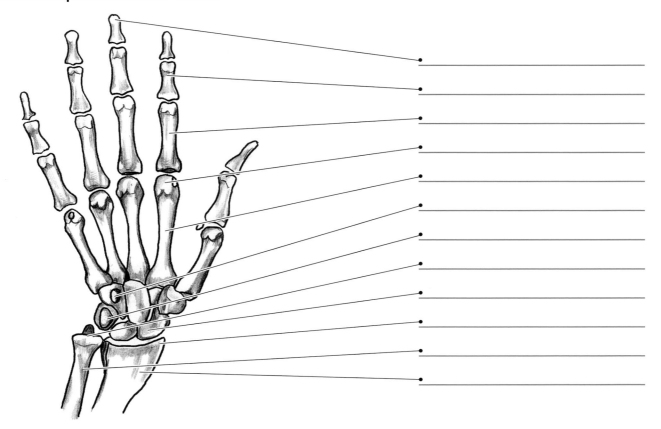

Fig. 2.4 (b) Bones of the right hand (anterior view)

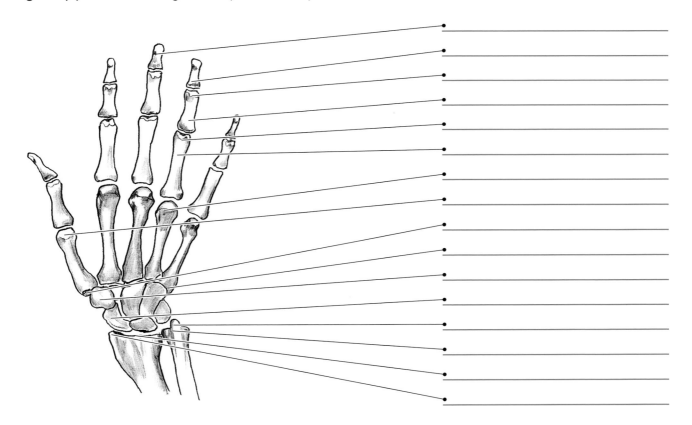

Fig. 2.5 (b) Bones of the right hand (posterior view)

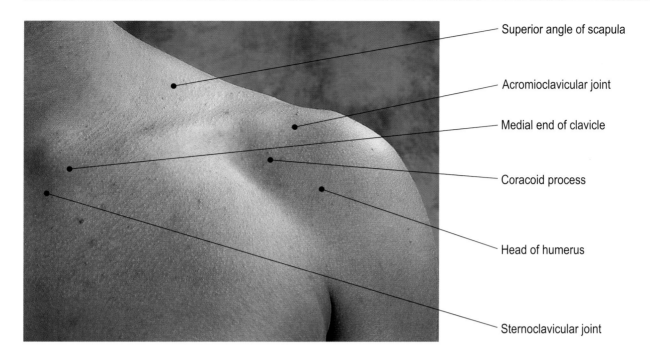

Superior angle of scapula

Acromioclavicular joint

Medial end of clavicle

Coracoid process

Head of humerus

Sternoclavicular joint

Fig. 2.6 (a)
The shoulder region (anterior view)

JOINTS

Joints of the pectoral girdle

The sternoclavicular joint [Fig. 2.6]

At its medial end the clavicle articulates with the clavicular notch of the manubrium. The joint is synovial, being surrounded by a capsule lined with synovial membrane, except where it is attached to the edges of a fibrous disc which divides the joint space into two separate cavities. It is a modified saddle (sellar) joint and its capsule is supported by ligaments, the intercostal above and medially, the costoclavicular laterally below the clavicle and the anterior and posterior across the front and back of the joint. It is subcutaneous, allowing easy palpation of the joint line and a reasonable examination of joint movement.

Surface marking

The sternoclavicular joint can be palpated at the upper lateral corner of the manubrium sterni, as a curved line concave laterally. It is approximately 1 cm in length, extending over the lower half of the medial surface of the clavicle, passing inferolaterally for approximately 0.5 cm.

Palpation

Run your fingers down the front of the neck until you reach the sternal notch. Below you will feel the manubrium sterni and laterally the medial end of the clavicle with the sternoclavicular joint between the two.

Immediately lateral to the joint, between the clavicle and the first rib, is the costoclavicular ligament. This is not palpable, but acts as the fulcrum for movements of the clavicle at the joint. Thus when the lateral end of the clavicle is drawn backwards (retraction), the medial end can be observed gliding forward, projecting anterior to the plane of the manubrium. Similarly, when the

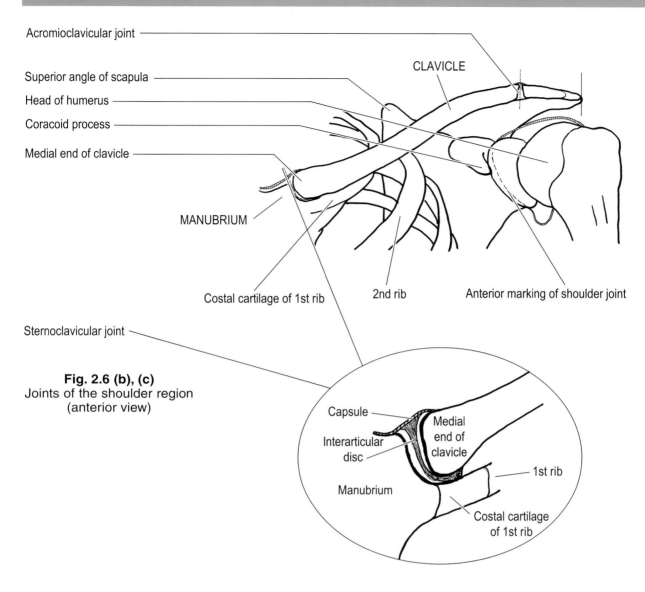

Acromioclavicular joint

Superior angle of scapula

Head of humerus

Coracoid process

Medial end of clavicle

CLAVICLE

MANUBRIUM

Costal cartilage of 1st rib

2nd rib

Anterior marking of shoulder joint

Sternoclavicular joint

Fig. 2.6 (b), (c)
Joints of the shoulder region
(anterior view)

Capsule

Interarticular disc

Manubrium

Medial end of clavicle

1st rib

Costal cartilage of 1st rib

lateral end of the clavicle is brought forwards (protraction), the medial end can be palpated moving backwards behind the plane of the manubrium. If the pectoral girdle is raised (elevation), the medial end of the clavicle glides downwards on the clavicular notch of the manubrium until it is level with the superior border of the manubrium. If the pectoral girdle is pulled downwards (depression), the medial end of the clavicle rises on the clavicular notch. All these movements can be observed occurring around the attachment of the costoclavicular ligament.

When the upper limb is raised above the head, the scapula laterally rotates against the chest wall, and the lateral end of the clavicle is elevated until, during the final few degrees of movement, it is accompanied by a backward rotation of the whole clavicle so that the anterior surface faces more superiorly. This rotation is due to the tension developed in the coracoclavicular ligament.

Accessory movements

Gliding of the medial end of the clavicle either forwards, backwards, upwards or downwards, or rotating its articular surfaces upwards, are all normal movements. Pressure applied to the medial end of the clavicle will produce little movement, as the stress is taken by the costoclavicular ligament which usually remains taut and reasonably inflexible. If, however, similar pressures are applied to the medial end of the clavicle, with the pectoral girdle in an appropriate position to aid the movement, then additional movement can be achieved. For example, if the pectoral girdle is protruded, pressure applied anteroposteriorly will augment the movement of the medial end of the clavicle. Pressure to raise the anterior surface of the medial end of the clavicle, as in the final stages of elevation, is best applied when the upper limb is as near to full elevation as possible.

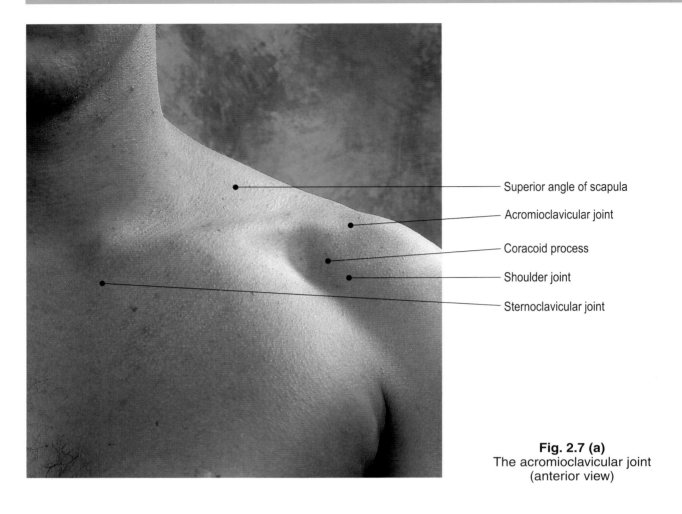

Superior angle of scapula

Acromioclavicular joint

Coracoid process

Shoulder joint

Sternoclavicular joint

Fig. 2.7 (a)
The acromioclavicular joint
(anterior view)

The acromioclavicular joint [Fig. 2.7]

The acromioclavicular joint is immediately lateral to the anterior concavity at the lateral one-third of the clavicle, approximately 1.5 cm medial to the lateral border of the acromion process. It can be marked from above by drawing a line in an anteroposterior direction just lateral to a small tubercle on the upper surface of the lateral end of the clavicle. It is a plane synovial joint lying in a paramedian plane of the body. It is surrounded by a joint capsule supported above by the superior acromioclavicular ligament. It does rely for its stability, however, on the costoclavicular and the coracoclavicular ligaments which act as accessory ligaments to this joint. The two oval facets, one on the lateral end of the clavicle and the other on the medial aspect of the acromion process, are not congruent and rely on a small disc or part of a disc which fills the upper part of the joint space.

Palpation

Stand facing the model's left shoulder. Run your right hand up over the beautiful shape of the deltoid muscle on the lateral aspect of the shoulder. At the top you will feel the lateral border of the acromion process marked posteriorly by its angle. Now trace along the anterior border of the acromion for 1.5 cm and you will feel a small indentation where the clavicle joins the acromion. A very faint groove passes posteriorly to another small indentation on the posterior surface. The joint is quite difficult to palpate unless movement is occurring. Slight twisting or gapping of the acromion against the clavicle can be identified with movements of the pectoral girdle, but even then only with careful palpation. On full elevation of the pectoral girdle the acromion process rotates backwards against the lateral end of the clavicle until the final few degrees of elevation when the clavicle also rotates backwards, producing an upward movement of the anterior surface of the clavicle in its entire length. This is partly due to

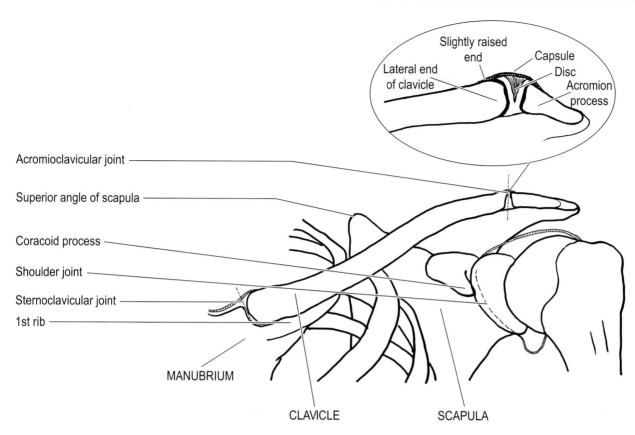

Acromioclavicular joint

Superior angle of scapula

Coracoid process

Shoulder joint

Sternoclavicular joint

1st rib

MANUBRIUM

CLAVICLE   SCAPULA

Fig. 2.7 (b), (c)
The acromioclavicular joint
(anterior view)

the tension of the coronoid part of the coraco-clavicular ligament pulling down the posterior aspect of the clavicle, and partly due to the costo-clavicular ligament at the medial end of the clavicle attaching to its posterior aspect. This movement is also facilitated by the thickness of the disc in the sternoclavicular joint allowing a longitudinal rotation to occur.

The superior surface of the acromioclavicular joint is usually quite tender on palpation, due to pressure on the superior acromioclavicular liga-ment. This tenderness is increased after prolonged activity involving the pectoral girdle or after carrying heavy loads on the shoulder.

Accessory movements

This joint is capable of slight gliding movements, these being forwards, backwards, upwards and downwards. It is also able to rotate, with one surface pivoting on the other, as well as allowing a certain amount of gapping anteriorly and poste-riorly. All these movements are normal but, as with the sterno-clavicular joint, the end-range can be increased by addition of pressure in the appro-priate direction. These again are best performed at the end of normal range, so that, for example, an increase in posterior gliding of the acromion is best achieved with the pectoral girdle retracted. Movement can be achieved by applying pressure, with the thumbs, either to the lateral end of the clavicle or the anterior aspect of the acromion. The former appears to be easier to apply.

Although the acromioclavicular and sterno-clavicular joints may appear to be insignificant, stiffness of either will reduce the range of move-ment of the pectoral girdle, resulting in serious functional loss in the range of movement of the upper limb, and may be misdiagnosed as shoulder joint stiffness.

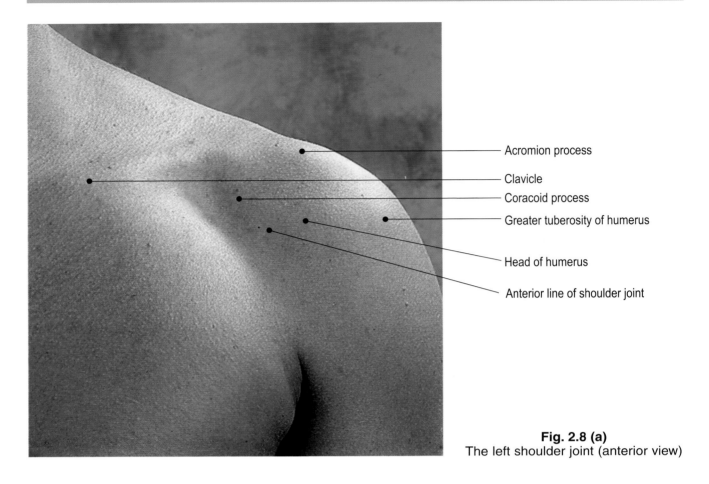

Acromion process

Clavicle

Coracoid process

Greater tuberosity of humerus

Head of humerus

Anterior line of shoulder joint

Fig. 2.8 (a)
The left shoulder joint (anterior view)

The shoulder joint [Fig. 2.8]

This is a synovial joint of the ball-and-socket type. The head of the humerus is slightly less than half a sphere, but is more ovoid in shape. The glenoid cavity is shallow and is estimated to have only one-third the articular surface of the head of the humerus. Both surfaces are covered with articular cartilage. The joint is capable of a large range of movements which are essential for full functional activity of the upper limb. The apparent range of the joint is further increased by the movements of the shoulder (pectoral) girdle, allowing the glenoid cavity to be directed more upwards than laterally.

The joint is surrounded by a loose capsule which is lined by synovial membrane and is supported by ligaments, in front by the glenohumeral, above and posteriorly by the coracohumeral and across the bicipital groove by the transverse ligament. Around the outer rim of the glenoid cavity of the scapula, deep to the joint capsule, is attached a fibrous ring, which is triangular in cross-section and named the glenoidal labrum.

Surface marking

The anterior joint line is a shallow curve concave laterally; its upper boundary is just lateral to and above the coracoid process passing downwards and slightly laterally for approximately 2–3 cm. The head of the humerus can also be identified lying lateral to the joint line.

Palpation

The joint is deep, being surrounded by strong, thick muscles, and is therefore not easy to palpate. Its anterior aspect is the nearest to the surface, and with careful palpation the head of the humerus and the anterior rim of the glenoid fossa can be identified. The rounded anterior part of the head can be palpated with comparative ease; traced upwards it is masked by the anterior part of the acromion, while below it becomes lost in the axilla. Laterally it is bounded by the lesser tubercle, projecting forwards, which forms the medial lip of the bicipital (inter-tubercular) groove. The long head of the biceps brachii can be palpated running

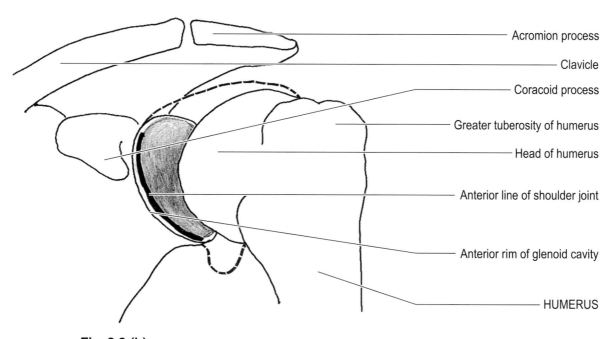

Fig. 2.8 (b)
The left shoulder joint (anterior view)

Labels: Acromion process, Clavicle, Coracoid process, Greater tuberosity of humerus, Head of humerus, Anterior line of shoulder joint, Anterior rim of glenoid cavity, HUMERUS

up the groove and on to the anterolateral aspect of the humeral head.

When the upper limb is laterally rotated, more of the head becomes palpable: on medial rotation it can be felt sliding backwards against the glenoid fossa, eventually disappearing. The lesser tubercle can also be palpated, moving laterally and medially with the movement of rotation of the humerus.

On abduction of the arm, the anterior part of the humeral head can be felt gliding downwards, with the reverse happening when the arm is returned to the side. Palpation of the head in this case, however, is made more difficult by the contraction of the anterior fibres of the deltoid which pass across the anterior aspect of the joint.

Posteriorly (see Fig. 2.8e,f), the shoulder joint is estimated to be at the same level and in the same sagittal plane as it is anteriorly, being just below the spine of the scapula 2–3 cm medial to the angle of the acromion. Laterally (see Fig. 2.8c,d), the centre of the joint is approximately 2 cm below the anterior half of the lateral border of the acromion.

Although the lateral border, angle and posterior border are easily palpable and useful for calculating the position of the shoulder joint from the back, the joint itself is set so deeply in muscle that it is impossible to recognise in normal subjects.

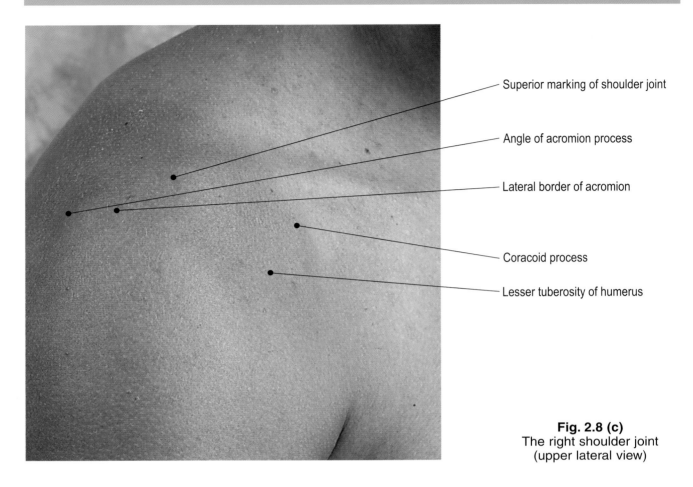

— Superior marking of shoulder joint

— Angle of acromion process

— Lateral border of acromion

— Coracoid process

— Lesser tuberosity of humerus

Fig. 2.8 (c)
The right shoulder joint
(upper lateral view)

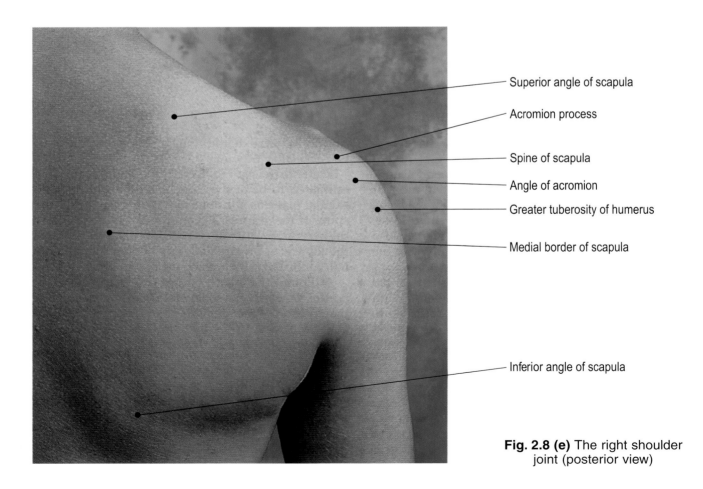

— Superior angle of scapula

— Acromion process

— Spine of scapula

— Angle of acromion

— Greater tuberosity of humerus

— Medial border of scapula

— Inferior angle of scapula

Fig. 2.8 (e) The right shoulder
joint (posterior view)

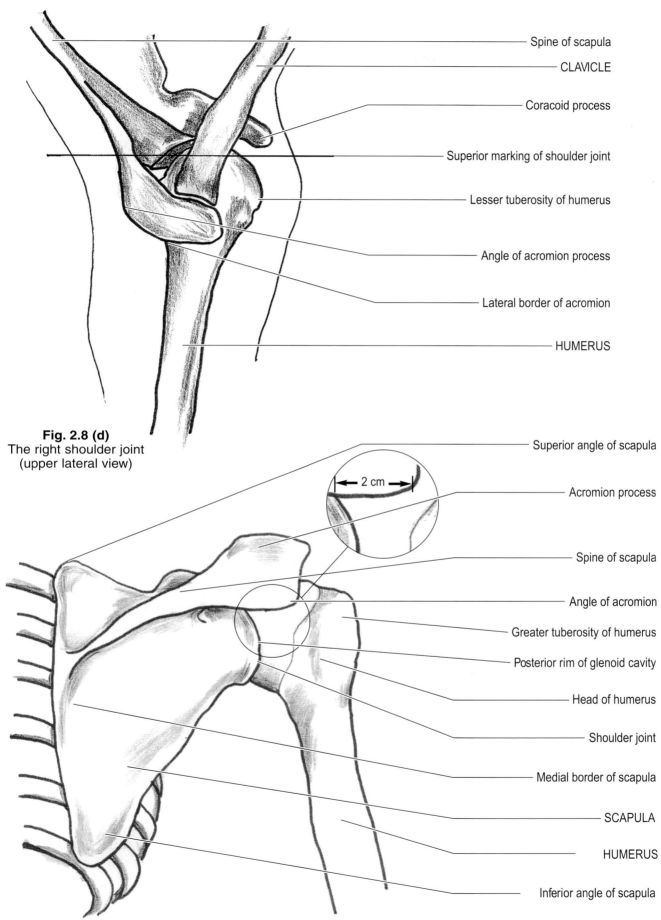

Spine of scapula

CLAVICLE

Coracoid process

Superior marking of shoulder joint

Lesser tuberosity of humerus

Angle of acromion process

Lateral border of acromion

HUMERUS

Fig. 2.8 (d)
The right shoulder joint
(upper lateral view)

Superior angle of scapula

2 cm

Acromion process

Spine of scapula

Angle of acromion

Greater tuberosity of humerus

Posterior rim of glenoid cavity

Head of humerus

Shoulder joint

Medial border of scapula

SCAPULA

HUMERUS

Inferior angle of scapula

Fig. 2.8 (f) The right shoulder joint
(posterior view)

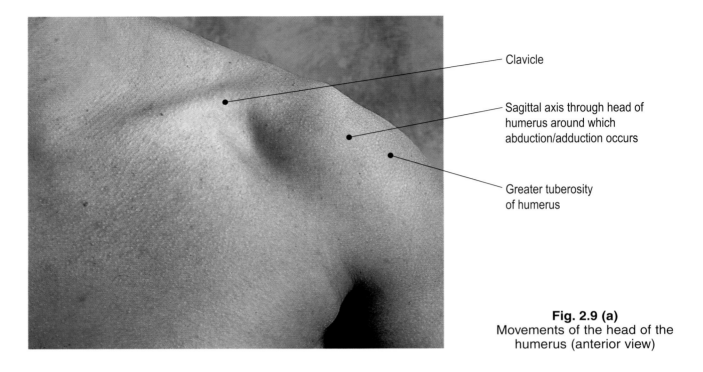

Clavicle

Sagittal axis through head of humerus around which abduction/adduction occurs

Greater tuberosity of humerus

Fig. 2.9 (a)
Movements of the head of the humerus (anterior view)

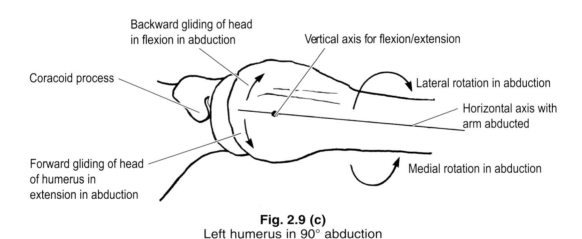

Backward gliding of head in flexion in abduction

Vertical axis for flexion/extension

Coracoid process

Lateral rotation in abduction

Horizontal axis with arm abducted

Forward gliding of head of humerus in extension in abduction

Medial rotation in abduction

Fig. 2.9 (c)
Left humerus in 90° abduction (superior view)

Movements of the head of the humerus

As the axis of movement of the shoulder joint is through the centre of the head of the humerus (Palastanga, Field and Soames 1998), movements of the distal end of the humerus produce an opposite gliding of the head against the glenoid fossa. Thus, abduction causes a downward gliding and an upward rolling of the head of the humerus on the glenoid cavity around a sagittal axis (Fig. 2.9b). Flexion and extension (Fig. 2.9d), however, produce rotation or spin of the head around a frontal axis within the glenoid fossa, similar to that produced by rotating the limb in abduction (Fig. 2.9c). Rotation, with the arm by the side, however, produces a gliding forwards and rolling backwards of the head on lateral rotation and a gliding backwards and rolling forwards on medial rotation around a vertical axis. The combination of rolling in one direction and gliding in the other maintains the position of the centre of axis of the head (Fig. 2.9e). With the subject performing one movement at a time and with your fingers placed over the head of the humerus, these movements can be observed. It becomes even clearer if the palpation is performed with one hand and the humerus is carefully taken through the movement passively.

The shoulder joint has a loose joint capsule and relatively weak associated ligaments, relying to a large extent on muscular activity, especially in the 'rotator cuff' muscles (supraspinatus, infraspinatus, teres minor and subscapularis), for joint stability. It has an extensive range of movement together with a complementary range of accessory movements.

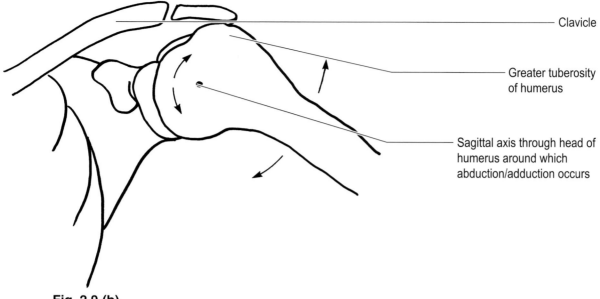

Fig. 2.9 (b)
Movements of the head of the
humerus (anterior view)

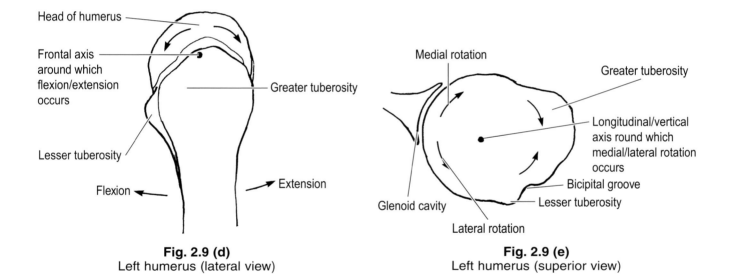

Fig. 2.9 (d)
Left humerus (lateral view)

Fig. 2.9 (e)
Left humerus (superior view)

Accessory movements

If the accessory movements are reduced, or lost, normal movement becomes reduced or occasionally eliminated.

The head of the humerus can be drawn laterally away from the glenoid fossa for approximately 1–2 cm, but only when the muscles are completely relaxed (distraction). This is usually possible when the humerus is between 0° and 90° of abduction. To palpate the gapping which occurs, it is best to ask the subject to lie either supine or on his or her side with a colleague actually performing the distraction. Place your fingers on the anterior aspect of the joint where the head and anterior rim of the glenoid fossa can be palpated (see page 40).

Other accessory movements at the joint are: a gliding of the head of the humerus either downwards or upwards by pulling down or pushing up on the arm; and a gliding of the head either forwards or backwards on the glenoid fossa by direct pressure on the upper end of the humerus. Again, it is better to ask a colleague to move the head of the humerus, in the way described above, while you gently palpate using several fingers on the area at the front of the joint where the head and glenoid fossa can be palpated.

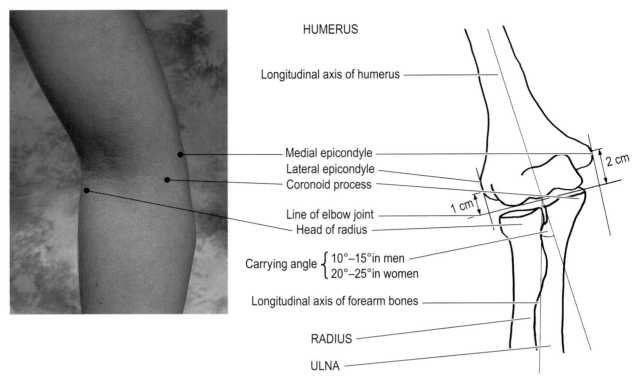

Fig. 2.10 (a), (b)
The right elbow joint (anterior view)

The elbow joint [Fig 2.10]

The elbow joint is basically a hinge joint between the humerus above and the ulna and radius below. The articular surfaces are, medially, the trochlea above and the trochlear notch of the ulna below, and laterally the capitulum above and the upper surface of the head of radius below.

The articular surfaces of the trochlea, capitulum, trochlear notch and the head of the radius are all covered with articular cartilage. The joint is surrounded by an extensive capsule which extends up onto the front and back of the humerus above the radial, coronoid and olecranon fossae. It is supported on either side by two strong ligaments. The ulna collateral, triangular, joining the medial epicondyle to the medial side of the olecranon and coronoid processes, and the lateral, again triangular, joining the lateral epicondyle to the annular ligament surrounding the head of the radius. The capsule is lined with synovial membrane.

Surface marking

The joint line is drawn from a point 2 cm below the tip of the medial epicondyle to a point 1 cm below the tip of the lateral epicondyle of the humerus (Fig. 2.10a,b). The line passes downwards and medially due to the medial margin of the trochlea projecting down further than the lateral. When viewed from the front, this produces an angle at the elbow where the long axis of the ulna deviates laterally from that of the humerus by approximately 10–15° in men and 20–25° in women (Palastanga, Field and Soames 1998). The angle at the elbow is only apparent on full extension and supination of the forearm and is commonly termed the 'carrying angle' (Fig. 2.10b).

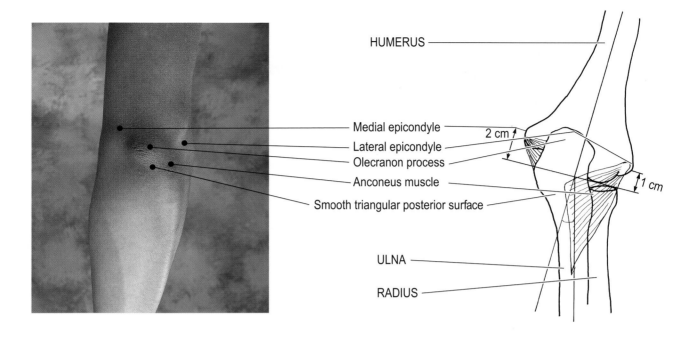

HUMERUS

Medial epicondyle
2 cm
Lateral epicondyle
Olecranon process
Anconeus muscle
1 cm
Smooth triangular posterior surface

ULNA

RADIUS

Fig. 2.10 (c), (d)
The right elbow joint (posterior view)

Palpation

The joint is easily identified on the lateral side between the lateral epicondyle of the humerus and the lateral side of the head of the radius (see page 20). However, moving anteriorly the joint line is difficult to follow as it disappears under the superficial extensor muscles which arise from the lateral epicondyle. Posteriorly, it can be traced as far as the radial notch of the ulna at the posterior aspect of the superior radioulnar joint (Fig. 2.10d).

Anteriorly, the elbow joint is not palpable as it lies deep to muscles: the extensor muscles laterally and the strong flexor muscles anteromedially, with brachialis and biceps between. Posteriorly, however, with the elbow flexed to 90°, the anterior edge of the olecranon can be palpated and can be traced down either side until hidden by anconeus laterally and by the medial collateral ligament medially (Fig. 2.10d).

Accessory movements

With the elbow flexed approximately 15°, the ulna and radius can be rocked from side to side. This is achieved by stabilizing the arm just above the medial and lateral supracondylar ridges with one hand and applying a side-to-side force just above the wrist. The correct angle is critical for the movement to take place and varies from individual to individual.

The elbow can also be distracted, provided that the muscles are relaxed, by applying a force in the direction of the long axis of the humerus on a flexed elbow. This may need considerable force and is best achieved with the subject lying supine or on their side.

With the elbow at a right angle and the upper arm stabilized, the forearm can be moved very slightly in its long axis, producing a gapping at the anterior and posterior aspect of the joint. These techniques are best studied from the mobilization and manipulation literature.

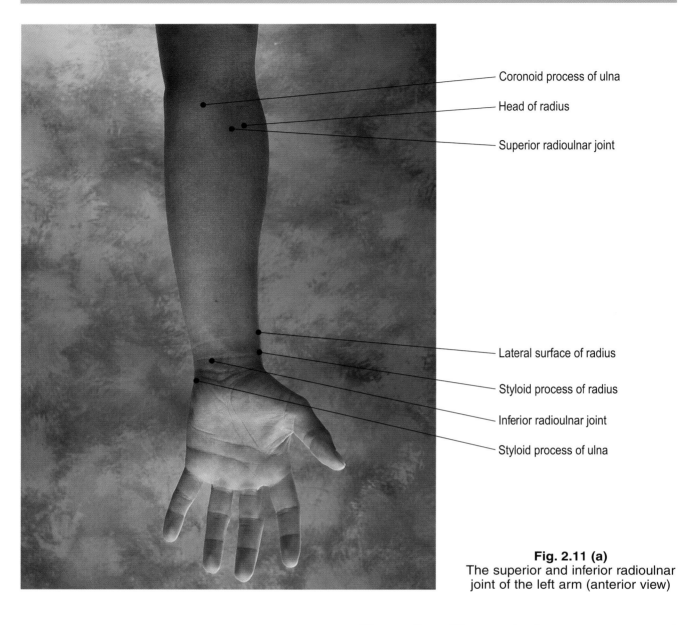

Coronoid process of ulna

Head of radius

Superior radioulnar joint

Lateral surface of radius

Styloid process of radius

Inferior radioulnar joint

Styloid process of ulna

Fig. 2.11 (a)
The superior and inferior radioulnar
joint of the left arm (anterior view)

The radioulnar union

The movements of pronation and supination occur between the radius and ulna. They involve a type of rotation movement at the superior and inferior radioulnar joint and a twisting movement between the shafts of both bones. This latter region is often referred to as the radioulnar union, as the two bones are held together by the interosseous membrane.

The superior radioulnar joint

The superior radioulnar joint is a synovial pivot joint between the medial one-fifth of the head of the radius and the radial notch on the lateral side of the coronoid process of the ulna.

Both surfaces are covered with hyaline cartilage and are reciprocally curved. The head is surrounded by the annular ligament, which is attached in front and behind the radial notch of the ulna and forms the other four-fifths of the ring and is lined with

fibrocartilage. The annular ligament is supported from above by the capsule and the triangular radiocollateral ligament of the elbow joint and from below by the quadrate ligament attaching it to the ulna. The joint is further stabilized by the interosseous membrane which binds the radius and ulna together.

Synovial membrane lines the inner surface of the annular ligament in a double fold attaching to the edges of the articular facets of ulna and radius and emerges just below the annular ligament as a loose fold. It is continuous with that of the elbow joint, although functionally it is a completely separate joint.

Surface marking

The surface marking for the joint anteriorly and posteriorly is a vertical line, 1 cm long, drawn downwards from the line of the elbow joint (see above), 2 cm medial to the lateral edge of the head of the radius (Fig. 2.11).

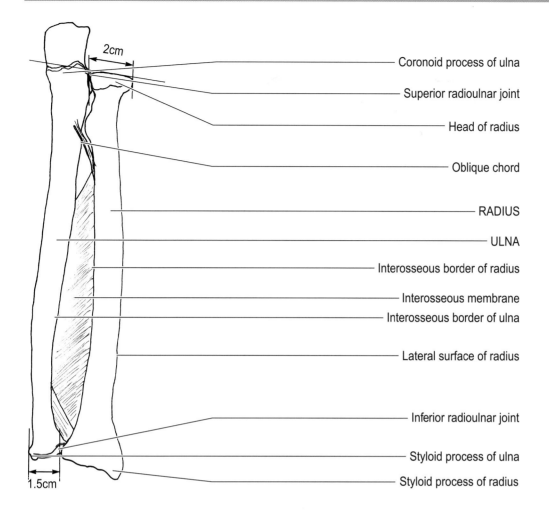

Fig. 2.11 (b)
The superior and inferior radioulnar
joint of the left arm (anterior view)

Palpation

Locate the head of the radius just below the lateral epicondyle of the humerus. Trace backwards around the radial head until the movement is arrested by contact with the lateral side of the ulna. The joint space is usually hidden by the anconeus muscle. Anteriorly, the surface marking is covered by muscle and is not palpable.

When the forearm is pronated and supinated, the head of the radius can be felt rotating under the fingers.

Accessory movements

If the head of the radius is firmly gripped between the fingers and thumb of one hand and the upper end of the ulna is stabilized by the other, slight backwards and forwards gliding of the head can be produced.

Traction on the lower part of the radius can produce a slight gliding up and down of the head of the radius against the radial notch of the ulna. Note that if too much traction is applied to the radius in younger children, as in lifting the child by the forearm, the head of the radius may dislocate out of the annular ring causing much pain and discomfort.

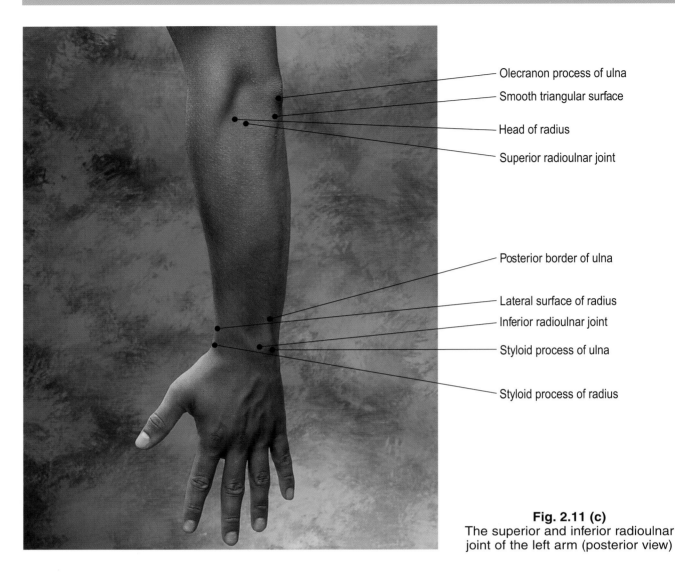

Olecranon process of ulna
Smooth triangular surface
Head of radius
Superior radioulnar joint

Posterior border of ulna
Lateral surface of radius
Inferior radioulnar joint
Styloid process of ulna

Styloid process of radius

Fig. 2.11 (c)
The superior and inferior radioulnar
joint of the left arm (posterior view)

The inferior radioulnar joint

This joint is also a synovial pivot joint, being between the ulnar notch on the medial side of the distal end of the radius and the lateral rim of the head of the ulna. Both surfaces are covered with articular cartilage and the joint is surrounded by a capsule which is thicker front and back. A triangular interarticular disc is situated between the lower end of the ulna and the carpus, which attaches medially to the base of the styloid process of the ulna and laterally to the medial edge of the inferior surface of the radius. At this joint, the radius moves around the head of the ulna in conjunction with the rotation of the head of the radius against the ulna at the superior radioulnar joint.

The mid radioulnar union

The radius and the ulna are joined together for most of their length by the interosseous membrane, which attaches to the interosseous borders of both bones, except for a small space at the upper part. This thin collagenous sheet, broader at its middle, is made up of fibres which pass downwards and medially from the radius to the ulna. Its fibres help to bind the two bones together whilst allowing movement between them. It gives support to the superior and inferior radioulnar joints and, owing to the direction of its fibres, transmits weight from the radius to the ulna. If you examine both the radius and the ulna you will note that the lower end of the radius is large and takes any force transmitted from the carpus, whereas its head is relatively small and obviously transmits very little, if any, force to the capitulum. The ulna, on the other hand, has a very small head at its lower end, which takes very little force from the carpus, whereas its upper end is large and obviously transmits most of the force through to the trochlea of the humerus.

There is an oblique cord running downwards and laterally which attaches the tubercles at the upper part of the ulna with the radius just below its tuberosity. It is distinct from the interosseous membrane.

The interosseous membrane and oblique cord cannot be palpated.

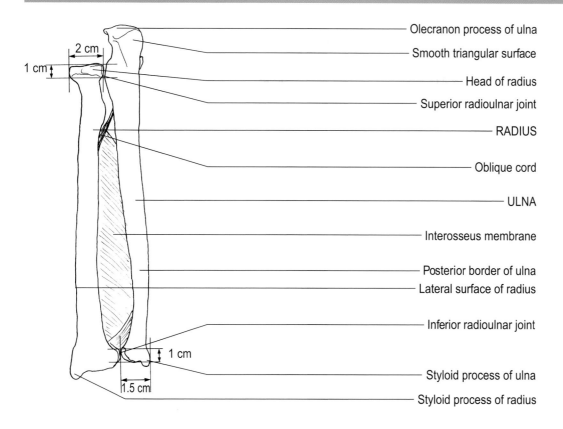

Olecranon process of ulna
Smooth triangular surface
Head of radius
Superior radioulnar joint
RADIUS
Oblique cord
ULNA
Interosseus membrane
Posterior border of ulna
Lateral surface of radius
Inferior radioulnar joint
Styloid process of ulna
Styloid process of radius

Fig. 2.11 (d)
The superior and inferior radioulnar
joint of the left arm (posterior view)

Surface markings

The joint line is 1.5 cm lateral to the medial rim of
the head of the ulna running 1 cm upwards from
the line of the wrist joint (Figs 2.11 and 2.12).

Palpation

The joint can more easily be palpated posteriorly,
where there is a vertical depression for 1 cm immediately above the line of the wrist joint 1.5 cm
lateral to the ulnar styloid process (Fig. 2.11). The
tendon of extensor digiti minimi crosses the posterior aspect of the joint and if the little finger is
extended it can be identified. Anteriorly the joint
is much more difficult to palpate, as the fingers
must be slipped under the thick tendon of flexor
carpi ulnaris from the medial side.

On pronation and supination the radius can be
felt moving around the lateral side of the head
of the ulna, which itself in turn moves slightly
laterally on pronation and medially on supination.

Accessory movements

If the head of the ulna is gripped firmly between
fingers and thumb of one hand and the lower end
of the radius is stabilized by the other hand, slight
forwards and backwards gliding of the ulnar head
can be achieved.

In pronation of the forearm the radius rotates
around the head of the ulna. At the same time
the lower end of the ulna moves slightly laterally.
In supination the reverse occurs. These movements can be observed by holding the forearm in
a loose hand, with the elbow flexed, and allowing
the model to pronate and supinate. Loss of this
movement will limit the range. With the forearm
in full pronation, lateral movement can be achieved
by applying pressure to the anteromedial aspect
of the head of the ulna with the thumbs. With
the forearm fully supinated, medial movement of
the head of the ulna can be achieved by applying
pressure with the thumbs to the posterolateral side
of the head of the ulna. Both these manoeuvres
achieve slight movement of the head of the ulna.

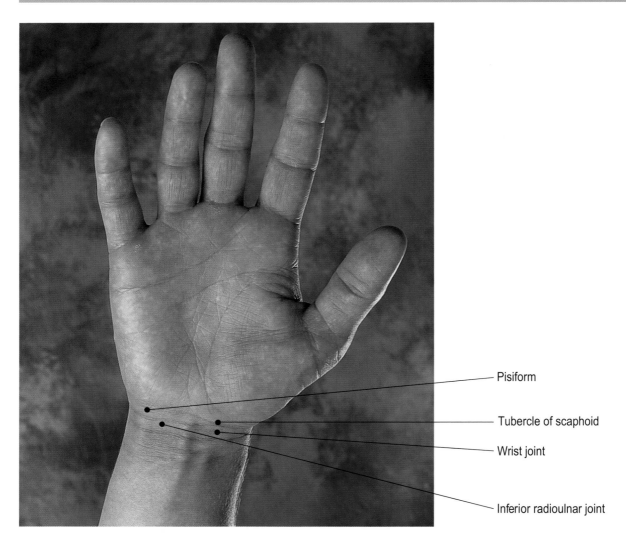

Pisiform

Tubercle of scaphoid

Wrist joint

Inferior radioulnar joint

Fig. 2.12 (a)
The right wrist joint (radiocarpal joint)
(anterior view)

The wrist (radiocarpal) joint [Fig. 2.12]

The wrist joint is formed by the inferior surface of the lower end of the radius and an interarticular disc superiorly, and the proximal surfaces of the scaphoid, lunate and triquetral inferiorly, which together with the ulnar and radius styloid processes form a synovial ellipsoid joint. All joint surfaces are covered with articular cartilage and the joint is surrounded by a capsule, lined with synovial membrane, and supported by the palmar and dorsal radiocarpal, ulnocarpal, radial and ulnar collateral ligaments. The interarticular disc lies between the inferior surface of the head of the ulna and the triquetral bone.

Surface marking

The surface marking of the wrist joint is a line drawn between the tips of the two styloid processes, being slightly concave distally, with the line becoming increasingly curved as it approaches the styloid processes (Fig. 2.12).

Palpation

The joint is covered both anteriorly and posteriorly by tendons running from the forearm into the hand. There are, however, areas, mainly on the medial side, where the joint space of the wrist can be palpated.

Locate the ulnar styloid process on the postero-medial side of the wrist and trace along both the medial and posterior edges of the head of the ulna. The gap just distal, which is clearly observable medially, contains the interarticular disc, the inferior surface of which takes part in the wrist joint articulation.

On the lateral side of the wrist, the joint line can clearly be palpated just proximal to the radial styloid process posteriorly and, with a little more difficulty, anteriorly. If the fingers are pressed between the extensor tendons, the joint line can be traced just distal to the dorsal tubercle across the back of the wrist as far as the head of the ulna. The joint line cannot be palpated anteriorly; however, its line can be drawn horizontally just

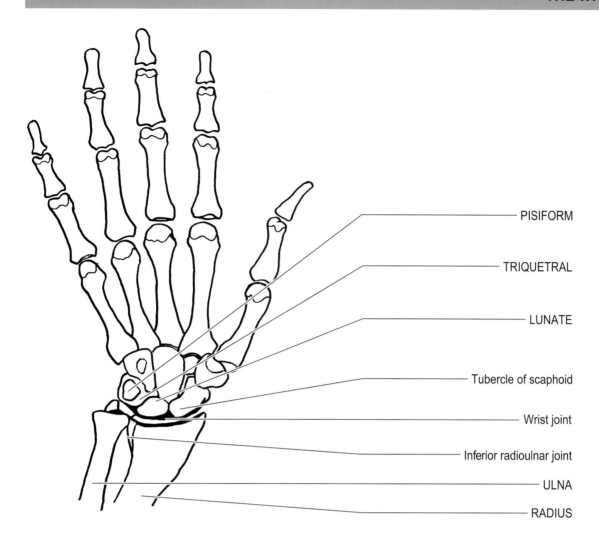

PISIFORM

TRIQUETRAL

LUNATE

Tubercle of scaphoid

Wrist joint

Inferior radioulnar joint

ULNA

RADIUS

Fig. 2.12 (b)
The right wrist joint (radiocarpal joint)
(anterior view)

proximal to the tubercle of the scaphoid. A crease across the anterior of the wrist between the flattened lower end of the forearm and the elevations of the thenar and hypothenar eminences marks the anterior line of the joint. This crease is made more obvious by slight flexion of the wrist.

Accessory movements

With the subject's forearm pronated, grip the dorsum of the lower end of the radius and ulna with one hand and the carpal bones with the other, so that the radial sides of your index fingers and thumbs are nearly touching. The carpus can now be moved forwards and backwards, from side to side and even rotated slightly. Take care not to bend the wrist, but to glide one surface on the other in a transverse plane. It will be difficult to prevent some movement occurring between the bones of the midcarpal joint. As in nearly all joints, distraction is also possible at the wrist. Adopting the same hold as above, draw the two hands apart, taking care to grip the bones tightly, not allowing too much slide of the skin and fascia. Accessory movement at the wrist, if performed correctly, is quite dramatic, producing considerable movement in unusual directions. It must be remembered, however, that some of this occurs at the intercarpal and carpometacarpal joints. It is possible, with practice, to move the bones of the carpus individually on each other or on the lower end of the radius and disc. This is achieved by gripping one bone between finger and thumb of one hand, while stabilizing its neighbour as above, or with the finger and thumb of the other hand.

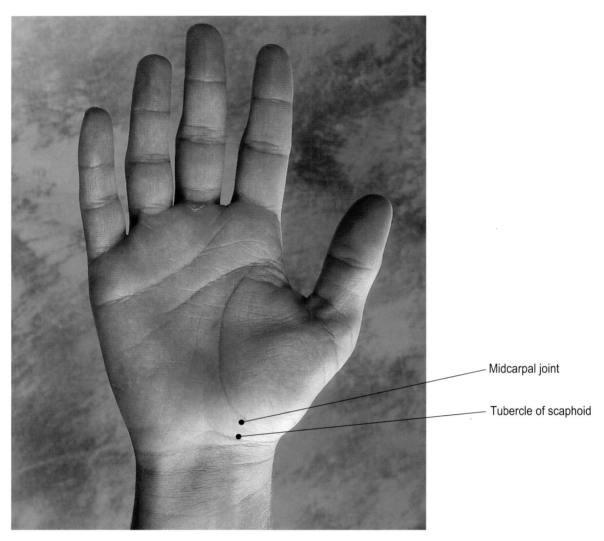

Midcarpal joint

Tubercle of scaphoid

Fig. 2.13 (a)
The intercarpal and midcarpal
joints (anterior view)

The hand

The intercarpal joints [Fig. 2.13]

These are all synovial, plane joints with their surfaces covered with articular cartilage and their capsules lined with synovial membrane. With the exception of the pisotriquetral joint, the capsule is supported by the palmar and dorsal ligaments, and radial and ulnar collateral carpal ligaments. There are also some interosseous ligaments between the proximal ends of the proximal row and distal ends of the distal row of carpal bones.

The pisotriquetral joint is also a synovial plane joint, but it has a distinct capsule which is supported by the tendon of flexor carpi ulnaris proximally and pisohamate and pisometacarpal ligaments distally.

With the exception of the joint between the pisiform and triquetral, the joints between the carpal bones are very difficult to palpate with any degree of accuracy. The posterior aspects of the carpal bones can be identified either by relating their position to the metacarpals or by noting any

particular features (see page 26). Each carpal bone can be gripped between finger and thumb and moved against the adjacent bone, but the joint line remains elusive to the touch.

The pisotriquetral joint. The joint between the pisiform and the triquetral is easier to identify medially. The joint line can be palpated by running the fingers dorsally for 1 cm from the anterior point of the pisiform on its medial side. Slight movement of the pisiform will emphasize the joint line.

The midcarpal joint. The joint between the two rows of carpal bones is known as the midcarpal joint. It permits gliding forwards, backwards and from side to side, augmenting the movements of flexion, extension, abduction and adduction at the wrist joint. It can be marked by a line drawn across the carpus just below the tips of the radial and ulna styloid processes concave downwards, slightly more concave than that of the wrist joint.

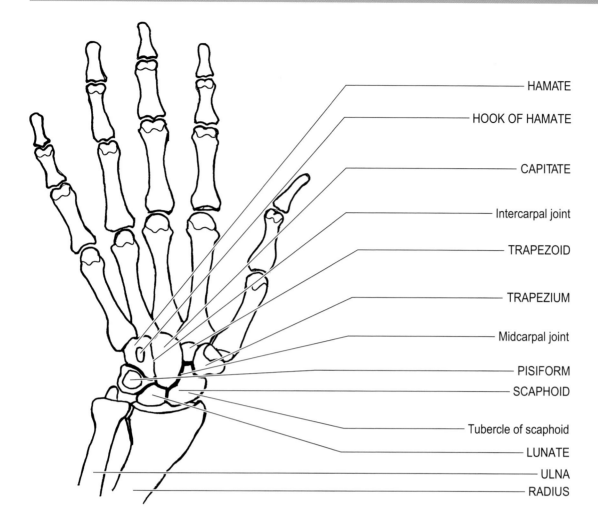

Fig. 2.13 (b)
The intercarpal and midcarpal joints
(anterior view)

Accessory movements

With the wrist slightly flexed, ulnar deviated, and the flexor carpi ulnaris relaxed, the pisiform can easily be moved from side to side with respect to the triquetral. If the capitate, situated at the base of the third metacarpal, is stabilized, by gripping it between the index finger anteriorly and thumb posteriorly, the surrounding carpal bones can be made to glide anteriorly and posteriorly using a similar grip with the other hand on each bone in turn. The trapezium is clearly palpable at the lateral side of the distal row. Using the same hold as above and stabilizing the rest of the carpus, it can also be moved anteriorly and posteriorly. A good knowledge of the carpal bones is essential, and should be combined with practise of this

type of movement. It is advisable to consult the literature on mobilization and manipulations for therapeutic techniques.

Passive movement can be produced between the two rows of carpal bones (the midcarpal joint) by applying a similar hold to that described for producing accessory movements of the wrist joint, but in this case one hand stabilizes the proximal row while the other moves the distal row. The index finger and thumb of the stabilizing hand should grip the proximal row of carpal bones just distal to the radial and ulnar styloid processes. During the anterior, posterior, lateral and medial gliding, however, it is impossible to prevent some movement occurring in the neighbouring joints.

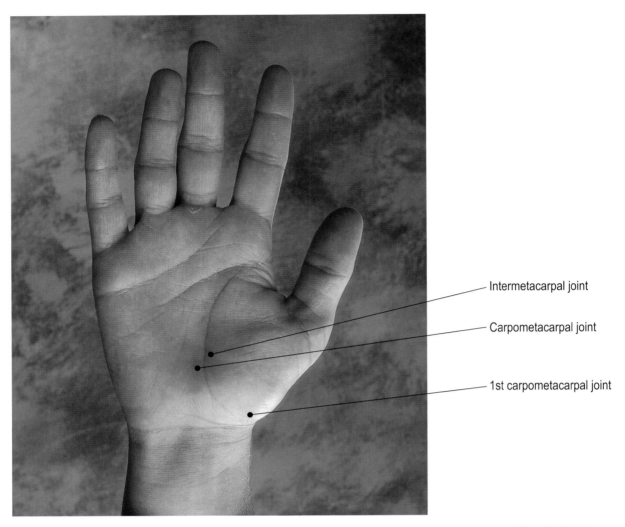

Fig. 2.14 (a)
Carpometacarpal and intermetacarpal
joints (anterior view)

The carpometacarpal joints [Fig. 2.14]

The **first metacarpal** articulates with the **trapezium** by means of a synovial saddle (sellar) joint and is separate from the remaining **carpometacarpal joints**. It is surrounded by a capsule which is lined with synovial membrane and supported by the radial carpometacarpal, anterior and posterior oblique ligaments. The second articulates mainly with the trapezoid, having small facets on either side for the trapezium laterally and the **capitate** medially. The third metacarpal articulates only with the capitate, while the fourth and fifth articulate with the **hamate**. Except for that of the thumb, they are all plane synovial joints having a capsule lined with synovial membrane and supported by palmar and dorsal ligaments. As stated previously (see page 54) between the distal ends of the hamate, capitate and trapezoid there is normally an interosseous ligament.

Palpation

These joints are only palpable from the posterior aspect. Trace proximally along the back of the first metacarpal to its enlarged base, beyond which is a depression. There, the joint line can be palpated either side of the tendon of extensor pollicis longus.

Dorsally, just proximal to the bases of the second, third, fourth and fifth metacarpals, 2 cm distal to the line of the wrist joint, is a line of depressions between the extensor tendons. These represent the surface marking of the common carpometacarpal joint.

On flexion, extension, abduction and adduction of the thumb, the base of the first metacarpal can be seen and felt moving on the trapezium. There is little movement at the common carpometacarpal joint, except a slight gliding of the surfaces against each other accompanying movements of the hand.

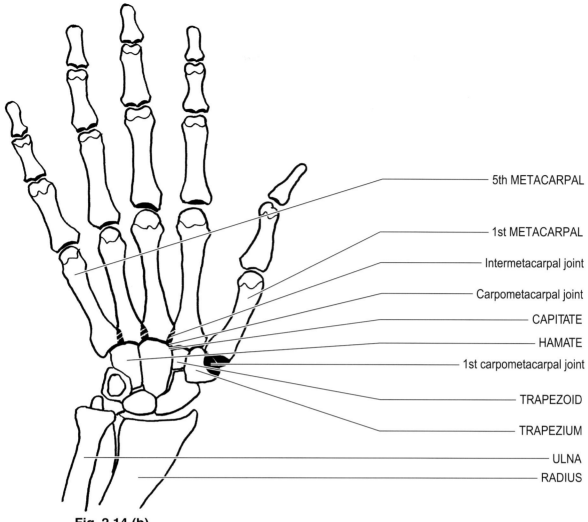

5th METACARPAL

1st METACARPAL

Intermetacarpal joint

Carpometacarpal joint

CAPITATE

HAMATE

1st carpometacarpal joint

TRAPEZOID

TRAPEZIUM

ULNA

RADIUS

Fig. 2.14 (b)
Carpometacarpal and
intermetacarpal joints (anterior view)

Accessory movements

With the finger and thumb of one hand stabilizing the trapezium and the other hand gripping the first metacarpal, anterior, posterior, medial and lateral gliding of the metacarpal base against the trapezium can be produced, as can a limited amount of rotation (i.e. rotation of the metacarpal about its long axis). Slight distraction of the joint is possible. If the remaining carpus is stabilized with one hand, and each metacarpal is gripped in turn between fingers and thumb of the other, each metacarpal base can be moved forwards and backwards slightly.

The intermetacarpal joints [Fig. 2.14]

Between the bases of the second to fifth metacarpals are small plane synovial joints surrounded by a capsule lined with synovial membrane and supported by palmar, dorsal and interosseous ligaments. These allow them to be moved individually, giving the hand more mobility and thus more dexterity.

Palpation

On the posterior aspect of the hand, trace proximally up the spaces between the second and third, third and fourth, and fourth and fifth, metacarpal bones until you feel the two bones touching. The joint line can be palpated running vertically for approximately 1 cm from the line of the carpometacarpal joint (see above).

Accessory movements

It is extremely difficult to move the base of one metacarpal against another, except when they are used as levers. With the subject's forearm pronated, grip one metacarpal head between the index finger and thumb of one hand and its neighbour similarly in the other, and move them up and down against each other. There may be up to a centimetre of movement at the level of the heads, with a much smaller twisting movement of one base against its neighbour.

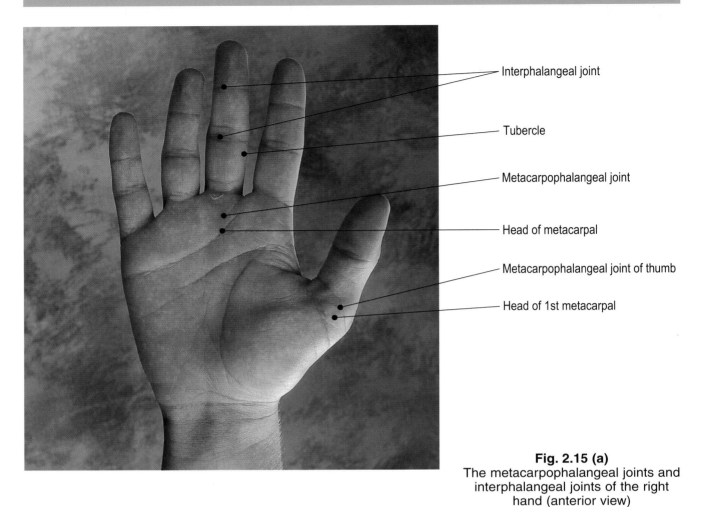

Interphalangeal joint

Tubercle

Metacarpophalangeal joint

Head of metacarpal

Metacarpophalangeal joint of thumb

Head of 1st metacarpal

Fig. 2.15 (a)
The metacarpophalangeal joints and
interphalangeal joints of the right
hand (anterior view)

The metacarpophalangeal joints

Metacarpophalangeal joints are synovial ellipsoid joints between the head of each metacarpal and the proximal end of each associated proximal phalanx. Each joint is surrounded by a fibrous capsule enclosing the head of the metacarpal and the proximal surface of the phalanx.

The capsule is lined with synovial membrane and is supported by strong, cord-like collateral ligaments and a dense palmar ligament. The posterior of the joint is protected by the dorsal expansion of the extensor digitorum longus tendon. The palmar ligaments of the 2nd to 5th metacarpophalangeal joints are linked by the deep transverse metacarpal ligament. It is worth noting (a) that flexion of the metacarpophalangeal joint of the thumb is only 45°, whereas that of the fingers is 90°, and (b) that this movement occurs at right angles to that in the other metacarpal joints taking the thumb across the palm.

Palpation

The metacarpophalangeal joints of each finger can be palpated just distal to the head of the metacarpal. With the finger flexed to 90°, the joint line appears to be beyond the knuckles, on the anterior surface of the head of the metacarpal (Fig. 2.15). It is easily palpable dorsally on either side of the extensor digitorum longus tendons.

The metacarpophalangeal joint of the thumb is clearly palpable posteriorly, just beyond the metacarpal head.

Accessory movements

With the metacarpal stabilized by one hand and the digit gripped by the other, the base of the proximal phalanx can be moved forwards, backwards and from side to side. The digit can also be rotated about its long axis, producing spin between the two surfaces and distracted sufficiently to produce the 'pop' which some children enjoy doing as a party trick. This is not normally possible at the metacarpophalangeal joint of the thumb.

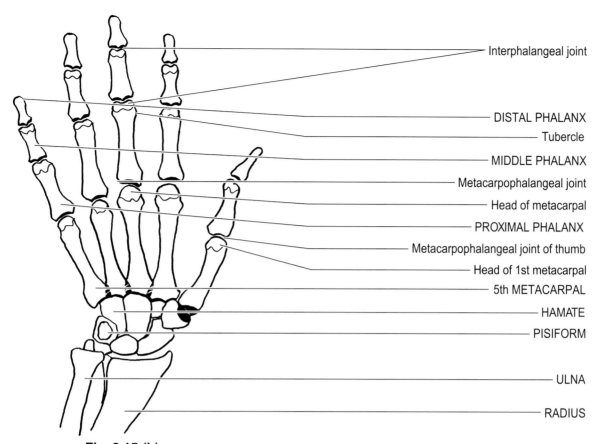

Fig. 2.15 (b)
The metacarpophalangeal joints and
interphalangeal joints of the right
hand (anterior view)

Labels in figure:
- Interphalangeal joint
- DISTAL PHALANX
- Tubercle
- MIDDLE PHALANX
- Metacarpophalangeal joint
- Head of metacarpal
- PROXIMAL PHALANX
- Metacarpophalangeal joint of thumb
- Head of 1st metacarpal
- 5th METACARPAL
- HAMATE
- PISIFORM
- ULNA
- RADIUS

The interphalangeal joints

Each finger has two interphalangeal joints, whereas the thumb has only one. They are synovial hinge joints between the head of the more proximal phalanx and the base of the more distal phalanx. These joints are surrounded by a capsule which is lined with synovial membrane and supported by collateral and palmar ligaments.

Palpation

The joints are easier to palpate posteriorly. With the joint flexed to 90°, trace distally down the back of each phalanx. Just beyond the slightly expanded head, the joint line can be palpated, covered centrally by the expansion of extensor digitorum (dorsal digital expansion).

Accessory movements

With the subject's forearm and hand pronated and the joint flexed to approximately 30°, stabilize the more proximal phalanx with one hand and grip the more distal phalanx between fingers and thumb of the other. The base of the more distal phalanx can now be rocked from side to side, often giving rise to a 'cracking' sound. It is also possible to produce a slight forwards and backwards gliding of the base on the head, not easy to palpate, but useful in mobilizing stiff finger joints. Finally, all the interphalangeal joints can be distracted, but owing to their tight collateral ligaments the space gained between the articular surfaces is only a fraction of that gained at the metacarpophalangeal joints.

SELF ASSESSMENT

Page 36

1. Name the joint at the medial end of the clavicle.

2. What class and type is this joint?

3. Which supporting ligament joins the two clavicles together?

4. Which ligament joins the clavicle to the upper part of the first rib?

5. Does this joint contain a disc?

6. Give the surface markings of this joint.

7. Name the notch between the two clavicles.

8. Which ligament acts as a fulcrum for movements of the clavicle?

9. If the lateral end of the clavicle is drawn backward, what happens to the medial end?

Page 37

10. When the lateral end of the clavicle is raised, what happens to the medial end?

11. What happens to the clavicle on the last few degrees of elevation of the upper limb?

12. What is an accessory movement and can such movement be produced at this joint?

13. If so, how is this movement produced?

Page 38

14. Give the surface marking of the acromioclavicular joint.

15. Describe and explain planes of movement and identify in which plane this joint lies.

16. What class and type of joint is it?

17. Which ligament supports the joint from above?

18. Name the two accessory ligaments of this joint.

Please complete the labels below.

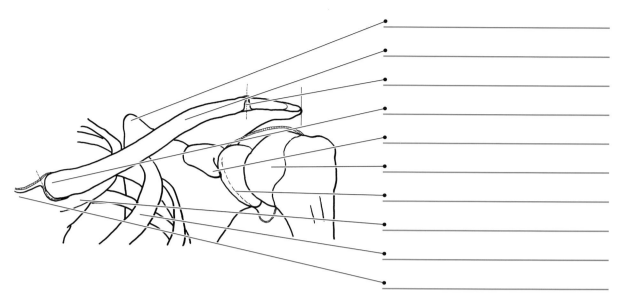

Fig. 2.6 (b) Joints of the shoulder region (anterior view)

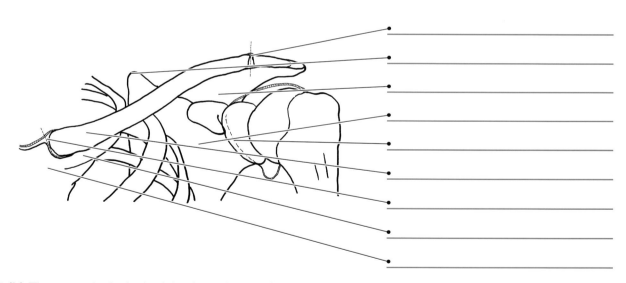

Fig. 2.7 (b) The acromioclavicular joint (anterior view)

19. Does the acromioclavicular joint contain a disc?

20. Name and demonstrate the movements which occur at the acromioclavicular joint.

21. Describe how these movements are produced.

Page 39

22. Which ligament is considered to assist in the rotation of the clavicle?

23. Can any accessory movements be produced at the acromioclavicular joint?

Page 40

24. What is the class and type of the shoulder joint?

25. Name the bony surfaces which take part in this joint.

26. How much of the articular surface of each bone is in contact at any one time?

27. Name the substance with which both surfaces are covered and explain the reasons for its existence (fr).

28. What movement of which structures apparently increases the range of movement of the shoulder joint?

29. Name the material which lines the shoulder joint and explain the reasons for its presence (fr).

30. Which ligament supports the anterior aspect of the shoulder joint?

31. Identify the ligament which supports the joint posterosuperiorly.

32. Name the ligament which crosses the bicipital (intertubercular) groove.

33. Describe the glenoidal labrum.

34. Name and palpate the bony structure which protects the joint superiorly.

35. Which components of this joint can be palpated anteriorly?

36. Between which two bony landmarks does the bicipital groove lie?

Please complete the labels below.

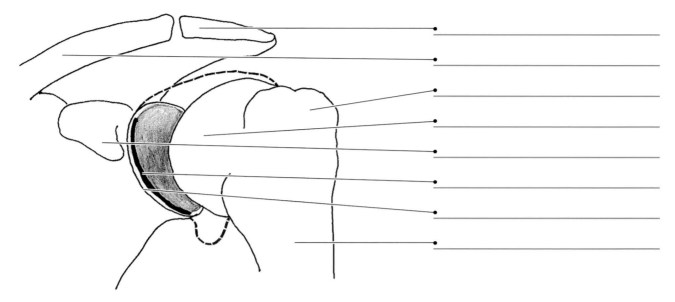

Fig. 2.8 (b) The left shoulder joint (anterior view)

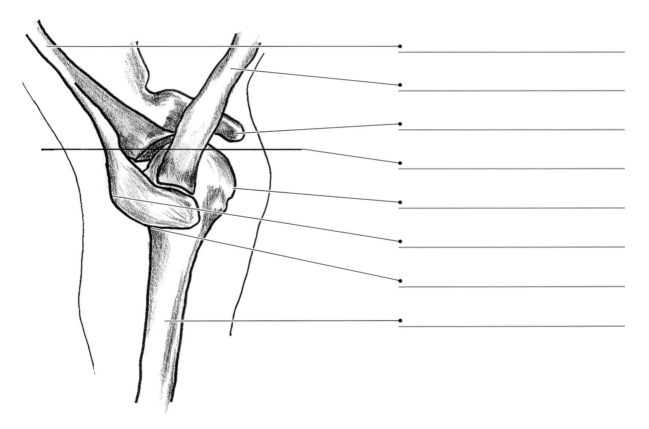

Fig. 2.8 (d) The right shoulder joint (upper lateral view)

Page 41

37. Name and identify the muscle tendon which passes down this groove.

38. Describe what happens to the head of the humerus when the upper limb is rotated laterally.

39. When the upper limb is rotated medially, what movement occurs at the head of the humerus?

40. Describe what movement occurs at the head when the arm is abducted.

41. When the upper limb is lowered, what movement occurs at the head of the humerus?

42. Which fibres of what muscle pass across the anterior surface of this joint?

43. Give the surface markings of the joint anteriorly.

44. Give the surface markings of the joint posteriorly.

45. What is the surface marking of the joint from the lateral side?

Page 44

46. Explain the meaning of the term 'axis'.

47. Where is the axis of the shoulder joint located?

48. Around which axis does abduction and adduction occur?

49. Identify the structures upon which the shoulder joint mainly depends for its stability.

50. Name and palpate the rotator cuff muscles.

Page 45

51. Explain what is meant by the term 'accessory movements'.

52. Describe and demonstrate the accessory movements which can be produced at the shoulder joint.

53. What is the optimum position for the production of accessory movements?

Please complete the labels below.

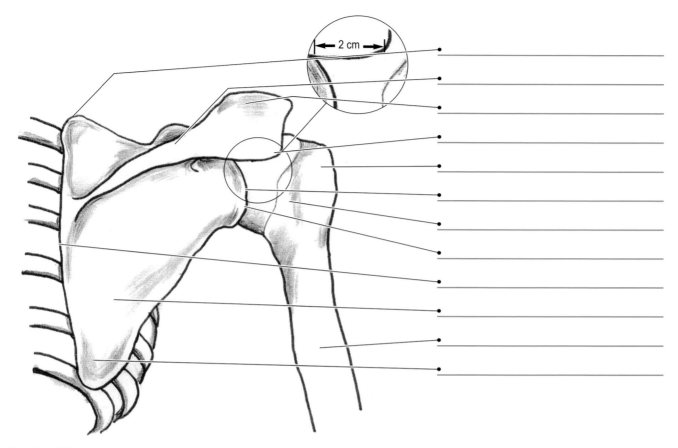

Fig. 2.8 (f) The right shoulder joint (posterior view)

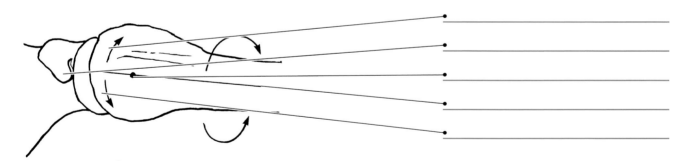

Fig. 2.9 (c) Left humerus in 90° abduction (superior view)

Page 46

54. Name the class and type of the elbow joint.

55. Identify the articular surfaces which take part in this joint.

56. What structure covers the articular surfaces?

57. Which three fossae are covered by the synovial membrane?

58. Identify and palpate the two collateral ligaments of the joint.

59. Describe the shape of these ligaments.

60. Give the surface markings of the elbow joint.

61. Name and identify the humeral condyle which extends furthest.

62. Name and demonstrate the angle between the arm and the forearm when the arm is extended.

63. What is the angle, in degrees, in men?

64. What is the angle in women?

Page 47

65. Name the two bony landmarks lateral to the elbow joint.

66. Indicate the muscle which prevents the anterior aspect of the elbow joint from being palpated.

67. What accessory movements are possible at the elbow joint?

Page 48

68. Name the class and type of the superior radioulnar joint.

69. Describe the articular surfaces which participate in the joint.

70. With what substance are these surfaces covered?

71. Name and palpate the ligament which surrounds the head of the radius.

72. What type of cartilage lines this ligament?

73. Identify the structure which supports this ligament from above.

74. Describe how this ligament is supported inferiorly.

Please complete the labels below.

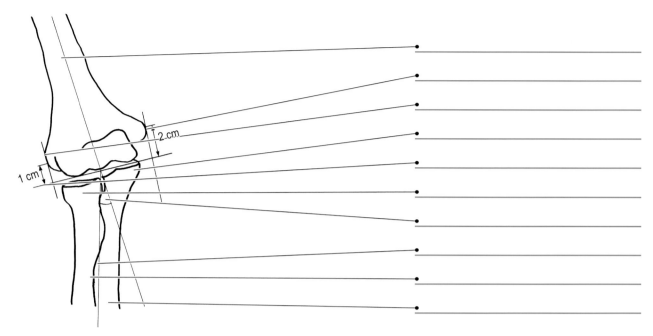

Fig. 2.10 (b) The right elbow joint (anterior view)

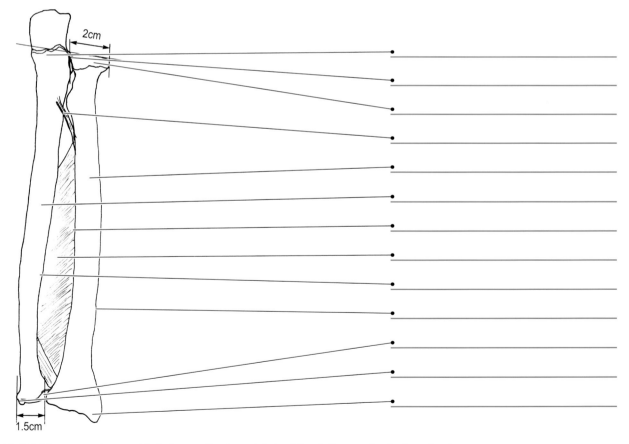

Fig. 2.11 (b) The superior and inferior radioulnar joint of the left arm (anterior view)

75. What binds the two bones together?

76. Does this joint communicate with the elbow joint?

77. Give the surface markings of the superior radioulnar joint.

Page 49

78. Name and palpate the muscle which covers the posterior aspect of this joint.

79. Demonstrate pronation and supination and describe what happens to the radial head during these movements.

80. What accessory movements are possible at this joint?

Page 50

81. Name the class and type of the inferior radioulnar joint.

82. Describe the bony surfaces taking part in this joint.

83. What substance covers the articular surfaces?

84. Name and palpate the ligament which separates the lower end of the ulna from the carpus.

85. Name the sheet of tissue which binds the radius and ulna together.

86. Where does it attach to each bone?

87. In which direction do the fibres of this tissue pass from the radius to the ulna?

88. What is its function?

89. Describe the means by which weight is transmitted from the carpus, through the forearm, to the elbow.

Page 51

90. What is the surface marking of the inferior radioulnar joint?

91. The tendon of which muscle crosses the posterior aspect of this joint?

92. Is the joint more palpable anteriorly or posteriorly?

93. Describe the movement which occurs between the radius and the ulna at the lower end during pronation and supination.

94. What accessory movements can be produced at the inferior radioulnar joint?

Please complete the labels below.

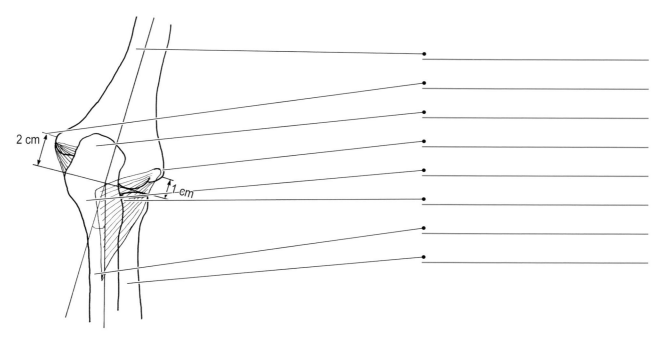

Fig. 2.10 (d) The right elbow joint (posterior view)

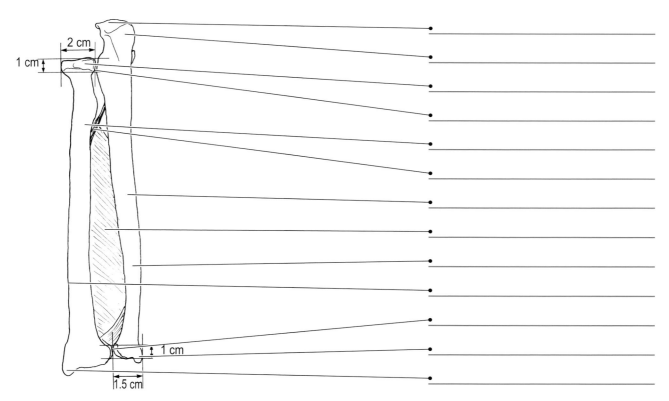

Fig. 2.11 (d) The superior and inferior radioulnar joint of the left arm (posterior view)

Page 52

95. Name the class and type of the wrist joint.

96. Which bony surfaces take part in this joint?

97. Name the bony process which projects downwards lateral to the joint.

98. Which bony process projects downwards posteromedial to the joint?

99. What substance covers the joint surfaces?

100. Name the ligaments which support the joint anteriorly.

101. Which ligaments support the joint posteriorly?

102. Name and palpate the ligaments which support the joint on either side.

103. Give the surface markings of the wrist joint.

Page 53

104. Describe the relationship between the surface marking of the wrist joint and the dorsal tubercle of the radius.

105. Explain why it is difficult to palpate this joint.

106. Can the joint be palpated anteriorly?

107. What accessory movements are possible at the wrist joint?

108. Describe and demonstrate a technique for producing one of the accessory movements.

Page 54

109. Name the class and type of the intercarpal joints.

110. Identify the ligaments which support the anterior and posterior aspects of the majority of these joints.

111. Name the joint which is distinct from the other joints.

112. On what does this joint rely for its stability?

Please complete the labels below.

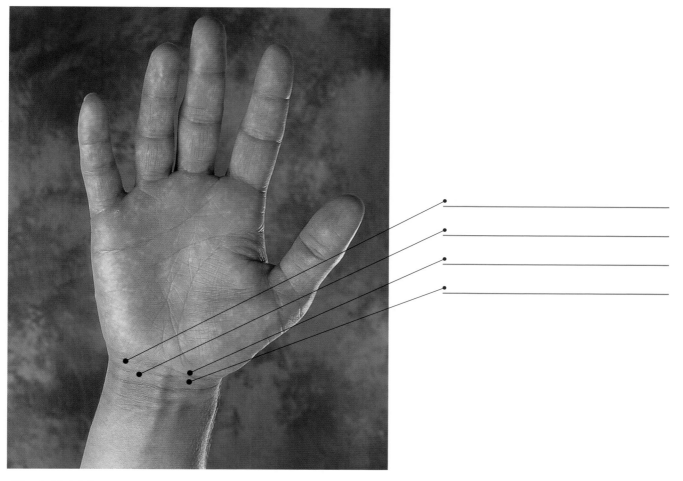

Fig. 2.12 (a) The right wrist joint (radiocarpal joint) (anterior view)

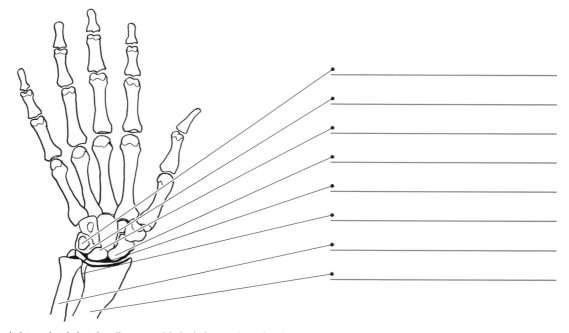

Fig. 2.12 (b) The right wrist joint (radiocarpal joint) (anterior view)

113. Which surfaces take part in the pisotriquetral joint?

114. What is its class and type?

115. Which ligaments support the joint?

116. Give the surface markings of this joint.

Page 55

117. What accessory movements can be produced between the pisiform and triquetral bones?

Page 56

118. Name the class and type of the carpometacarpal joint of the thumb.

119. Describe its bony components.

120. Name the ligaments of the joint.

121. Describe the position of these ligaments.

122. With which bones does the second metacarpal articulate proximally?

123. The third metacarpal bone articulates with which carpal bone proximally?

124. With which bone do the fourth and fifth metacarpals articulate proximally?

125. Give the class and type of the second, third, fourth and fifth carpometacarpal joints.

126. Where are interosseous ligaments found between the bones?

127. What movements occur at the first carpometacarpal joint?

Page 57

128. What accessory movements can be produced at the first carpometacarpal joint?

129. What accessory movements can be produced at the second, third, fourth and fifth carpometacarpal joints?

Please complete the labels below.

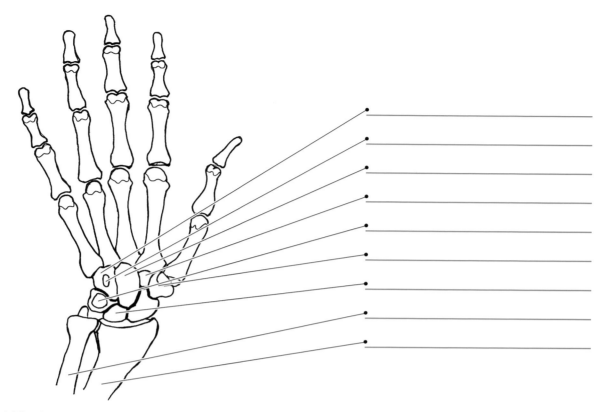

Fig. 2.13 (b) The intercarpal and midcarpal joints (anterior view)

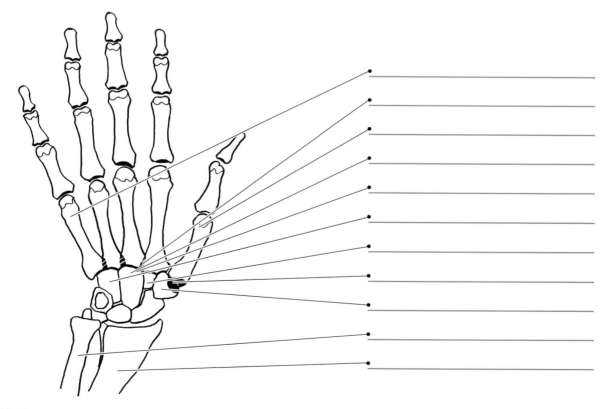

Fig. 2.14 (b) Carpometacarpal and intermetacarpal joints (anterior view)

130. Give the class and type of the intermetacarpal joints.

131. Name the ligaments which support the joints.

132. How can accessory movements be best produced at these joints?

Page 58

133. Name the class and type of the metacarpophalangeal joints.

134. Describe the articular surfaces which take part in these joints.

135. Name and describe the ligaments which support these joints.

136. With what structure is the posterior aspect of each joint covered?

137. Name the ligament which links the joints together.

138. Describe how the movements of the first metacarpophalangeal joint differ from those of the other joints.

139. Choose the most effective palpation technique for these joints and explain your reasons for this choice.

140. What accessory movements can be produced at each of these joints?

Page 59

141. Name the class and type of the interphalangeal joints.

142. Describe the surfaces taking part in the joints.

143. Name the ligaments which support the joints.

144. Describe the arrangements of these ligaments.

145. What structure covers the posterior part of the joint?

146. What accessory movements can be produced at each of these joints?

Please complete the labels below.

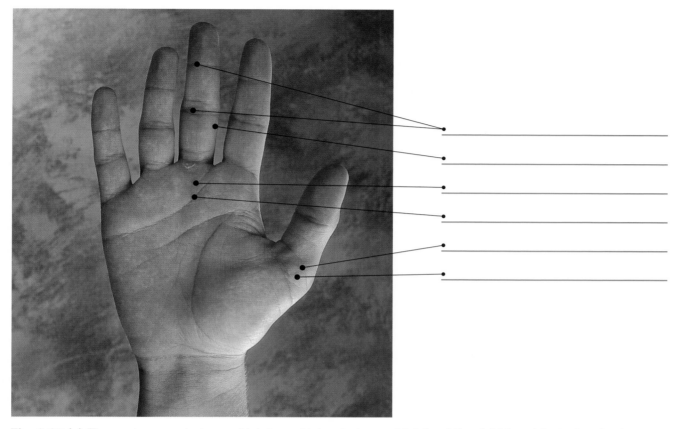

Fig. 2.15 (a) The metacarpophalangeal joints and interphalangeal joints of the right hand (anterior view)

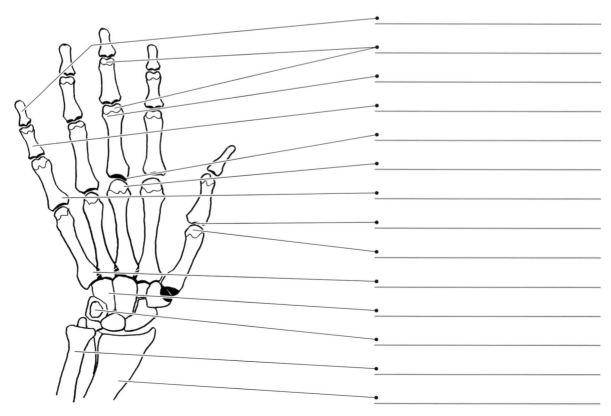

Fig. 2.15 (b) The metacarpophalangeal joints and interphalangeal joints of the right hand (anterior view)

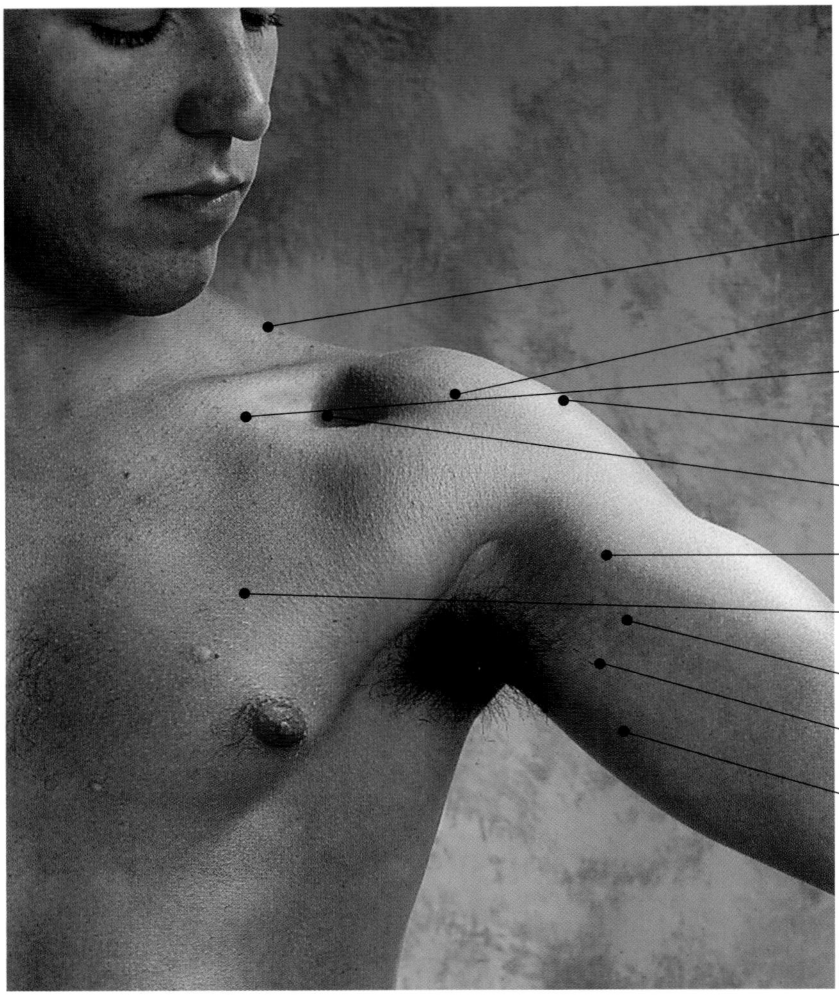
Upper fibres of trapezius
Deltoid, anterior fibres
Pectoralis major, clavicular fibres
Deltoid, middle fibres
Subclavian fossa
Biceps, long head
Pectoralis major, sternal fibres
Biceps, short head
Coracobrachialis
Triceps, long head

Fig. 2.16 (a)
Muscles on the anterior of the left chest, shoulder and arm

MUSCLES

The muscles that move the arm

Deltoid [Figs 2.16 and 2.17]

The **deltoid** is a triangular or delta-shaped muscle situated on the lateral aspect of the shoulder joint. It is made up of **anterior**, **middle** and posterior sections. These fibres arise above from the lateral end of the anterior border of the clavicle, anterior, lateral and posterior borders of the acromion process, and the lower lip of the spine of the scapula, respectively. They all unite below to attach to the deltoid tubercle on the lateral side of the humerus.

Below the pectoral girdle, the anterior fibres of the deltoid can be seen some 3 cm below the lateral lip of the acromion, level with the greater tuberosity of the humerus. This delta-shaped muscle also covers the anterior and posterior aspects of the shoulder joint and feels thick and well developed. If the upper limb is abducted, its anterior and posterior fibres can be identified as triangular sections with fascial septa separating them from the central fibres.

Palpation

The anterior and posterior fibres feel smooth and strap-like, whereas the middle fibres feel coarse with stringy fibrous bands running vertically. This is due to this middle section of the deltoid being composed of multipennate muscle fibres, which pass obliquely from one vertical tendinous intersection to another. These coarse strips of muscle pass vertically from the lateral border of the acromion downwards to the final common tendon of all three sections halfway down the lateral aspect of the humerus. If the shoulder is flexed or medially rotated, the anterior fibres stand clear and can be traced from clavicle above to humerus below. If the shoulder is extended or laterally rotated, the posterior fibres stand clear and can be traced from the lower lip of the spine of the scapula above to the humerus below.

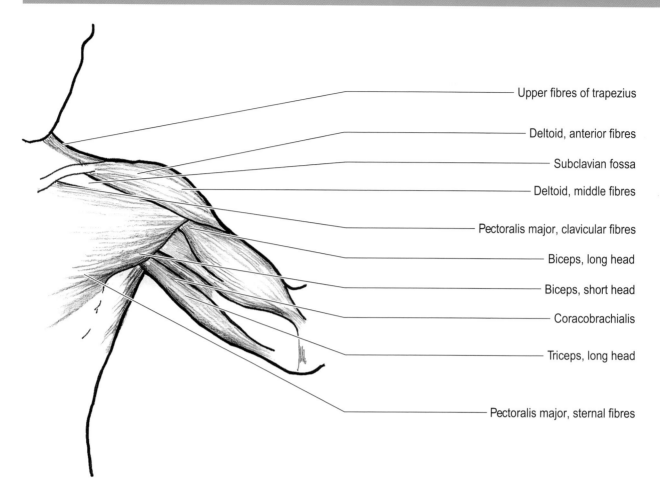

Upper fibres of trapezius

Deltoid, anterior fibres

Subclavian fossa

Deltoid, middle fibres

Pectoralis major, clavicular fibres

Biceps, long head

Biceps, short head

Coracobrachialis

Triceps, long head

Pectoralis major, sternal fibres

Fig. 2.16 (b)
Muscles on the anterior of the left
chest, shoulder and arm

Pectoralis major [Fig. 2.16]

Pectoralis major is a thick, strong, triangular muscle, which covers the upper anterior chest wall. It has its tendinous apex laterally. It comprises two functionally distinct groups of fibres: **clavicular** and **sternal**. The clavicular section attaches medially to the anterior surface of the medial half of the clavicle. The sternal fibres have an extensive attachment medially to the manubrium, body of the sternum, anterior surfaces of the upper six costal cartilages and ribs and the upper part of the aponeurosis of the external oblique muscle. Laterally, the muscle forms a broad tendon which attaches to the lateral lip of the bicipital groove. The lower border of the muscle appears thickened. This is due to its lower fibres being folded up behind its upper fibres and forming a bilaminal tendon at its insertion.

Palpation

If this muscle is traced laterally it passes across, and forms the anterior wall of the axilla. When the arm is flexed, its clavicular fibres can be palpated as a thick muscular column passing from the medial end of the clavicle to the humerus. If the arm is now extended, from a flexed position against resistance, the sternal fibres can be palpated from the lower ribs and sternum to the same insertion. In women, much of the muscular section is covered by the breast but contraction of the muscle is evident to see or palpate. In men, the whole of the muscle is clearly palpable and becomes hard and tense on adduction and medial rotation of the arm. Laterally a groove can be palpated between its upper border and the lower border of the deltoid.

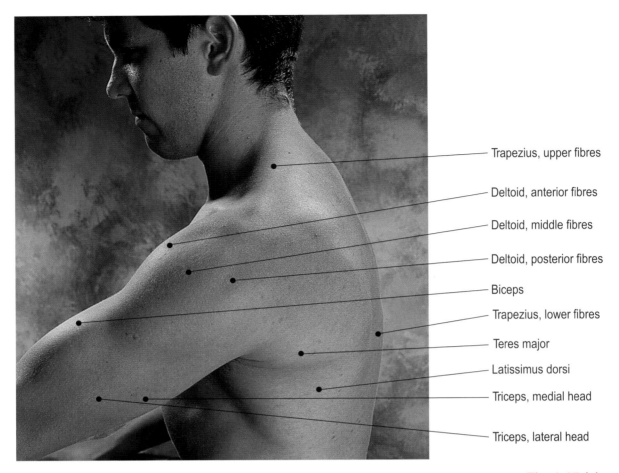

Trapezius, upper fibres

Deltoid, anterior fibres

Deltoid, middle fibres

Deltoid, posterior fibres

Biceps

Trapezius, lower fibres

Teres major

Latissimus dorsi

Triceps, medial head

Triceps, lateral head

Fig. 2.17 (a)
Muscles that move the arm and
forearm (lateral view of left arm)

Biceps brachii [Figs 2.16–2.18]

Biceps brachii is fusiform in shape, situated on the anterior aspect of the upper arm. Its upper end attaches by two heads, as its name implies, one from the supraglenoid tubercle, the other from the tip of the coracoid process of the scapula. Below, it attaches by a strong tendon to the posterior aspect of the radial tubercle on the upper medial aspect of the radius and by an expansion from its medial aspect which blends with the fascia on the medial side of the forearm.

The fusiform shape of biceps brachii can be seen and palpated covering the front of the arm. It can be traced upwards, running deep to pectoralis major and splitting into two parts, both palpable: the long head passing as a tendon in the inter-tubercular groove, and the short head passing medially to the coracoid process. The tendon of the long head of biceps can be traced up the bicipital groove to pass over the head of the humerus to the supraglenoid tubercle. Below, the muscle forms a well-defined tendon which passes through the cubital fossa giving off an expansion (the bicipital aponeurosis) which blends with the fascia on the medial side of the forearm, reaching as far as the posterior border of the ulna, forming a sickle-shaped edge. On supination of the flexed forearm against resistance, the shape and tendons of biceps become more clearly defined and the aponeurosis can be palpated spreading medially from the tendon. In a well-developed model, the tips of the fingers can be slipped under the posterior border of the bicipital aponeurosis approximately 2 cm anteroinferior to the medial epicondyle (Fig. 2.18).

Brachialis

Brachialis is a thick, triangular muscle situated deep to the lower part of the biceps. It attaches above to the lower half of the anterolateral and anteromedial surfaces of the humerus, crosses the front of the elbow joint and attaches below to the anterior surface of the coronoid process of the ulna.

Palpation

Being deeply situated this muscle is difficult to palpate; however, contraction and relaxation of brachialis, during flexion and extension of the elbow, can be felt on deep palpation either side of the biceps tendon as the subject gently flexes and extends the elbow joint.

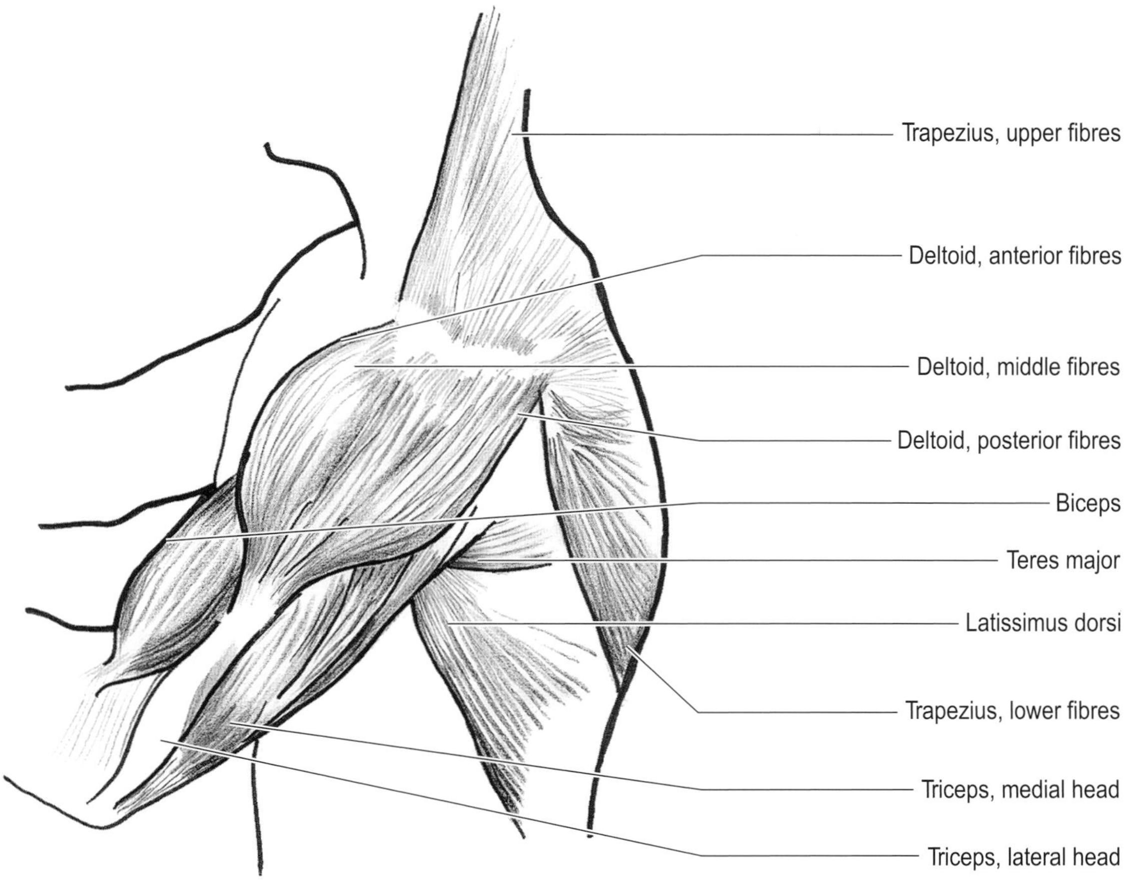
Trapezius, upper fibres
Deltoid, anterior fibres
Deltoid, middle fibres
Deltoid, posterior fibres
Biceps
Teres major
Latissimus dorsi
Trapezius, lower fibres
Triceps, medial head
Triceps, lateral head

Fig. 2.17 (b)
Muscles that move the arm and forearm (lateral view of left arm)

Triceps [Figs. 2.16a,b 2.17a,b]

On the posterior aspect of the arm, the thick muscular mass of the **triceps** is situated. As its name implies, it arises from three heads: (1) the long head, which is tendinous and passes upwards, below the shoulder joint to attach to the infraglenoid tubercle of the scapula; (2) the **lateral head**, which attaches to the upper lateral part of the posterior surface of the humerus above and lateral to the radial groove; and (3) the **medial head**, which attaches to the lower medial part of the posterior surface of the humerus below and medial to the radial groove. All three attach to the posterior part of the superior surface of the olecranon via the triceps tendon.

Palpation

Medially, the long head can be traced upwards as a tendon on the medial aspect of the arm passing up, under the posterior fibres of deltoid, infraspinatus, teres major and minor to lie in front of the posterior wall of the axilla. The medial and lateral heads form a much more fleshy mass down the posterior aspect of the whole of the arm. Just above the elbow joint, the three heads form a strong, thick tendon which attaches to the upper surface of the olecranon process. The muscle and its tendon are more easily palpated if the elbow is slightly flexed and then extended against resistance. The lateral and medial heads can readily be identified, with the former being slightly higher and lateral, while the latter is lower and more medial (Fig. 2.17).

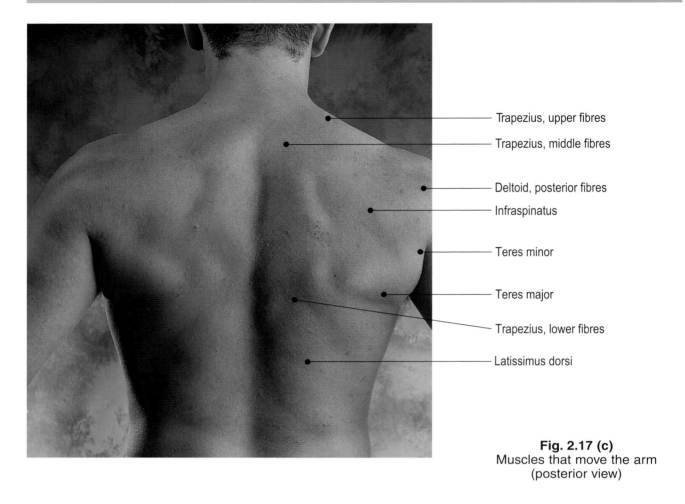

Trapezius, upper fibres

Trapezius, middle fibres

Deltoid, posterior fibres

Infraspinatus

Teres minor

Teres major

Trapezius, lower fibres

Latissimus dorsi

Fig. 2.17 (c)
Muscles that move the arm
(posterior view)

Latissimus dorsi [Fig. 2.17a,b,c and d]

The latissimus dorsi is a large triangular muscle situated on the lower, posterior part of the trunk but passes upwards and laterally to attach to the upper part of the upper limb.

This muscle has an extensive origin from the lower part of the thoracolumbar fascia, the spines of the lower six thoracic, all the lumbar and sacral vertebrae, from the supraspinous and interspinous ligaments which lie between the thoracic and lumbar vertebrae and from the outer lip of the posterior sixth of the crest of the ilium. As it passes upwards it also attaches to the lower three ribs and the posterior aspect of the inferior angle of the scapula.

It attaches above by a flattened tendon, which twists under the axilla and attaches to the floor of the intertubercular groove which lies on the anterior surface of the humerus.

Palpation

The tendon of the latissimus dorsi can be palpated as it passes under teres major, forming the posterior wall of the axilla. If extension and medial rotation of the arm is resisted, the tendon can be traced along the medial side of the humerus towards its insertion into the floor of the inter-tubercular groove of the humerus. The muscle fibres can also be palpated in the upper lumbar area, particularly if the subject is pulling down on a beam above his/her head (beam heaves) or is asked to cough.

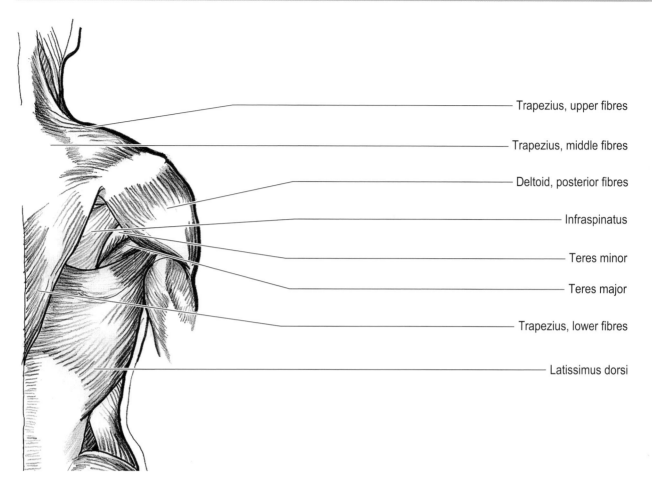

— Trapezius, upper fibres

— Trapezius, middle fibres

— Deltoid, posterior fibres

— Infraspinatus

— Teres minor

— Teres major

— Trapezius, lower fibres

— Latissimus dorsi

Fig. 2.17 (d)
Muscles that move the arm
(posterior view)

Coracobrachialis [Fig. 2.16a and b]

This is a long thin fusiform muscle situated on the upper medial area of the arm. It attaches above to the tip of the coracoid process by a tendon common to it and the biceps brachii. Below it attaches by a short tendon to a point halfway down the medial side of the humerus.

Palpation

During adduction of the upper limb, the belly of coracobrachialis (see Fig. 2.16a,b) can be palpated high up on the medial side of the arm, passing upwards and forwards towards the coracoid process. If the subject places the hand on the hip and adducts the arm with some force, the tendon can be traced to the posterior aspect of the short head of the biceps and can be identified blending with this tendon. Care must be taken when palpating this area as it contains numerous branches of the brachial plexus and major blood vessels to and from the upper limb.

The posterior aspect of the scapula [Fig. 2.17c and d]

Above the spine of the scapula, the muscle belly of supraspinatus can be palpated, particularly if the upper limb begins to abduct from the side.

Below the spine, the belly of infraspinatus can be palpated passing upwards and laterally to the humerus. This contracts during lateral rotation of the humerus.

The large bulk of muscle covering the lateral border of the scapula is made up of the fibres of teres major and minor and the upper part of latissimus dorsi. These all come into action in adduction of the humerus, the teres minor taking part in lateral rotation of the humerus whilst the teres major and latissimus dorsi take part in medial rotation.

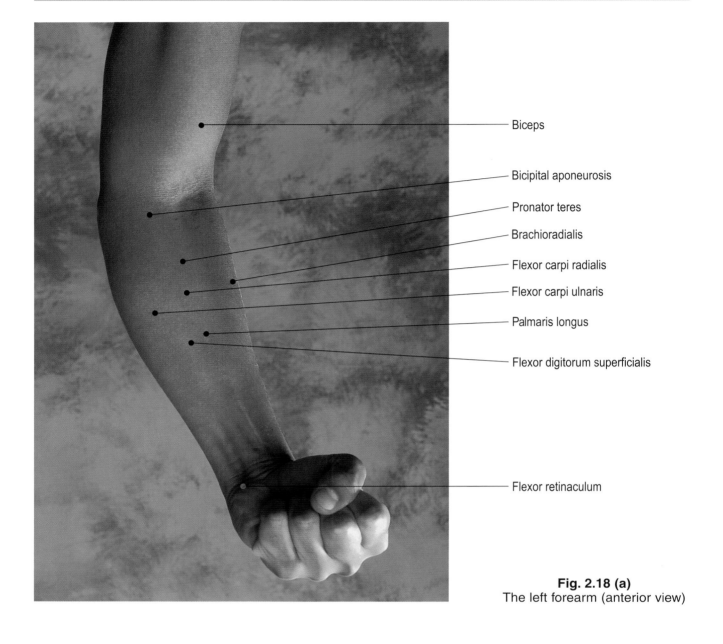

Biceps

Bicipital aponeurosis

Pronator teres

Brachioradialis

Flexor carpi radialis

Flexor carpi ulnaris

Palmaris longus

Flexor digitorum superficialis

Flexor retinaculum

Fig. 2.18 (a)
The left forearm (anterior view)

The anterior aspect of the forearm and wrist

Because of their close proximity, individual identification of the muscles of the forearm is difficult. The point of greatest clarity is where their tendons cross the wrist joint; consequently most muscles will be identified at this point and then traced proximally and distally.

Generally the forearm is greater in circumference in its upper half than in its lower half owing to the presence of the muscle bellies, whereas lower down the muscles give way to tendons (Fig. 2.18).

Brachioradialis is situated most laterally and gives shape to the upper part of the forearm. It appears strap-like and thicker near the elbow, narrowing to a broad tendon towards the lateral surface of the radius. If the elbow is flexed in the mid-prone position against resistance, the muscle stands clear, showing that its origin attaches to

the proximal part of the lateral supracondylar ridge of the humerus (Fig. 2.18).

On the anterior aspect of the wrist, approximately 1 cm medial to the styloid process of the radius, the tendon of flexor carpi radialis can be palpated. Distally, it passes in front of the scaphoid, being lost in the groove on the front of the trapezium. The tendon can, however, be traced halfway up the front of the forearm, becoming muscular in the upper part which attaches to the medial epicondyle of the humerus (Fig. 2.18).

If the wrist is slightly flexed and the base of the thumb and little finger are drawn together, a slim tendon (palmaris longus) can be seen and palpated (if present) medial to the tendon of flexor carpi radialis. Traced distally, the palmaris longus tendon blends with the palmar aponeurosis. Proximally, the narrow belly of palmaris longus

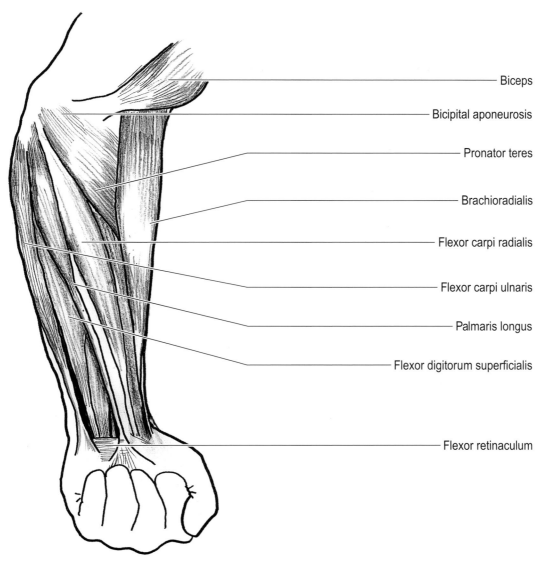

Biceps

Bicipital aponeurosis

Pronator teres

Brachioradialis

Flexor carpi radialis

Flexor carpi ulnaris

Palmaris longus

Flexor digitorum superficialis

Flexor retinaculum

Fig. 2.18 (b)
Muscles of the left forearm
(anterior view)

can be palpated on the medial side of the previous muscle.

On the anteromedial aspect of the wrist is the stout tendon of flexor carpi ulnaris. Distally it blends with the pisiform bone, while proximally it can be traced almost halfway up the forearm approximately 2 cm anterior to the posterior border of the ulna, being replaced by thick muscle which lies in front of the posterior border of the ulna.

Between the tendons of palmaris longus and flexor carpi ulnaris is a depressed area. If the subject flexes the fingers, particularly the middle and ring fingers, the tendons of flexor digitorum superficialis can be seen and palpated in that

groove. The tendons to the index and little fingers, and those of flexor digitorum profundus, lie deeper and are difficult to differentiate. If the fingers are flexed only at the metacarpophalangeal and proximal interphalangeal joints, flexor digitorum superficialis can be palpated immediately medial to the tendon of palmaris longus. If, however, the fingertips are pressed against the palm of the hand, flexor digitorum profundus can be palpated on the medial side of the forearm, deep to flexor carpi ulnaris. In the palm, the tendons of these muscles are well covered with fascia and are difficult to determine, except for an area just proximal to the metacarpophalangeal joints.

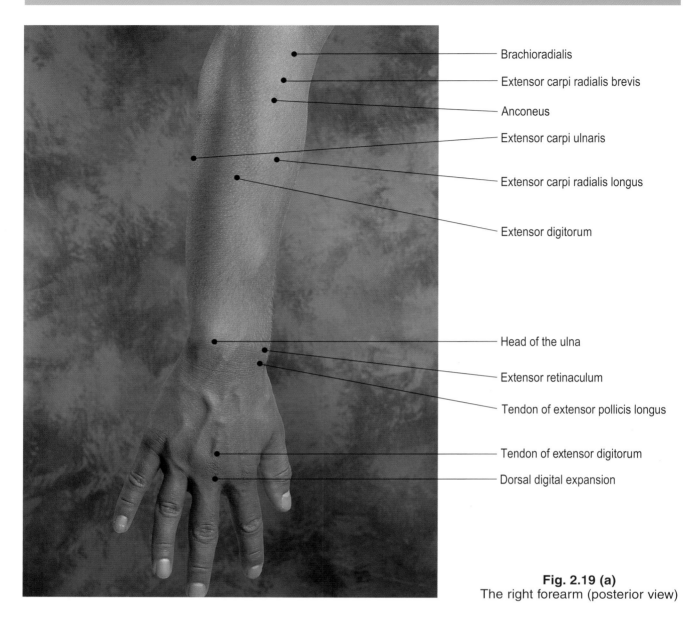

Brachioradialis

Extensor carpi radialis brevis

Anconeus

Extensor carpi ulnaris

Extensor carpi radialis longus

Extensor digitorum

Head of the ulna

Extensor retinaculum

Tendon of extensor pollicis longus

Tendon of extensor digitorum

Dorsal digital expansion

Fig. 2.19 (a)
The right forearm (posterior view)

The posterior aspect of the forearm and wrist

In order to identify muscles in this area, care must be taken to maintain the forearm in the anatomical position, i.e. the arm hanging loosely by the side with the palms facing forwards. Brachioradialis can be palpated most laterally (see page 82). About 1 cm medial to the radial styloid process, two tendons cross the wrist so close to each other that they are often mistaken as one: the lateral is extensor carpi radialis longus which can be traced distally to the base of the second metacarpal; the medial is extensor carpi radialis brevis, attaching to the base of the third metacarpal distally (see Fig. 2.21a). Proximally both muscles can be traced along the medial side of the bulk of brachioradialis to their attachment to, and just above, the lateral epicondyle of the humerus. These become much clearer if the wrist is gently extended.

Passing around the dorsal tubercle of the radius, the tendon of extensor pollicis longus can be palpated, particularly if the thumb is extended. The tendon can be followed to its insertion into the base of the distal phalanx of the thumb. Proximally the tendon is covered almost immediately by superficial muscles (Figs 2.19 and 2.21).

If all the fingers are extended, the tendon of extensor digitorum can be palpated immediately medial to the tendon of extensor pollicis longus (Fig. 2.19). It is broad and flat, dividing into four separate tendons distally. Each tendon can be traced over the back of the hand and along the posterior aspect of each finger, becoming slightly broader over the back of the metacarpophalangeal joint (dorsal digital expansion). Distally, each tendon can be traced to its attachment to the base of the distal phalanx. Proximally, the extensor digitorum can be traced up the middle of the

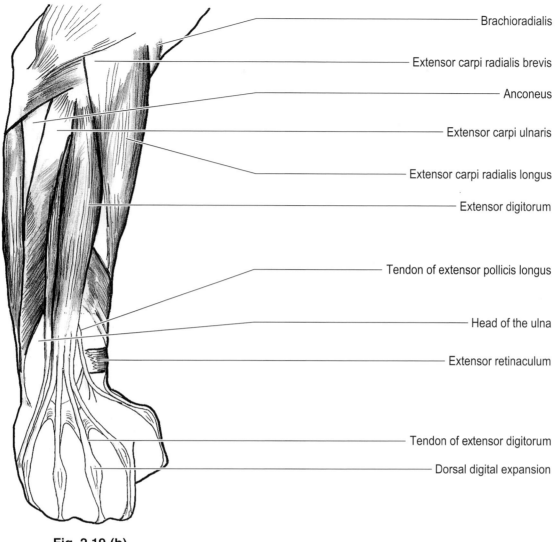

Fig. 2.19 (b)
Muscles of the right forearm
(posterior view)

Labels on the figure:
- Brachioradialis
- Extensor carpi radialis brevis
- Anconeus
- Extensor carpi ulnaris
- Extensor carpi radialis longus
- Extensor digitorum
- Tendon of extensor pollicis longus
- Head of the ulna
- Extensor retinaculum
- Tendon of extensor digitorum
- Dorsal digital expansion

forearm medial to the extensor carpi radialis longus and brevis to attach to the lateral epicondyle of the humerus. Often a separate muscle belly can be identified on the lateral side which passes to the index finger only.

Accompanying the extensor digitorum, across the back of the wrist, is the tendon of the extensor indicis, more easily identifiable as it joins the ulnar side of the extensor digitorum tendon to the index finger at the metacarpophalangeal joint.

Passing over the inferior radioulnar joint, the thin tendon of extensor digiti minimi can be traced towards the little finger, joining the tendon of the extensor digitorum at its dorsal digital expansion.

The tendon can be traced proximally to a thin fusiform belly which attaches to the lateral epicondyle. The tendon of extensor digiti minimi is much clearer when the little finger is rhythmically extended and relaxed.

Finally, crossing the posteromedial aspect of the wrist, just lateral to the styloid process of the ulna, is the thick tendon of the extensor carpi ulnaris, again becoming much clearer on extension of the wrist. This can be traced distally to the base of the fifth metacarpal and proximally, via its muscle belly, to the lateral epicondyle (Fig. 2.19). In the mid-forearm the muscle belly lies lateral to the posterior border of the ulna.

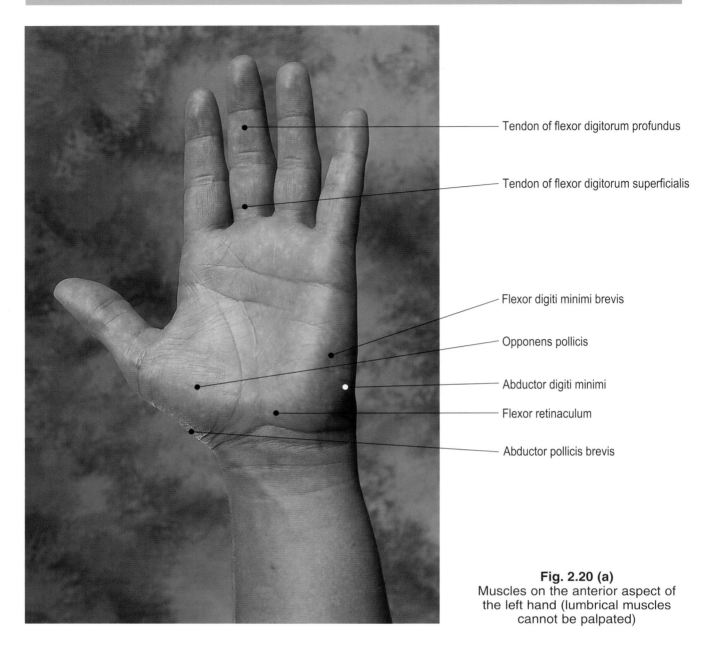

Tendon of flexor digitorum profundus

Tendon of flexor digitorum superficialis

Flexor digiti minimi brevis

Opponens pollicis

Abductor digiti minimi

Flexor retinaculum

Abductor pollicis brevis

Fig. 2.20 (a)
Muscles on the anterior aspect of
the left hand (lumbrical muscles
cannot be palpated)

The anterior aspect of the hand

The bones and joints of the hand are moved and controlled by two main groups of muscles: (a) those of the forearm, whose tendons pass over the wrist to attach to particular bony points in the hand and govern the relationships between the forearm and hand (the extrinsic muscles) (see pages 82–85); and (b) those within the hand which change the relationships of the component parts of the hand from within (the intrinsic muscles).

The palm appears to have a flattened central portion with muscular masses on either side which are closer together proximally and diverge distally

(Fig. 2.20a). The lateral mass, the thenar eminence, is the larger of the two and consists of muscles responsible for producing movements of the thumb. The medial mass, the hypothenar eminence, consists of muscles responsible for producing movements of the little finger.

It must be remembered that movements of the thumb take place in a plane at right angles to the palm of the hand. Consequently, abduction is movement of the thumb anteriorly away from the index finger, while flexion is movement of the thumb medially across the palm of the hand.

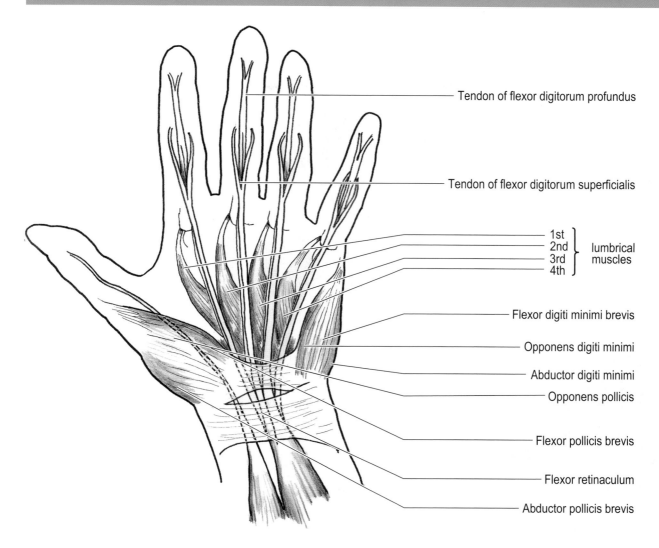

Fig. 2.20 (b)
Muscles on the anterior aspect of
the left hand (lumbrical muscles
cannot be palpated)

Palpation

If the thumb is abducted, the muscle belly of abductor pollicis brevis can be palpated on the lateral side of the thenar eminence, with its tendon passing distally to the lateral side of the proximal phalanx of the thumb (Fig. 2.20). In opposition, i.e. when the pad of the thumb is made to oppose the pad of the fingers, the opponens pollicis contracts, causing the whole central section of the thenar eminence to contract and become hard. If the thumb is flexed, against resistance, at the metacarpophalangeal joint, flexor pollicis brevis, on the medial aspect of the thenar eminence, will be felt contracting.

On abduction of the little finger, i.e. moving it away from the ring finger, abductor digiti minimi can be palpated on the medial side of the hypothenar eminence, which can be traced via a short tendon to the medial side of the base of the proximal phalanx of the little finger (Fig. 2.20). By opposing the little finger to the thumb, the whole of the hypothenar eminence hardens due to the contraction of opponens digiti minimi. With the little finger flexed against resistance, flexor digiti minimi brevis can be palpated, with some difficulty, on the lateral side of opponens digiti minimi (Fig. 2.20).

The central section of the palm of the hand is covered by the strong and thick palmar aponeurosis, making palpation of muscles such as adductor pollicis (transverse head), the palmar interossei or the lumbrical muscles impossible. The long tendons of the flexor digitorum superficialis and profundus can be traced, particularly over the fronts of the metacarpophalangeal joints, but again with difficulty. They become more evident if the fingers are flexed against resistance.

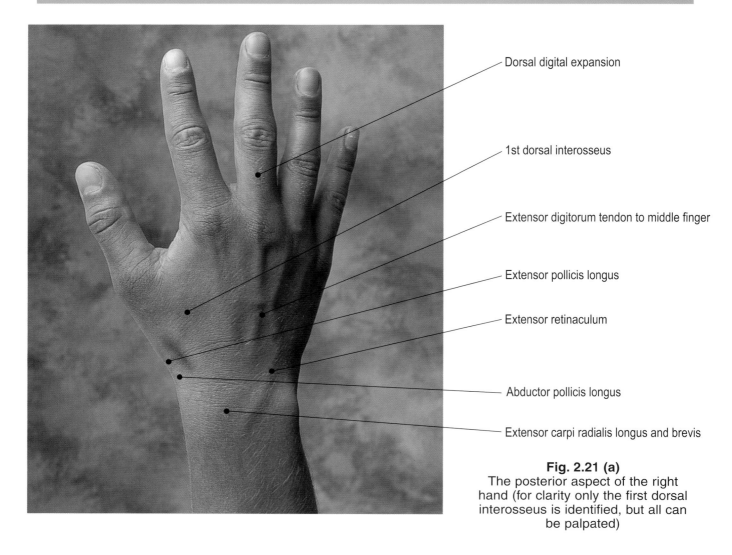

Dorsal digital expansion

1st dorsal interosseus

Extensor digitorum tendon to middle finger

Extensor pollicis longus

Extensor retinaculum

Abductor pollicis longus

Extensor carpi radialis longus and brevis

Fig. 2.21 (a)
The posterior aspect of the right hand (for clarity only the first dorsal interosseus is identified, but all can be palpated)

The posterior aspect of the hand [Fig. 2.21a–g]

The skin and fascia on the posterior aspect of the hand are thin and relatively loose, giving easy access for palpation of muscles that are present. As the main function of the hand is to manipulate and hold implements and tools, often with great care and precision, most of the muscles are situated anteriorly. Releasing the grip tends to be left to the long extensor muscles whose muscle bellies lie in the forearm, with their connection to the hand being through long tendons which cross the back of the wrist (see muscles on the posterior aspect of the forearm, page 00–00). Nevertheless, there are a few muscles which can be palpated and are worthy of note.

Palpation

On the lateral side of the thumb the posterior part of abductor pollicis brevis can be palpated (see page 87), lying just lateral to the tendon of extensor pollicis longus. Its short tendon can be palpated attaching to the lateral side of the proximal phalanx of the thumb, while its proximal

attachment can be traced to the tubercle of the scaphoid. With the thumb abducted and extended, two tendons can be identified crossing the wrist just in front of the radial styloid. These are the abductor pollicis longus and extensor pollicis brevis. The abductor can be traced to the base of the metacarpal and the extensor to the base of the proximal phalanx. Proximal to the radial styloid both tendons wrap posteriorly around the lateral surface of the radius and disappear deep between the other muscles.

In the cleft between the thumb and index finger there is the large muscle mass of the first dorsal interosseus. When the index finger is abducted, i.e. drawn laterally away from the middle finger, contraction of the muscle becomes clear. The muscle belly can be traced from its origin to both the first and second metacarpals, to its tendon which attaches distally to the lateral side of the base of the proximal phalanx of the index finger (Fig. 2.21a). The muscle can easily be demonstrated and identified by placing the fingers on the upper surface of a table with the thumb over the edge running down the vertical section. If the index finger is now abducted, the muscle becomes hard and its belly and tendon easily palpable.

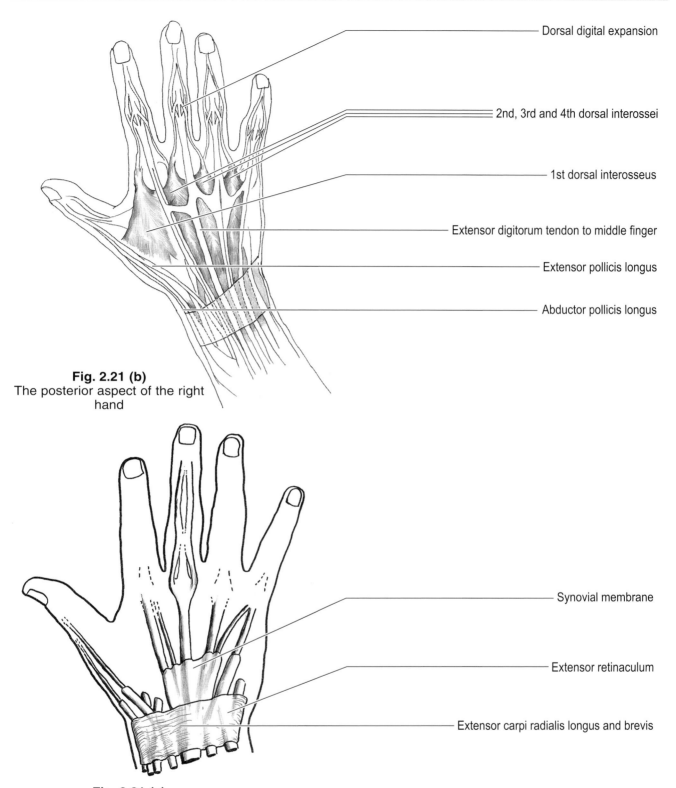

Dorsal digital expansion

2nd, 3rd and 4th dorsal interossei

1st dorsal interosseus

Extensor digitorum tendon to middle finger

Extensor pollicis longus

Abductor pollicis longus

Fig. 2.21 (b)
The posterior aspect of the right hand

Synovial membrane

Extensor retinaculum

Extensor carpi radialis longus and brevis

Fig. 2.21 (c)
The posterior aspect of the right hand

When the middle finger is abducted laterally, i.e. towards the index finger, the second dorsal interosseus can be palpated, its fibres bulging between the proximal half of the second and third metacarpals. If the same finger is now abducted medially, i.e. towards the ring finger, the third dorsal interosseus can be palpated between the proximal half of the third and fourth metacarpals (Fig. 2.21d).

Abducting the ring finger, the fourth dorsal interosseus can be palpated between the proximal half of the fourth and fifth metacarpals. In addition, abductor digiti minimi can also be seen and palpated on the medial side of the hand (see page 87).

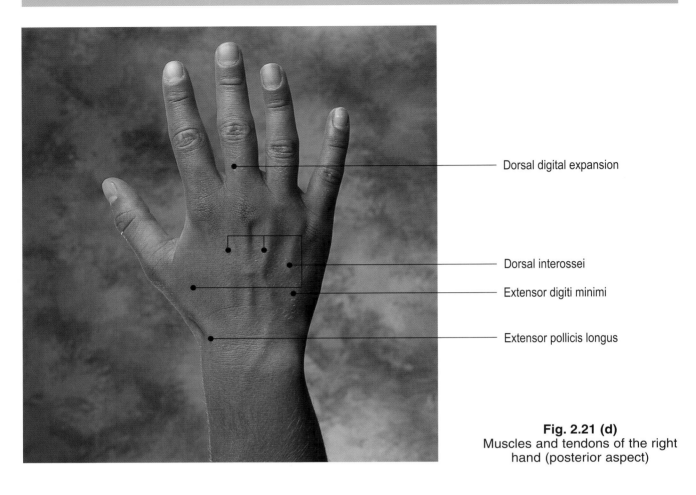

Dorsal digital expansion

Dorsal interossei

Extensor digiti minimi

Extensor pollicis longus

Fig. 2.21 (d)
Muscles and tendons of the right
hand (posterior aspect)

Fig. 2.21 (f)
The posterior aspect of the right
hand

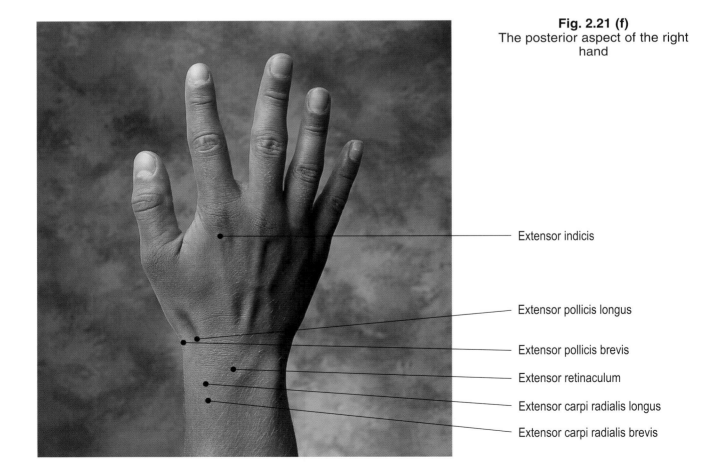

Extensor indicis

Extensor pollicis longus

Extensor pollicis brevis

Extensor retinaculum

Extensor carpi radialis longus

Extensor carpi radialis brevis

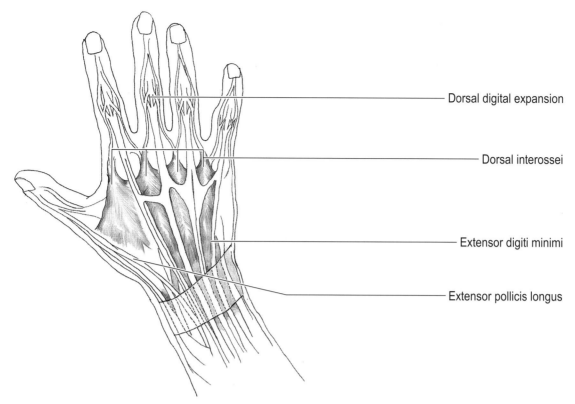

— Dorsal digital expansion

— Dorsal interossei

— Extensor digiti minimi

— Extensor pollicis longus

Fig. 2.21 (e)
Muscles and tendons of the right
hand (posterior aspect)

Fig. 2.21 (g)
The posterior aspect of the right
hand

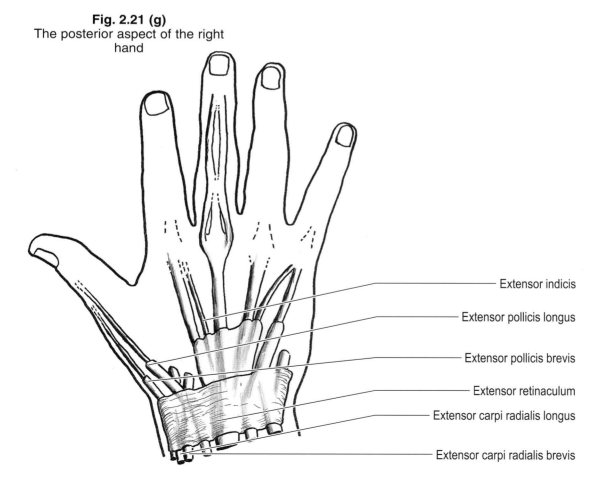

— Extensor indicis

— Extensor pollicis longus

— Extensor pollicis brevis

— Extensor retinaculum

— Extensor carpi radialis longus

— Extensor carpi radialis brevis

SELF ASSESSMENT

Page 76

1. Describe the shape of the deltoid muscle.

2. Name the three components of the muscle.

3. Identify the upper attachment of the deltoid.

4. Where does the common tendon attach below?

5. Describe how the fibres of the central section differ from the others.

6. Describe the arrangement of the fibres in this central portion.

7. Name and demonstrate the movements which are produced by the anterior fibres.

8. Name and demonstrate the movements produced by contraction of the posterior fibres.

9. When all fibres of deltoid contract together, what movement is produced?

Page 77

10. Describe and outline the shape of the pectoralis major.

11. Describe the general location of this muscle.

12. Name the two sections of the muscle.

13. Where does the upper section attach centrally?

14. To what do the lower fibres attach centrally?

15. Describe the arrangement of the tendon as it passes laterally.

16. Indicate the bony process of the bone to which the tendon of pectoralis major attaches.

17. This muscle forms the anterior wall of which space?

18. Name and demonstrate the movement which is produced by the upper fibres of pectoralis major.

19. The inferior fibres produce what movement when they contract?

Please complete the labels below.

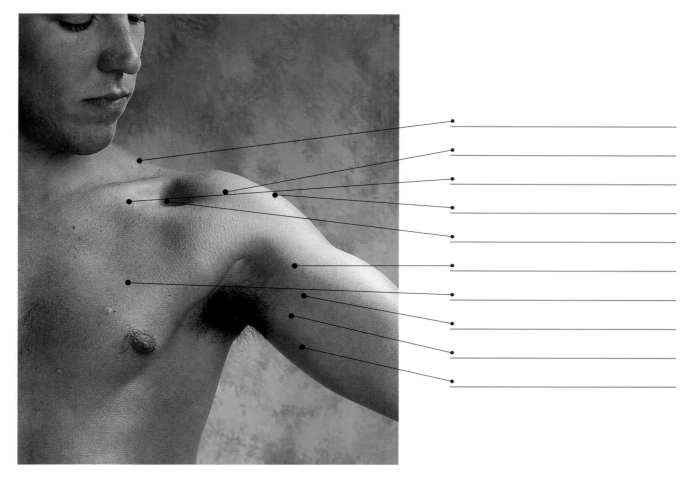

Fig. 2.16 (a) Muscles on the anterior of the left chest, shoulder and arm

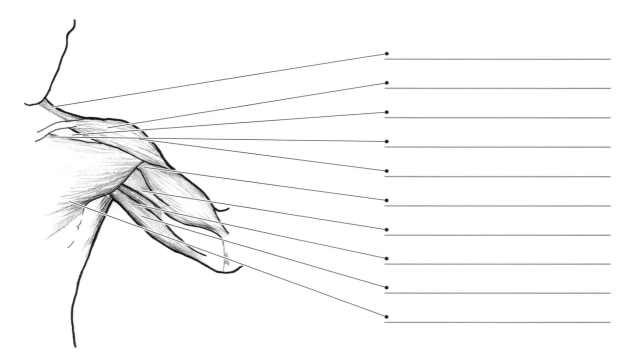

Fig. 2.16 (b) Muscles on the anterior of the left chest, shoulder and arm

Page 78

20. Describe the shape of the biceps brachii.

_____

21. Where is this muscle situated?

_____

22. List its bony attachments proximally.

_____

23. Name its lower attachment: bony and fascial.

_____

24. Describe the actions of biceps brachii.

_____

25. What shape is the brachialis muscle?

_____

26. Where is the brachialis situated?

_____

27. To which part of the humerus is brachialis attached?

_____

28. To which process of what bone does it attach below?

_____

29. How and where can the brachialis be palpated?

_____

Page 79

30. What are the components of the triceps muscle?

_____

31. How many attachments does it have proximally?

_____

32. List the attachments of the heads of triceps.

_____

33. What is the distal attachment of this muscle?

_____

Page 80

34. Describe the general shape of the latissimus dorsi muscle.

_____

35. Where is latissimus dorsi located?

_____

36. Describe the extensive lower attachment of this muscle.

_____

37. To what does it attach as it passes over the thorax?

_____

Please complete the labels below.

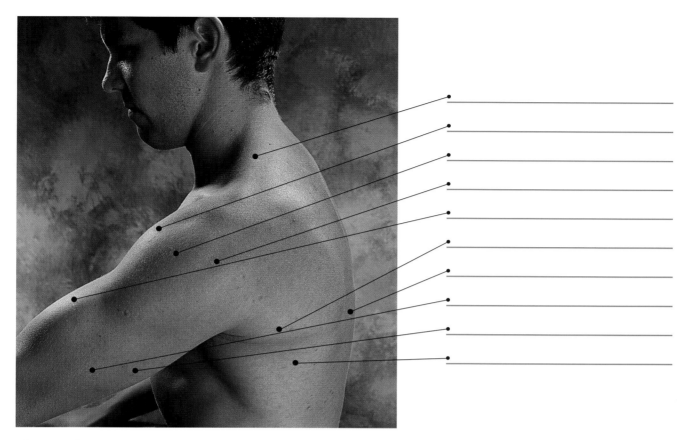

Fig. 2.17 (a) Muscles that move the arm and forearm (lateral view of left arm)

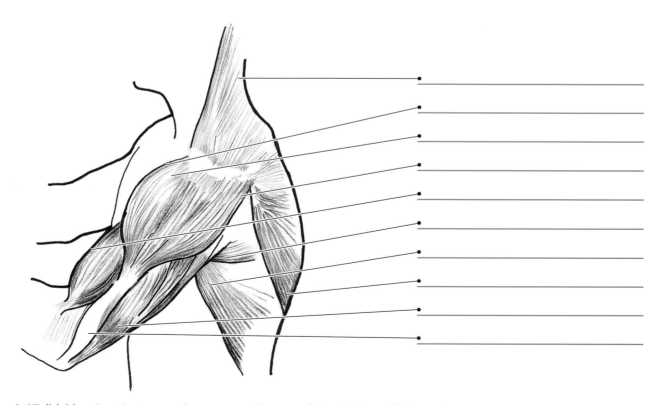

Fig. 2.17 (b) Muscles that move the arm and forearm (lateral view of left arm)

38. Describe what happens to the tendon as it passes under the axilla.

39. To what does the latissimus dorsi attach superiorly?

40. List the actions produced by contraction of the latissimus dorsi.

41. Describe a functional activity in which the latissimus dorsi takes part.

42. This muscle forms the posterior wall of which space?

Page 81

43. Describe the shape of the coracobrachialis.

44. Where is corocobrachialis located?

45. Its attachment proximally is to which process of what bone?

46. What is its distal attachment.

47. Where and how can this muscle be palpated?

48. Explain the reasons why care must be taken when palpating in this region.

49. Which muscle belly is found above the spine of the scapula?

50. Name the muscle which can be palpated below the spine of the scapula.

51. What movement can be produced by contraction of the muscle above the scapula spine?

52. Contraction of the muscle below the spine produces what movement?

53. Name the muscles situated around the lateral border of the scapula.

54. What action is produced by contraction of each of the above muscles?

Please complete the labels below.

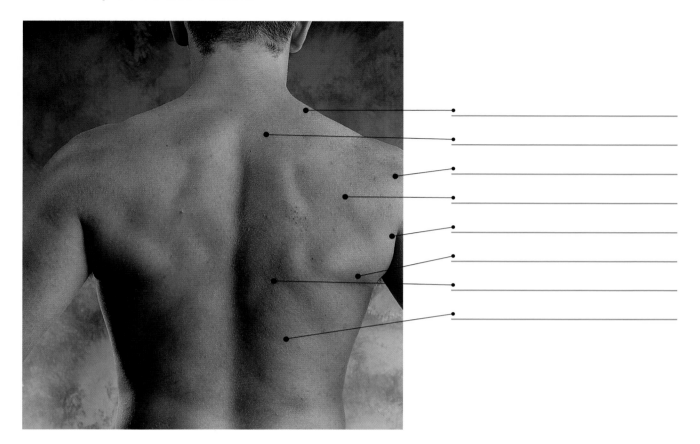

Fig. 2.17 (c) Muscles that move the arm (posterior view)

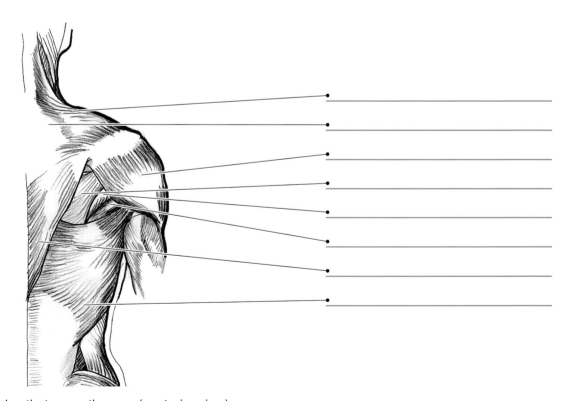

Fig. 2.17 (d) Muscles that move the arm (posterior view)

Page 82

55. Name the muscle which is situated most laterally in the forearm.

___

56. Where is its proximal attachment?

___

57. The tendon of which muscle lies 1 cm medially to the styloid process of the radius, anteriorly?

___

58. What is the action of palmaris longus?

___

59. To what structure does palmaris longus attach?

___

Page 83

60. Name the muscle whose tendon passes over the medial side of the anterior aspect of the wrist.

___

61. What is its distal attachment?

___

62. The tendons of which muscles lie in the groove just medial to the palmaris longus?

___

63. Describe how these two muscles vary in their distal attachment.

___

Page 84

64. How do the extensor carpi radialis longus and brevis vary in their distal attachment?

___

65. The tendon of which muscle passes round the dorsal tubercle of the radius?

___

66. What is the distal attachment of this muscle?

___

67. Into how many slips does the tendon of the extensor digitorum split?

___

68. What is the action of extensor digitorum?

___

69. Describe what is meant by 'the extensor expansion'.

___

70. Where do the tendons of the extensor digitorum attach distally?

___

Page 85

71. Where does the extensor digitorum attach proximally?

___

72. The tendon of which muscle accompanies the extensor digitorum as it crosses the wrist?

___

73. Which tendon crosses the wrist posterior to the inferior radioulnar joint?

___

74. To which structure does this tendon attach distally?

___

Please complete the labels below.

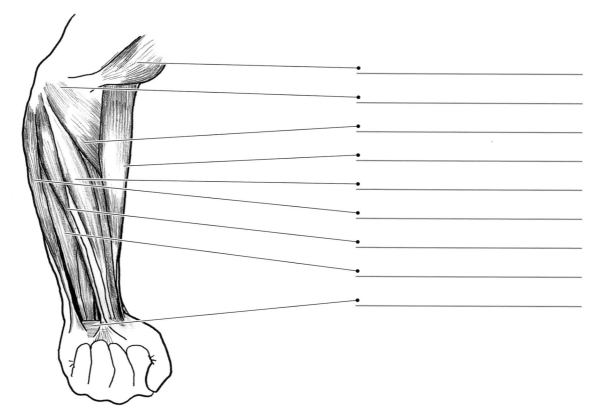

Fig. 2.18 (b) Muscles of the left forearm (anterior view)

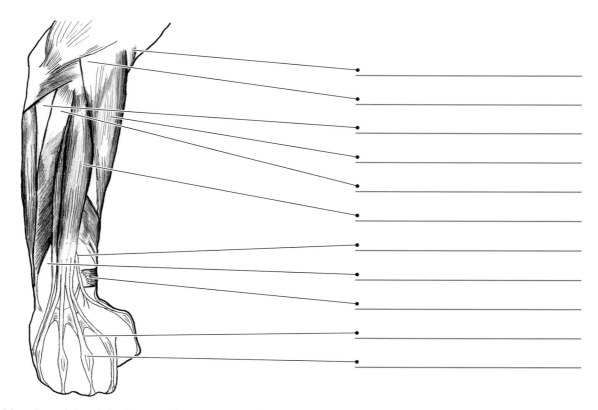

Fig. 2.19 (b) Muscles of the right forearm (posterior view)

75. Name the muscle whose tendon crosses the wrist just posterior to the ulnar styloid process.

_____

76. Where is the distal attachment of this muscle?

_____

Page 86

77. Name the bulk of muscle on the anterolateral aspect of the palm.

78. With which movements are these muscles mainly concerned?

79. Name the bulk of muscle on the anteromedial aspect of the palm.

80. With which digit are these muscles mainly concerned?

81. Describe the movements of the thumb.

82. Name the planes in which these movements occur.

Page 87

83. Which muscle is situated on the lateral side of the lateral bulk of muscle?

84. What is its action?

85. Name the muscle which produces opposition of the thumb and demonstrate this movement.

86. Describe the movement of abduction of the little finger.

87. Name the muscle responsible for this movement.

88. Where is the distal attachment of this muscle?

89. Can the little finger be opposed to the thumb?

90. What structure covers the central portion of the palm of the hand?

Page 88

91. Name the muscle which forms the mass between the first and second metacarpal.

92. What action does this muscle perform?

93. How is it best demonstrated?

Page 89

94. Which muscles lie between the second and third, third and fourth and fourth and fifth metacarpals?

95. Describe the action of each.

Please complete the labels below.

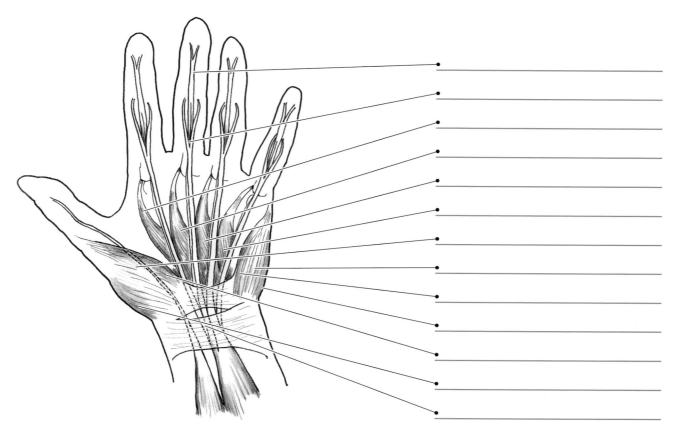

Fig. 2.20 (b) Muscles on the anterior aspect of the left hand (lumbrical muscles cannot be palpated)

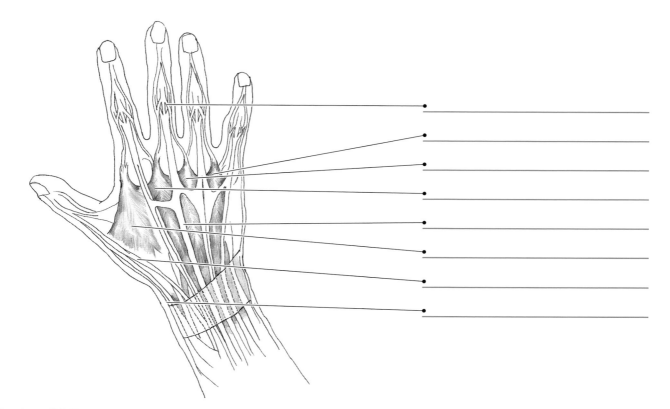

Fig. 2.21 (b) The posterior aspect of the right hand

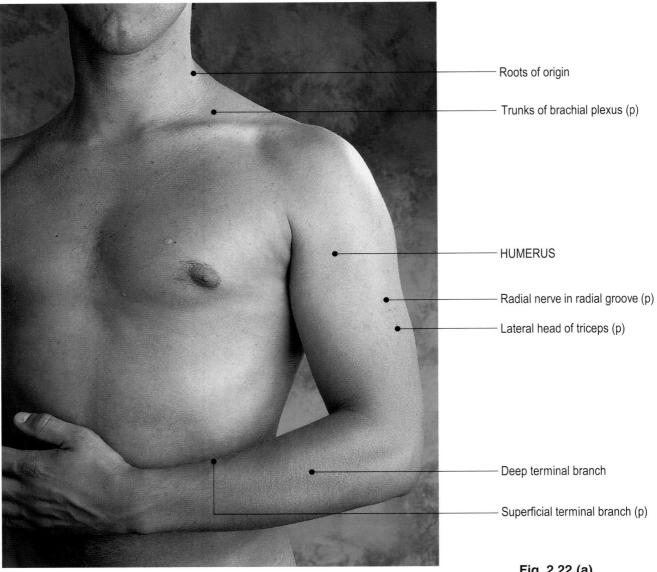

Roots of origin

Trunks of brachial plexus (p)

HUMERUS

Radial nerve in radial groove (p)

Lateral head of triceps (p)

Deep terminal branch

Superficial terminal branch (p)

Fig. 2.22 (a)
The radial nerve of the left upper
limb (p, palpable)

NERVES [Figs 2.22 and 2.23]

Most of the upper limb is innervated by nerves via the brachial plexus. The nerve roots contributing to this plexus are C5, 6, 7 and 8 and T1. The root of C5 may receive a contribution from C4 (pre-fixed plexus), while the T1 root may receive a contribution from T2 (post-fixed plexus). The roots combine to form trunks. The upper, middle and lower trunks, each of which divides into anterior and posterior divisions, combine to form the lateral, medial and posterior cords. It is from the cords that the majority of branches arise to be distributed to the whole of the upper limb. For a more detailed description see Palastanga, Field and Soames (1998).

Palpation

Palpation of nerves must be performed with care. To the palpator, nerves appear as slippery cord-like structures, which only occasionally become superficial, being mostly buried deep to other structures for protection. To the palpated, pressure on a nerve may evoke localized pain, but may also produce a tingling sensation, pain or numbness over the area of its distribution. The accurate location of nerves is important, but over-palpation must be avoided as this may lead to interference, with possible signs and symptoms.

Press the fingers into the depression above the medial end of the clavicle, just lateral to the sterno-cleidomastoid, and the trunks of the brachial plexus appear as a bundle of tense cords running downwards and laterally. Palpation in this area can be uncomfortable if you apply too much pressure.

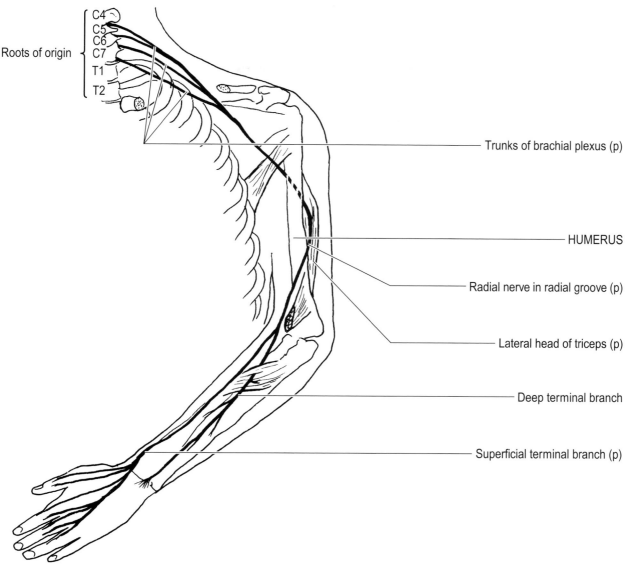

Roots of origin

C4
C5
C6
C7
T1
T2

Trunks of brachial plexus (p)

HUMERUS

Radial nerve in radial groove (p)

Lateral head of triceps (p)

Deep terminal branch

Superficial terminal branch (p)

Fig. 2.22 (b)
The radial nerve of the left
upper limb (p, palpable)

The radial nerve

Approximately halfway down the lateral side of the arm, below the insertion of deltoid, a groove can be palpated running downwards and forwards. Again, with careful palpation, particularly just behind the groove, the radial nerve can be rolled against the humerus just anterior to the lateral head of triceps. Anteriorly it enters a muscular groove between brachioradialis and brachialis, passing anterolateral to the elbow joint but too deep to be palpated.

On the lateral side of the radius, at variable points on its lower half, the superficial branch of the radial nerve can be rolled against the bone as it passes from under brachioradialis to its distribution on the back of the lateral side of the hand. Sometimes the nerve is single, whereas in others it splits into five divisions (Fig. 2.22).

With the subject's right forearm in your left hand and the thumb uppermost, glide the radial side of your right thumb up and down the lower end of the radius. The branch(es) of the radial nerve can be felt rolling against the bone. Even though they are lying superficially on the back of the hand, they are still difficult to trace. The subject is likely to experience similar sensations in the distribution of these superficial branches to the posterolateral aspect of the hand and lateral three-and-a-half digits as those experienced on tapping the median nerve on rolling of the superficial branches of the ulnar nerve over the hook of the hamate.

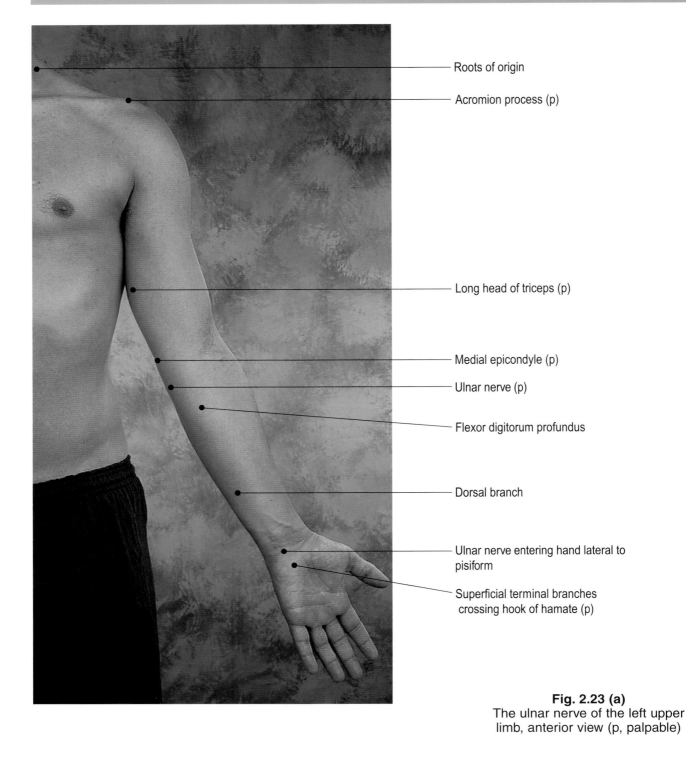

— Roots of origin

— Acromion process (p)

— Long head of triceps (p)

— Medial epicondyle (p)

— Ulnar nerve (p)

— Flexor digitorum profundus

— Dorsal branch

— Ulnar nerve entering hand lateral to pisiform

— Superficial terminal branches crossing hook of hamate (p)

Fig. 2.23 (a)
The ulnar nerve of the left upper limb, anterior view (p, palpable)

Palpation

Press the pads of the fingers against the lateral wall of the axilla (the upper medial surface of the arm), and more cord-like structures can be palpated extending down the medial aspect of the arm. Numerous branches of the brachial plexus, including the ulnar and median nerves, are palpable on the medial side of the arm but they are not easily identifiable. The axillary/brachial artery can, however, be recognized pulsating between them.

The ulnar nerve

Continue down the medial side of the arm until you can palpate the medial supracondylar ridge with the medial epicondyle projecting medially. Move the tips of your fingers to the posterior of this structure. The ulnar nerve can be palpated behind the medial epicondyle as it passes from the medial aspect of the arm, over the medial collateral ligament of the elbow joint, to enter the forearm between the two heads of flexor carpi ulnaris. The whole medial aspect of the arm is tender to palpation, so employ great care here.

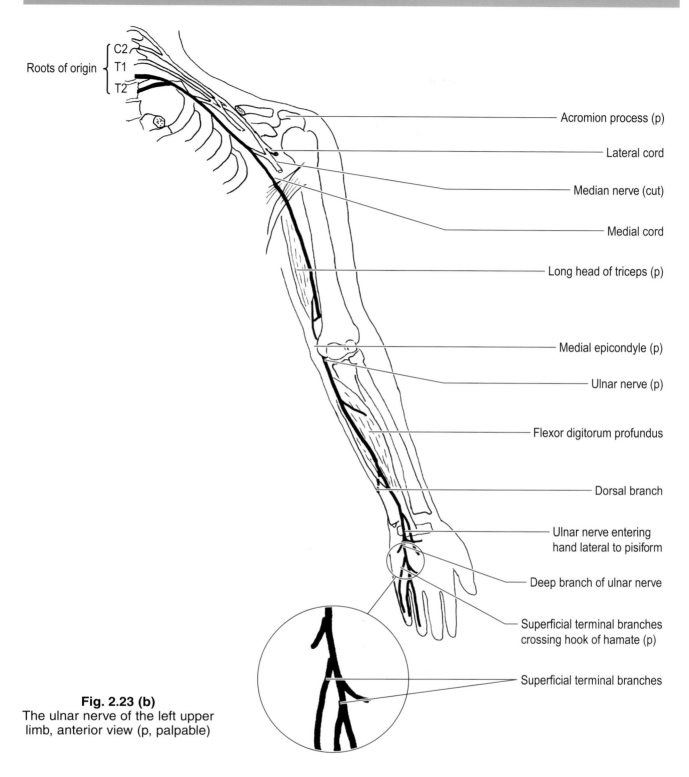

Roots of origin
- C2
- T1
- T2

Acromion process (p)

Lateral cord

Median nerve (cut)

Medial cord

Long head of triceps (p)

Medial epicondyle (p)

Ulnar nerve (p)

Flexor digitorum profundus

Dorsal branch

Ulnar nerve entering hand lateral to pisiform

Deep branch of ulnar nerve

Superficial terminal branches crossing hook of hamate (p)

Superficial terminal branches

Fig. 2.23 (b)
The ulnar nerve of the left upper limb, anterior view (p, palpable)

The nerve (Fig. 2.23a,b) can be traced from the groove behind the medial epicondyle down the medial aspect of the elbow joint and medial side of the olecranon until it disappears under the fibrous arch of the flexor carpi ulnaris. It passes down the medial aspect of the forearm deep to this muscle until approximately 7 cm above the wrist, where it appears on the lateral side of the tendon before passing over the flexor retinaculum to enter the medial side of the hand. It can be palpated with some difficulty, as it lies lateral to the tendon of flexor carpi ulnaris, often covered with a layer of fascia obscuring it from palpation. Its two superficial terminal branches, however, can be rolled against the hook of the hamate just distal to the pisiform, deep in the hypothenar muscle (see page 24). This procedure will give the subject a sensation of tingling over the anterior surface of the medial one-and-a-half digits.

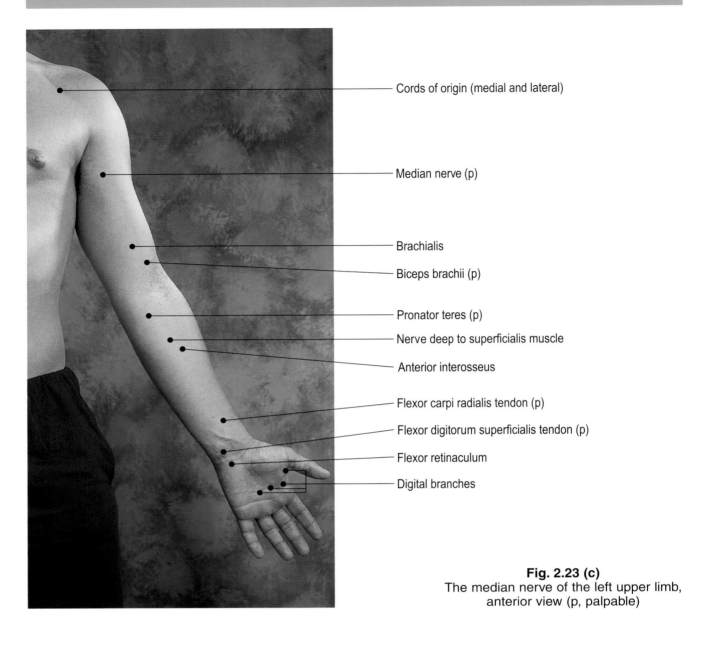

Cords of origin (medial and lateral)

Median nerve (p)

Brachialis

Biceps brachii (p)

Pronator teres (p)

Nerve deep to superficialis muscle

Anterior interosseus

Flexor carpi radialis tendon (p)

Flexor digitorum superficialis tendon (p)

Flexor retinaculum

Digital branches

Fig. 2.23 (c)
The median nerve of the left upper limb,
anterior view (p, palpable)

The median nerve [Fig. 2.23c and d]

The median nerve derives its fibres from the anterior primary rami of the fifth, sixth, seventh and eighth cervical and the first thoracic roots. The nerve is formed in front of the axillary artery after passing through all three trunks and the lateral and medial cords. It passes down the medial side of the arm accompanying the brachial artery, passing across the elbow joint superficial to the brachialis, but deep to biceps. It passes into the forearm between the two heads of pronator teres and passes down towards the front of the wrist under the flexor digitorum superficialis. It crosses the wrist joint under the flexor retinaculum on the radial side between the tendons of flexor carpi radialis and flexor digitorum superficialis, with which it shares a tunnel under the flexor retinaculum. For its distribution throughout the upper

limb the reader should refer to *Anatomy and Human Movement* (Palastanga, Field and Soames 1998).

Palpation

Although the cord-like structures of nerves can be palpated around the pulsating brachial artery on the medial side of the arm, identification of any particular nerve is virtually impossible. The only place that the median nerve can be palpated in the arm is on the medial side of the biceps just before it forms its tendon. The nerve then passes under the biceps tendon and retinaculum to enter the forearm. It is too well covered by the flexor digitorum superficialis to be palpated in the upper forearm, but becomes superficial as it emerges from the lateral side of the muscle, to cross the

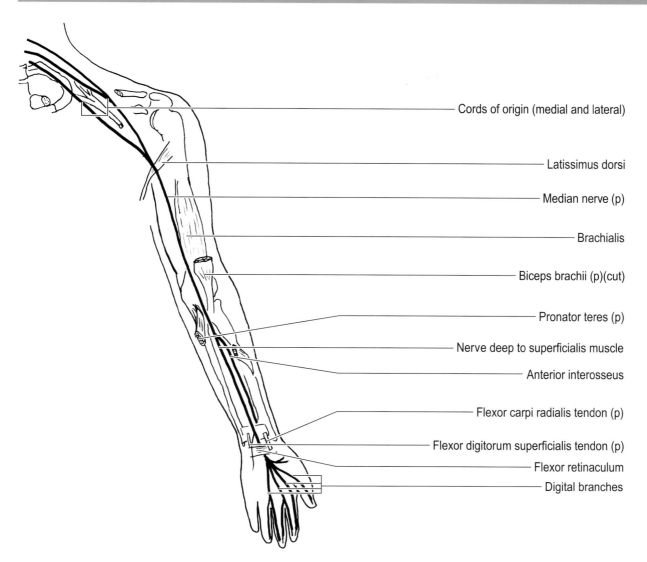

Cords of origin (medial and lateral)

Latissimus dorsi

Median nerve (p)

Brachialis

Biceps brachii (p)(cut)

Pronator teres (p)

Nerve deep to superficialis muscle

Anterior interosseus

Flexor carpi radialis tendon (p)

Flexor digitorum superficialis tendon (p)

Flexor retinaculum

Digital branches

Fig. 2.23 (d)
The median nerve of the left upper limb,
anterior view (p, palpable)

wrist. Here it can be palpated as a cord-like structure between the tendons of the above muscle and the flexor carpi radialis. It then disappears into the thenar muscles on the lateral side of the hand.

Because the median nerve passes through the same compartment as the tendons of flexor digitorum superficialis and profundus it can become compressed. This is commonly due to tightening of the flexor retinaculum or swelling of the synovial sheath surrounding the flexor tendons. This condition is referred to as 'carpal tunnel syn-

drome' and may be tested by tapping the nerve as it passes through the tunnel, which causes a tingling sensation over its distribution in the hand.

Sometimes the patient can suffer severe pain over the distribution of the nerve in the hand and may even lose the ability to use the muscles of the thenar eminence. Permanent dysfunction could occur if the pressure on the nerve is not quickly released. This is normally achieved by an operative procedure.

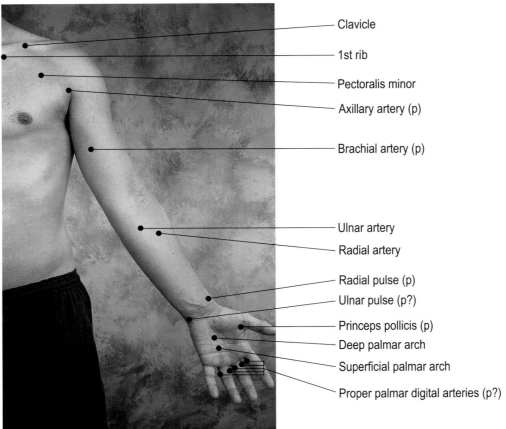

Clavicle

1st rib

Pectoralis minor

Axillary artery (p)

Brachial artery (p)

Ulnar artery

Radial artery

Radial pulse (p)

Ulnar pulse (p?)

Princeps pollicis (p)

Deep palmar arch

Superficial palmar arch

Proper palmar digital arteries (p?)

Fig. 2.24 (a)
Arteries of the left upper limb,
anterior view (p, palpable)

ARTERIES [Fig. 2.24]

A different approach must be made to the palpation of arteries. As stated earlier, when the tissue to be palpated is moving, the fingers should remain stationary. When palpating arteries, the fingertips should be used, never the thumb, as the palpator could be misled by the pulse in his or her own thumb. This is due to the presence of the relatively large artery (princeps pollicis) which supplies its pulp. Although the index finger is commonly used, all the fingertips are extremely sensitive. Sometimes the fingers are placed along the line of the artery, as it may be concealed for a short distance by another structure. Very gentle, sensitive touch must be employed because too much pressure may compress the artery and prevent its pulsations.

Palpation

Palpation of arteries throughout the limb varies from individual to individual, being modified by the texture of the skin, the thickness or tightness of fascial coverings, the bulk of muscles, the quantity of subcutaneous fat, etc. It is also dependent on the size of the artery and the patency of its walls. This varies enormously and may be affected by age and disease, *particularly* of the cardiovascular system.

The blood supply to the upper limbs is via the left subclavian artery, directly from the arch of the aorta, and the right subclavian, via the brachiocephalic trunk. All of these arteries are too deep to palpate, except where the subclavian passes over the first rib. With careful palpation just posterior to the mid-point of the clavicle, behind the insertion of scalenus anterior to the first rib, the pulsations of the subclavian artery can be felt. The artery, now named the axillary artery, then passes into the axilla and can be palpated behind the anterior and against the lateral wall by pressing gently upwards and laterally with the fingers. This may prove uncomfortable for the subject as the cords of the brachial plexus may intervene.

With careful palpation, the pulsations of the brachial artery can be traced down the medial side of the arm lying in a furrow anterior to coracobrachialis, in the upper part, and on the medial side of biceps and its tendon, in the lower part. The whole length of the artery is uncomfortable if too much pressure is applied, as the ulnar nerve lies superficial to it in the upper half, and the median nerve in the lower half of its course. It becomes easier to palpate just prior to passing under the bicipital aponeurosis in front of the elbow joint, but even here it can remain quite elusive. It is here that the pulsation of the brachial artery is auscultated with a stethoscope when taking blood pressure.

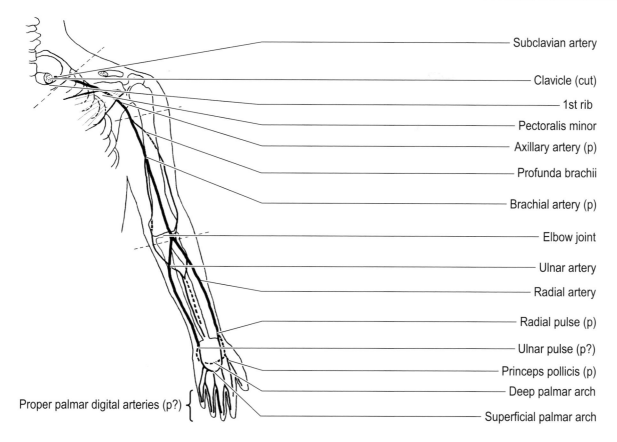

Subclavian artery

Clavicle (cut)

1st rib

Pectoralis minor

Axillary artery (p)

Profunda brachii

Brachial artery (p)

Elbow joint

Ulnar artery

Radial artery

Radial pulse (p)

Ulnar pulse (p?)

Princeps pollicis (p)

Deep palmar arch

Superficial palmar arch

Proper palmar digital arteries (p?)

Fig. 2.24 (b)
Arteries of the left upper limb,
anterior view (p, palpable)

The brachial artery divides into the radial and ulnar arteries just below the line of the elbow joint. These are both well covered by muscle and difficult to palpate until they emerge from between the tendons proximal to the wrist.

The radial artery is by far the easier to palpate, lying in a groove between flexor carpi radialis and the anterior border of the radius. This is best approached by wrapping your hand around the back of the subject's wrist with the fingertips resting on the lower end of the anterior border and styloid process of the radius. The fingers are then allowed to move gently medially some 0.5 cm where the pulsation of the radial artery becomes clear. This should be practised regularly, as it is the most common pulse that is checked in the human body. The artery can again be palpated on the lateral side of the scaphoid deep in the 'anatomical snuff box', between the tendons of extensor pollicis longus medially, and extensor pollicis brevis and abductor pollicis longus laterally. This area is, however, quite tender if too much pressure is applied.

The ulnar artery is much more difficult to palpate in the region of the wrist and hand as it is covered by the palmar aponeurosis. Nevertheless, its pulsations are recognizable just lateral to the pisiform bone. It then passes deeply into the palm as the superficial palmar arch, too deep to be palpated.

Throughout the hand, small branches of the radial and ulnar arteries can be palpated by an experienced practitioner beyond the superficial and deep palmar and carpal arches. The posterior metacarpal arteries are palpable between the metacarpal bones, especially at their bases. On each side of the palmar aspect of each finger, the pulsation of the very slender proper palmar digital arteries can be felt. These become clearer beyond the cleft of the fingers. The dorsal digital arteries on either side of the dorsum of each finger are less obvious. In the cleft between the thumb and index finger, the pulsations of the princeps pollicis, a comparatively large artery, can be traced up the anteromedial side of the thumb, particularly opposite the proximal phalanx. On the lateral side of the metacarpal of the index finger, the radialis indicis artery is palpable running up the dorsolateral side of the finger. If the thumb is gently rested against a firm surface, the pulsations of the princeps pollicis can readily be felt by the subject. This is why it is important to use only the fingertips to palpate a pulse.

Sometimes, on a subject with good strong pulsations and thin fascia, the posterior carpal arch arteries can be palpated crossing the posterior aspect of the carpus just below the level of the wrist joint.

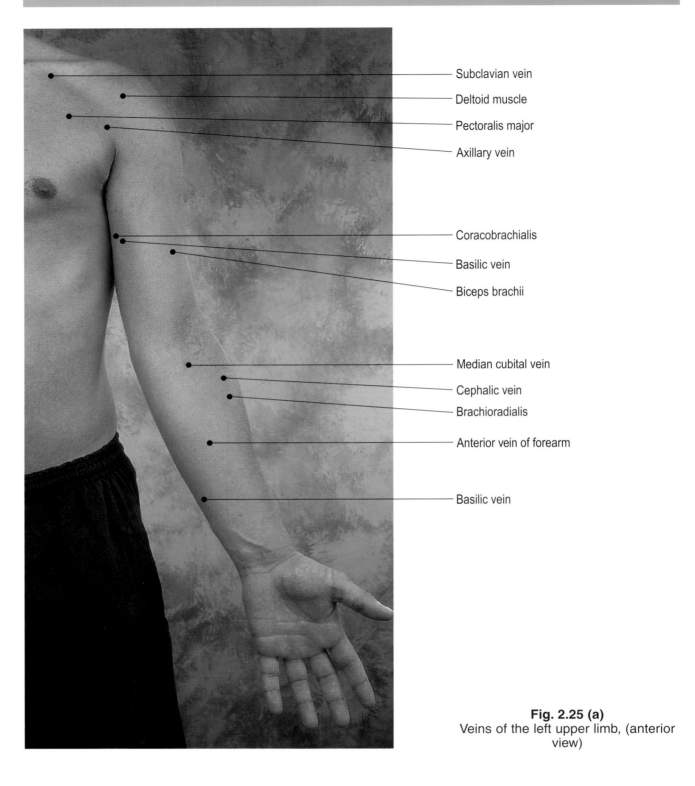

— Subclavian vein

— Deltoid muscle

— Pectoralis major

— Axillary vein

— Coracobrachialis

— Basilic vein

— Biceps brachii

— Median cubital vein

— Cephalic vein

— Brachioradialis

— Anterior vein of forearm

— Basilic vein

Fig. 2.25 (a)
Veins of the left upper limb, (anterior view)

VEINS

The veins of the upper limb are, for convenience of description, divided into two groups, deep and superficial. The deep veins tend to follow the arteries deep within the limb, whereas the superficial veins lie within the superficial fascia forming a variable network. All veins in the upper limb possess valves, more numerous in the deep than in the superficial veins, the function of which is to facilitate venous return to the heart.

Palpation

The superficial veins are extremely difficult to palpate as they are normally thin-walled, variable in position, concealed within the superficial fascia and possess low internal pressure. Thus, only a few of the superficial veins are palpable in the normal limb, the deep veins being impossible to palpate.

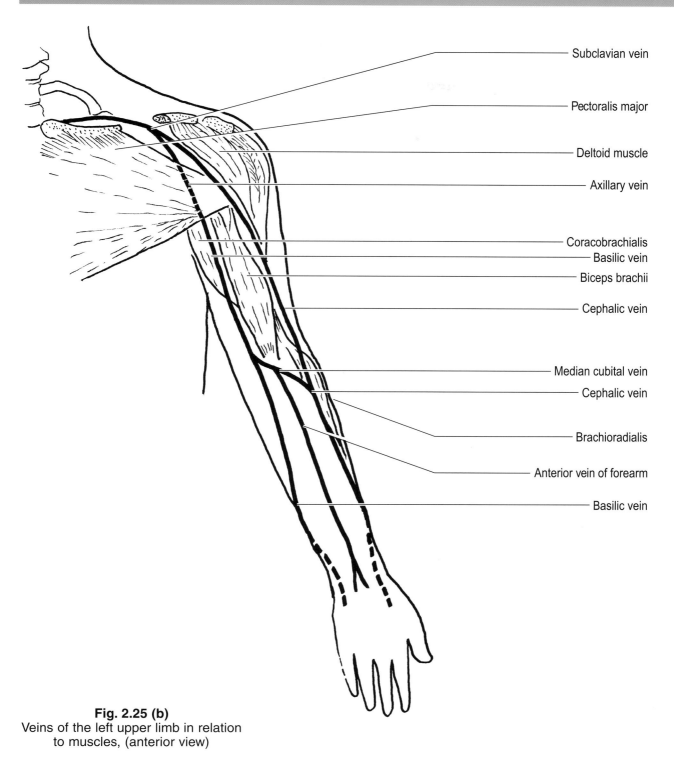

Subclavian vein

Pectoralis major

Deltoid muscle

Axillary vein

Coracobrachialis
Basilic vein
Biceps brachii
Cephalic vein

Median cubital vein
Cephalic vein

Brachioradialis

Anterior vein of forearm

Basilic vein

Fig. 2.25 (b)
Veins of the left upper limb in relation
to muscles, (anterior view)

Gentle brushing of the skin surface may be all that is required to indicate the course of superficial veins to the examiner. Some veins merely show as a bluish line just below the skin, while others are accompanied by raised areas. The appearance of the veins in individuals varies considerably, being dependent on factors such as sex, obesity and age. In males the veins are usually more prominent, whereas in the obese they are more difficult to find. Veins tend to show more clearly in the elderly, as the fascia becomes thinner and the veins themselves become tortuous and distended.

The venous network on the dorsum of the hand is palpable in most subjects, particularly if the arm hangs by the side and firm pressure is applied to the inner aspect of the arm anterior to the brachial artery (see page 108).

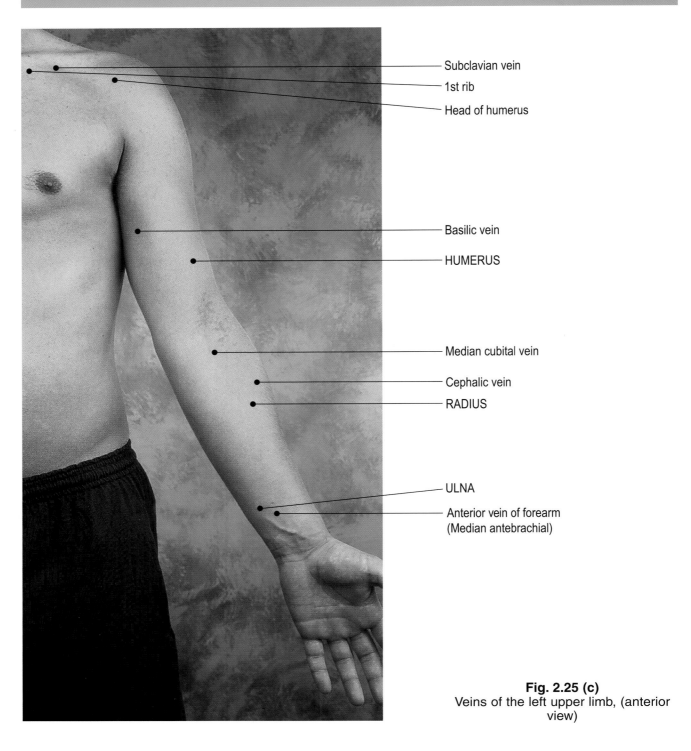

- Subclavian vein
- 1st rib
- Head of humerus
- Basilic vein
- HUMERUS
- Median cubital vein
- Cephalic vein
- RADIUS
- ULNA
- Anterior vein of forearm (Median antebrachial)

Fig. 2.25 (c)
Veins of the left upper limb, (anterior view)

Superficial drainage

The cephalic vein [Fig. 2.25]

The origin of the cephalic vein can be traced from the posterolateral aspect of the dorsal venous network, passing upwards around the lateral border of the forearm anterior to the head of the radius. It then ascends on the lateral side of biceps brachii to the groove between deltoid and pectoralis major (Fig. 2.25a,b) to end in the infraclavicular fossa, where it pierces the clavipectoral fascia to join the axillary vein. Proximal to the head of the radius the vein is more difficult to identify.

The basilic vein [Fig. 2.25]

The basilic vein begins on the medial side of the dorsal venous network and passes up the medial aspect of the forearm, coming to lie anterior to the medial condyle of the humerus. It continues up the medial side of the arm, piercing the deep fascia, near the insertion of coracobrachialis, to accompany the brachial vessels before becoming the axillary vein. The distal half of the vein can usually be palpated, whereas proximally it may only appear as a bluish line.

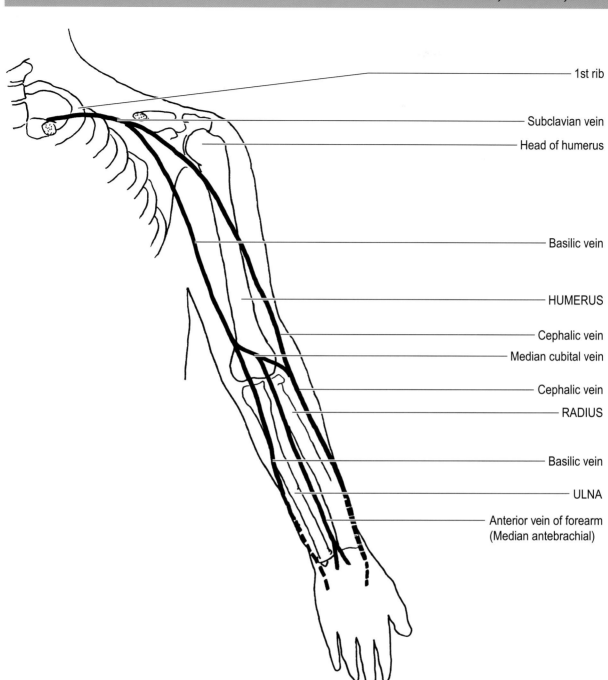

1st rib

Subclavian vein

Head of humerus

Basilic vein

HUMERUS

Cephalic vein

Median cubital vein

Cephalic vein

RADIUS

Basilic vein

ULNA

Anterior vein of forearm
(Median antebrachial)

Fig. 2.25 (d)
Veins of the left upper limb in
relation to bones, (anterior view)

On the front of the forearm there is normally a midline vein, the median antebrachial, which commonly joins with the median cubital vein. The median cubital vein itself passes across the cubital fossa, uniting the cephalic and basilic veins. All of these veins are normally palpable when pressure is applied to the inner aspect of the arm. However, they vary considerably in their position and size between individuals. Compression of these superficial veins is easily achieved by applying light pressure with a finger or thumb. This will emphasize the vein distal to the point of compression, and may, on larger veins, indicate the position of the valves.

SELF ASSESSMENT

Page 102

1. From which plexus is most of the upper limb innervated?

2. Identify the nerve roots contributing to this plexus.

3. Describe what is meant by a pre-fixed plexus.

4. Describe what is meant by a post-fixed plexus.

5. How many trunks are formed from the nerve roots?

6. Name the trunks.

7. From which cords are these trunks derived?

8. Explain why nerves are normally deep to other structures.

9. What appears as a bundle of tense cords in the supraclavicular fossa?

Page 103

10. Where can the radial nerve be palpated in the arm?

11. Name the two muscles which form the muscular groove through which the radial nerve enters the forearm.

12. Where can the superficial branches of the radial nerve be palpated in the forearm?

13. Which cutaneous area of the hand is supplied by these nerves?

14. Describe how the superficial nerves may be palpated on the lateral side of the forearm.

Page 104

15. Which artery lies between the nerves in the axilla?

16. Where can the ulnar nerve be palpated in the arm?

17. On which ligament does it lie as it passes over the elbow joint?

18. Describe how the ulnar nerve enters the forearm.

Please complete the labels below.

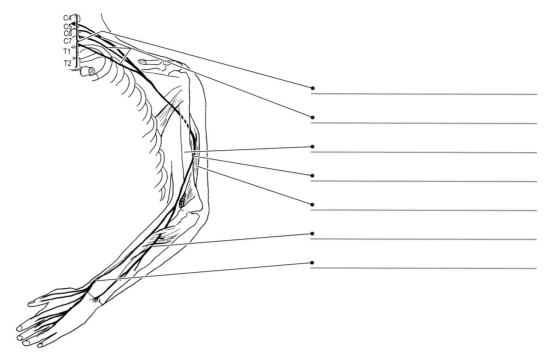

Fig. 2.22 (b) The radial nerve of the left upper limb (p, palpable)

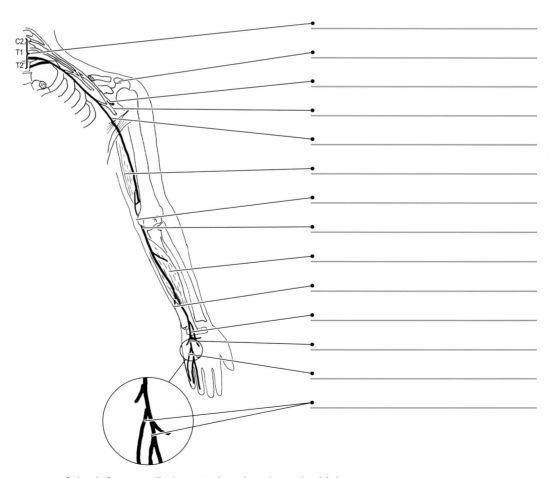

Fig. 2.23 (b) The ulnar nerve of the left upper limb, anterior view (p, palpable)

Page 105

19. How far above the wrist does the ulnar nerve become palpable?

20. Describe its relationship to the tendon of the flexor carpi ulnaris.

21. Does the nerve pass over or deep to the flexor retinaculum?

22. How many terminal branches does the ulnar nerve possess?

23. Where can these be palpated in the hand?

24. Describe how they can be palpated.

25. What is the cutaneous distribution of the ulnar nerve in the hand?

Page 106

26. From which roots does the median nerve derive its fibres?

27. Which artery does the median nerve accompany as it passes down the arm?

28. The median nerve crosses the elbow between which two muscles?

29. Describe how the median nerve passes into the forearm.

30. Under which muscle does it lie as it passes down the forearm?

31. Does it pass deep, or superficial to the flexor retinaculum as it crosses the wrist?

32. Between which two tendons does it lie as it crosses the wrist joint?

33. How can the median nerve can be palpated in the arm?

34. In which position can the median nerve be palpated in the forearm?

Page 107

35. Name the muscle group into which this nerve terminates.

36. Describe what is meant by the term 'carpal tunnel syndrome'.

37. By which methods may this condition be relieved? (fr)

Please complete the labels below.

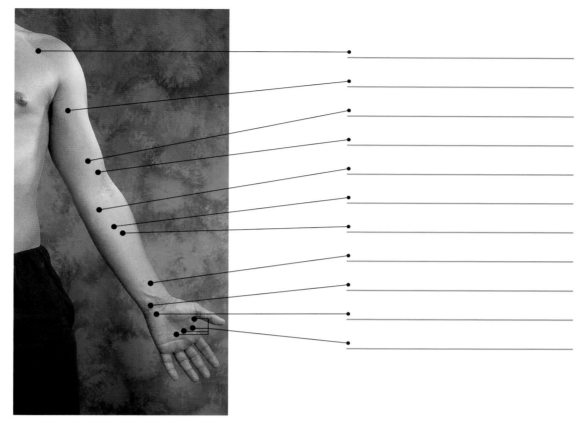

Fig. 2.23 (c) The median nerve of the left upper limb, anterior view (p, palpable)

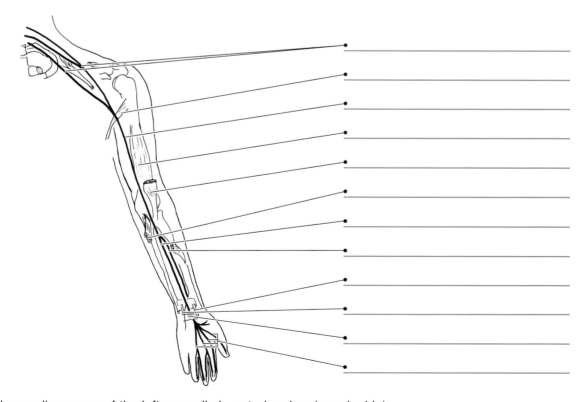

Fig. 2.23 (d) The median nerve of the left upper limb, anterior view (p, palpable)

SELF ASSESSMENT

Page 108

38. Describe the technique which should be employed when palpating arteries.

39. Explain the reasons why the thumb should never be used when palpating arteries.

40. Describe the factors on which palpation of the arteries are dependent.

41. By which root does the brachial artery of the left arm receive its blood from the heart?

42. By which root does the brachial artery of the right arm receive its blood from the heart?

43. Which artery can be palpated in the supraclavicular fossa?

44. Where can the brachial artery be palpated in the arm?

45. Explain the reasons why palpation of this artery may be tender.

46. Explain what is meant by the term 'auscultation' (fr).

Page 109

47. Name the two branches into which the brachial artery divides.

48. Where does this branching occur?

49. In which area can palpation of these two arteries be performed?

50. Where can the radial artery be palpated in the hand?

51. Name the arteries which can be palpated at the base of the fingers.

52. Which of the digits has an artery which is easiest to palpate?

53. How many arteries pass along each digit?

54. Name the artery which runs up the lateral side of the index finger.

Please complete the labels below.

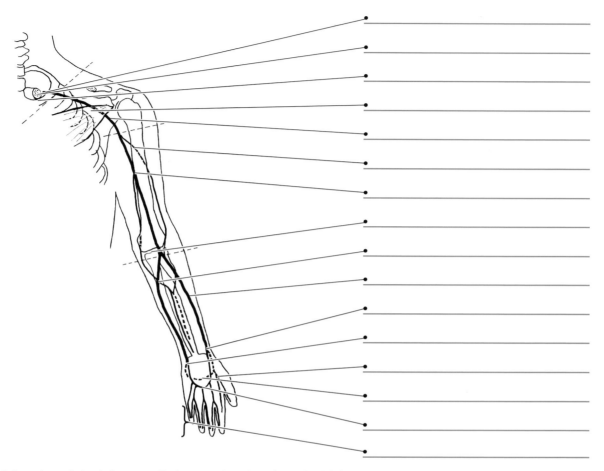

Fig. 2.24 (b) Arteries of the left upper limb, anterior view (p, palpable)

Page 110

55. There are two main groups of veins in the upper limb: where are they situated?

56. Do they communicate with each other?

57. Which venal structure facilitates venous return to the heart?

58. Are the deep veins palpable?

Page 111

59. In what groups of people are veins easier to see and palpate?

60. Name the group of veins on the posterior aspect of the hand.

61. How can these veins be made more prominent?

Page 112

62. Describe the course of the cephalic vein.

63. What is its relationship to the head of the radius?

64. Through which muscular groove does it pass?

65. Where does it pass into the axilla?

66. What structure does it pierce in order to enter the axilla?

67. Describe the route of the bacilic vein in the upper limb.

68. What does it pierce near the insertion of coracobrachialis?

69. By what name is it identified when it reaches the axilla?

Page 113

70. Which vein runs up the centre of the forearm anteriorly?

71. Where is the medial cubital vein?

72. Which two veins does it usually unite?

73. Describe how these veins may be made more visible and palpable.

Please complete the labels below.

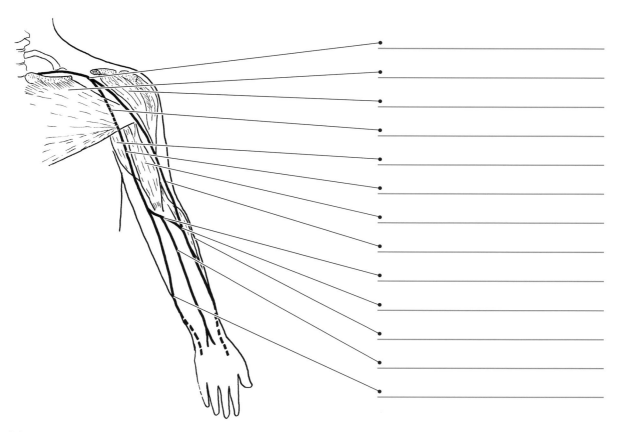

Fig. 2.25 (b) Veins of the left upper limb in relation to muscles, (anterior view)

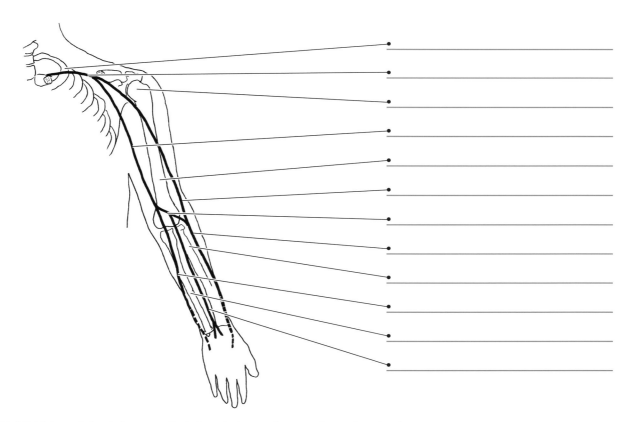

Fig. 2.25 (d) Veins of the left upper limb in relation to bones, (anterior view)

3

The lower limb

Contents

At the end of this chapter you should be able to:

A. Find, recognize the shape and position of the hip bone, femur, tibia, fibula, patella, tarsal, metatarsal bones and phalanges.
B. Recognize and palpate many of the bony features.
C. Name all the joints of the lower limb recognizing the bones which form them.
D. Palpate and trace the lines of the joints, where possible, indicating their bony landmarks and surface markings.
E. Describe or carry out any accessory movements possible noting the ranges in which they are most obvious.
F. Note the ranges of each of the joints and indicate the factors limiting the movement.
G. Give the class and type of each joint noting the axes of movement where possible.
H. Name and demonstrate the action of all the muscles palpable in the lower limb.
I. Draw the shape of the muscle on the surface and palpate its contraction.
J. Palpate tendons and attachments where possible.
K. Name all the main nerves supplying the lower limb.
L. Demonstrate the course and distribution of each of the main nerves of the lower limb.
M. Name the main arteries of the lower limb showing their course and giving their distribution.
N. Name the main veins of the lower limb noting their drainage areas and course.

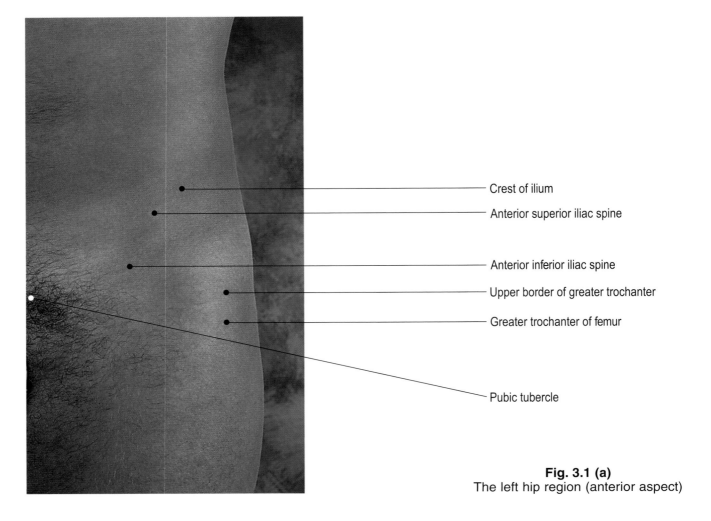

Crest of ilium

Anterior superior iliac spine

Anterior inferior iliac spine

Upper border of greater trochanter

Greater trochanter of femur

Pubic tubercle

Fig. 3.1 (a)
The left hip region (anterior aspect)

BONES

The hip region

The two hip bones on either side and the sacrum, posteriorly, form the pelvic girdle. In its lower section it forms a complete ring (the true pelvis) with the two pubic bones joined at the pubic symphysis, whereas in its upper part (the false pelvis) the two blades of the ilium leave a large space anteriorly.

The hip or innominate bone (*os innominatum* (L) = bone without a name), comprises the ilium, the ischium and the pubis. They are united at the acetabulum, a deep rounded hollow situated on the lateral side of the bone on the constricted area between two blades. That above and posterior is the ilium and that below and anterior is the pubis and ischium. The ilium has an inner and outer surface with a broad crest above a narrow border at the front and back and the upper part of the sciatic notch inferiorly just posterior to its junction with the ischium. The lower blade presents a large foramen, medial to which is the flattened bone of the body of the pubis with a superior ramus above and an inferior ramus passing downwards and laterally. The ischium is situated below the acetabulum and forms the lateral part of the

obturator foramen with its ramus passing from below upwards to join the inferior ramus of the pubis.

The upper end of the femur comprises the head, neck, greater and lesser trochanter. The head lies medially and articulates in the acetabulum, the greater trochanter lies at the lateral end of the neck and the lesser trochanter projects medially and backwards from just below the junction of the neck with the shaft.

Palpation

Owing to the size and thickness of muscle and fascia, this region is much more difficult to investigate than the shoulder. It is often covered by a layer of fat, particularly in women, and this also adds to the difficulty in observation and palpation.

Face the subject, who is standing, and place both hands around the waist. On sliding the hands downwards a bony ridge, the iliac [*ilium* (L) = the flank] crest, is encountered on either side. Each can be traced forwards to end in a well-defined projection, the anterior superior iliac spines (ASIS)

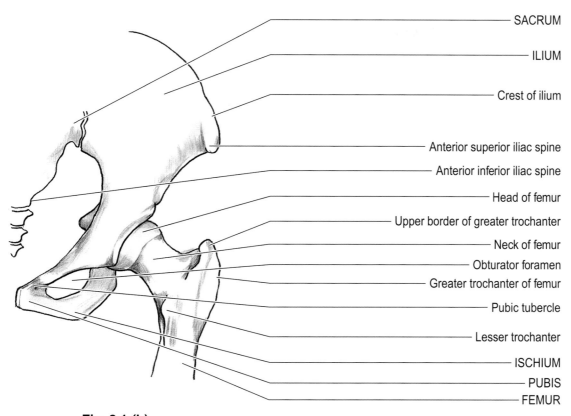

SACRUM

ILIUM

Crest of ilium

Anterior superior iliac spine

Anterior inferior iliac spine

Head of femur

Upper border of greater trochanter

Neck of femur

Obturator foramen

Greater trochanter of femur

Pubic tubercle

Lesser trochanter

ISCHIUM

PUBIS

FEMUR

Fig. 3.1 (b)
Bones of the left hip region (anterior
aspect)

(Fig. 3.1). In lean subjects the iliac crest is easily palpated from the ASIS to the posterior superior iliac spine (PSIS). In its anterior two-thirds it is convex laterally, broad and rounded, with inner and outer lips. Five to seven centimetres posterior to the ASIS, on its lateral lip, the tubercle of the crest is easily palpable, giving attachment to the upper end of the iliotibial tract. In its posterior third the iliac crest is concave laterally, less well defined and a little sharper on its superior border. The ASISs are set approximately 30 cm apart, a little more in the female, the abdomen usually protruding forwards between the two. From the ASIS, the sharp concave anterior border of the ilium can be traced downwards to another, less well-defined anterior projection, the anterior inferior iliac spine (AIIS), which lies approximately 2 cm above the rim of the acetablum (Fig. 3.1).

Now place the palm of your hand on the lower abdomen, moving it gently downwards; another ridge of bone can be palpated approximately 4 cm above the genitalia (Fig. 3.1). This is the anterior brim of the true pelvis. This ridge is depressed centrally where the two pubic bones join (the pubic [*pubes* (L) = the growth of hair in the region in adulthood] symphysis) and is marked superiorly on either side by the pubic tubercles. These are both palpable, approximately 1 cm on either side of the midline on the upper border of the pubis. This area is quite tender on palpation and is frequently covered with a fatty pad of tissue which may make positive identification of these tubercles difficult. Laterally, the superior ramus of the pubis can be palpated, gradually becoming hidden by muscle.

If the line of the pubic crest is extended laterally beyond the region of the hip joint to the lateral aspect of the upper thigh, a hard, bony prominence can be palpated; this is the greater trochanter of the femur (Fig. 3.1). It lies approximately 10 cm below the most lateral aspect of the iliac crest. The trochanters are quadrilateral in shape and, although surrounded by muscle, are easy to identify, being the most lateral bony part of the hip region. This tends to be the level around which the measurement of the hip circumference is erroneously taken.

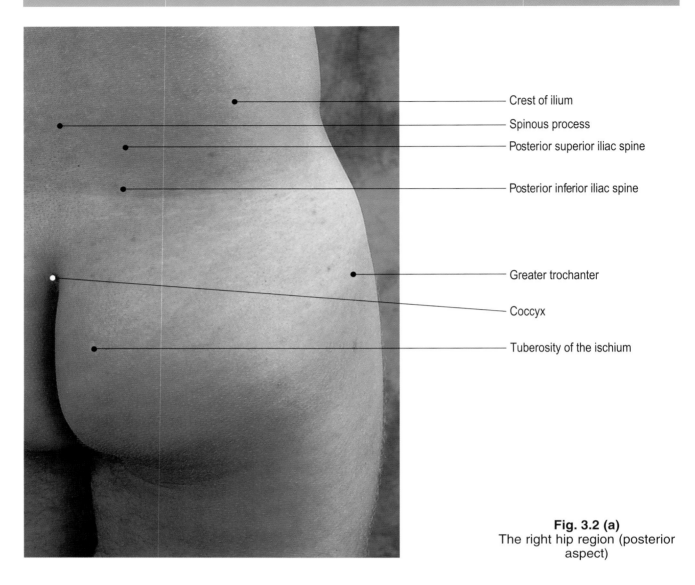

Crest of ilium
Spinous process
Posterior superior iliac spine

Posterior inferior iliac spine

Greater trochanter

Coccyx

Tuberosity of the ischium

Fig. 3.2 (a)
The right hip region (posterior aspect)

From the back, the ease of palpation depends to a large extent on the build of the subject. The region is often covered with a thick layer of fat, particularly in women, rendering precise identification of bony points extremely difficult.

Returning to the iliac crest, it can be traced backwards and medially until the PSIS is reached (Fig. 3.2). This is, however, less easy to identify than the ASIS. In women, it is often located in a small dimple characteristic of this region. From the PSIS the posterior border passes downwards and slightly medially, being concave posteriorly, to terminate approximately 2.5 cm below at the posterior inferior iliac spine (PIIS). From here the posterior border passes forwards, forming the upper boundary of the greater sciatic notch. The notch itself is difficult to identify, except in lean subjects.

The lower lateral border of the sacrum [*sacer* (L) = sacred; this is believed to be due to it being the only bone to survive a sacrifice] (S4,5) forms the medial component of the sciatic notch. It can easily be identified running downwards and medially to the cleft between the buttocks and terminating at the coccyx, which is often tucked forwards towards the anal canal. The upper part of the sacrum is held between the two ilia posteriorly, its upper border being on a line 2 cm above the level of the PSIS. If you run your hand down the centre of the sacrum posteriorly, a series of up to five tubercles, gradually diminishing in size, can be felt. These lie in line with the spines of the lumbar vertebrae and are termed spinous processes (Fig. 3.2). On either side of these spines, smaller tubercles can be palpated, in line with the articular processes of the vertebrae above. These are therefore known as the articular tubercles. This area is often covered with a fatty pad of tissue which may make positive identification of these tubercles difficult.

The ischial [*ischion* (Gk) = the socket in which the thigh bone turns] tuberosity is palpable in the standing or prone lying position, being anterolateral to the lateral border of the sacrum and posteromedial to the greater trochanter of the femur (Fig. 3.2). It is much easier, however, to identify these tuberosities if the subject either sits on your hands or is in the prone kneeling position. When sitting, large rounded processes can be felt

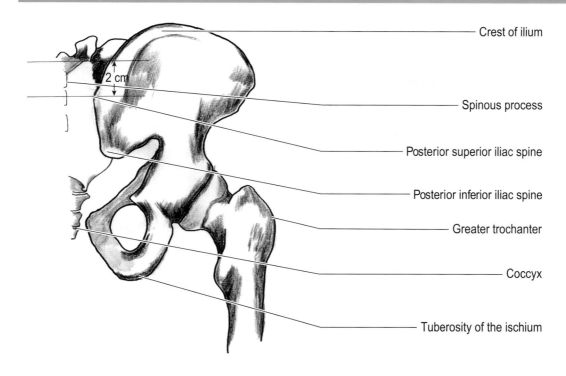

Crest of ilium

2 cm

Spinous process

Posterior superior iliac spine

Posterior inferior iliac spine

Greater trochanter

Coccyx

Tuberosity of the ischium

Fig. 3.2 (b)
Bones of the right hip
region (posterior aspect)

carrying most of the weight of the trunk to the supporting surface. If the subject is asked to move gently from side to side, the transference of weight from one tuberosity to the other can be observed. In sustained sitting on a hard surface, such as a wooden pew, these tuberosities become very tender and uncomfortable. The pressure is increased if the subject sits upright, preventing his or her sacrum sliding forward to take some of the weight. The lower area of the tuberosities are covered partially by a bursa medially, and the tendinous attachment of the adductor magnus laterally. The bursa may become inflamed after long periods of sitting upright, causing acute pain over the area (bursitis).

Palpation on movement

Once the position and shape of the pelvis has been established by palpation it is useful to know how its position may change during movements. One can normally consider the bony pelvis, i.e. the two hip bones and the sacrum, as one unit which moves as a whole.

Stand on the right side of the standing model and place your right hand on the upper anterior part of the ilium, place your left hand on the sacrum. If the model now drops the lower abdomen forwards by arching the lumbar spine the pelvis will be observed tilting forwards. If the model now pulls in the lower abdomen and flattens the lumbar spine the pelvis will be observed tilting backwards. Both movements occur around a frontal axis running through the heads of both femora.

Now stand facing the model, who is standing on one leg (the right). Place one hand on the crest of both ilia. The model can now draw up the left side of the pelvis by using the left trunk side flexors of the same side and the hip abductors of the standing leg. If these muscles are relaxed the pelvis will drop on the left side. This lateral tilting of the pelvis occurs around a sagittal axis through the right hip joint. Repeat the same procedure using the left leg as the standing leg.

Stand behind the standing model and place your fingers over the two greater trochanters. If the model flexes and extends the right hip rhythmically the trochanter will be observed rotating anticlockwise on flexion and clockwise on extension.

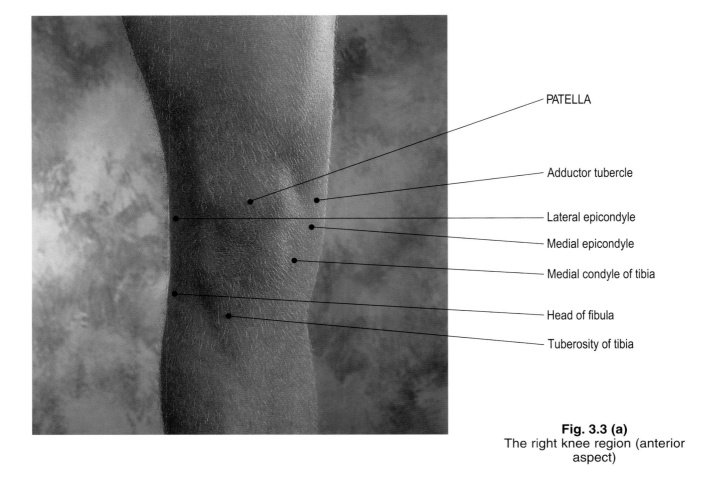

PATELLA

Adductor tubercle

Lateral epicondyle

Medial epicondyle

Medial condyle of tibia

Head of fibula

Tuberosity of tibia

Fig. 3.3 (a)
The right knee region (anterior aspect)

The knee region

There are four bones that can be palpated in this region: the femur, the tibia, the fibula and the patella.

The femur [*femur* (L) = a thigh] is the longest and strongest bone in the human body, taking the weight from the hip and transferring it through the knee joint to the tibia. This beautifully shaped bone narrows in its middle half, becoming more or less cylindrical with a very broad posterior border, the linea aspera. It broadens in its lower half, forming two large condyles at its lower end. These project backwards, being separated from each other by the intercondylar notch. The lateral condyle is stouter than the medial, which is slightly longer from front to back. Both condyles are smooth on their posterior, inferior and anterior surfaces, covered by hyaline cartilage in the living body. The smooth surfaces meet anteriorly at a triangular, patella, surface. The lateral surface of the lateral condyle is roughened and is marked just below its centre by a tubercle termed the lateral epicondyle. The medial condyle is also roughened on its medial side and marked just below its centre by a slightly larger tubercle termed the medial epicondyle. Each condyle has a sharp border above termed the medial and lateral supracondylar ridges, the medial presenting a tubercle at its lower end, the adductor tubercle.

The tibia [*tibia* (L) = a flute] is again a very strong stout bone carrying the body weight to the ankle joint and foot. It is broader above, having two large condyles, both flattened superiorly, being slightly depressed centrally. They are separated by the intercondylar eminence and a roughened area anteriorly and posteriorly. The shaft narrows as it descends, presenting a large tubercle anteriorly, the tibial tuberosity, just below the level of the knee joint. The sharp anterior border (shin) passes vertically down from this tubercle.

The patella [*patella* (L) = a small plate] is, as its name implies, a small flat bone situated on the front of the knee. It is triangular in shape with the apex downwards and has a roughened anterior surface and a smooth posterior surface divided into two articular facets with the roughened apex below.

The fibula [*fibula* (L) = a pin] is a long, thin bone situated lateral to the tibia, having complex surfaces and a border mainly produced by the muscles attaching to it. It is expanded above and below: the upper expansion, the head, articulates with the under surface of the lateral condyle of the tibia and takes no part in the knee joint. The lower expansion forms the lateral malleolus and takes part in the formation of the ankle joint.

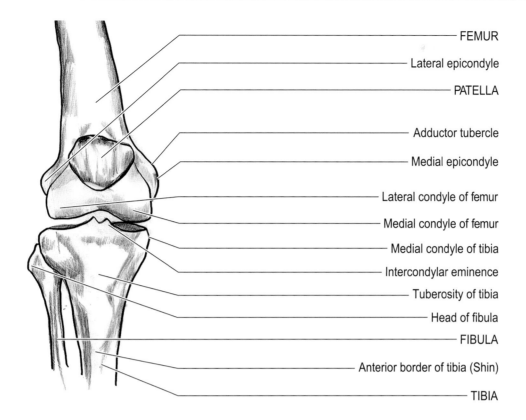

FEMUR
Lateral epicondyle
PATELLA
Adductor tubercle
Medial epicondyle
Lateral condyle of femur
Medial condyle of femur
Medial condyle of tibia
Intercondylar eminence
Tuberosity of tibia
Head of fibula
FIBULA
Anterior border of tibia (Shin)
TIBIA

Fig. 3.3 (b)
Bones of the right knee region
(anterior aspect)

Anterior aspect

Palpation

The obvious bony feature anteriorly is the patella. Place your fingers on its anterior surface and gently move them around, investigating its surfaces and borders. The patella is broader superiorly, narrowing to a rounded point below, where it is continuous with the ligamentum patellae. The borders are rounded, while the anterior surface, although appearing slippery due to the presence of the pre-patellar bursa, has rough vertical ridges in line with the fibres of the tendon of quadriceps femoris.

With the knee flexed to 90 degrees, the patella becomes more prominent, situated on the medial and lateral femoral condyles, each of which is clearly palpable either side. Each femoral condyle is convex forwards, and presents a strip either side of the patella. It is narrow superiorly, due to the breadth of the patella, but becomes broader below due to the comparative narrowness of the ligamentum patellae. These condylar surfaces pass posteriorly into the knee joint itself.

The medial and lateral tibial condyles are easily recognizable below the femoral condyles, with their flattened upper surfaces being marked by a sharp circumference separating them from the more vertical surfaces of the shaft.

Below and centrally the large tibial tuberosity is easily identified (Fig. 3.3); the lower part is smooth and slippery, due to the presence of the superficial infrapatellar bursa, while its upper part gives attachment to the ligamentum patellae. The tuberosity is particularly noticeable when the knee is extended. With the knee flexed to 90 degrees place your fingers in the small triangular fossae on either side of the ligamentum patellae. Here the upper surfaces of the tibial condyles can be felt below, the under surface of the femoral condyles above, while between your fingers lies the ligamentum patellae. Directly posteriorly is the cleft of the knee joint, with the medial and lateral menisci between. These are not always palpable, although the anterior edge of the medial meniscus can be observed bulging forwards on medial rotation of the tibia. The anterior edge of the lateral meniscus also becomes palpable, but to a lesser extent, on lateral tibial rotation.

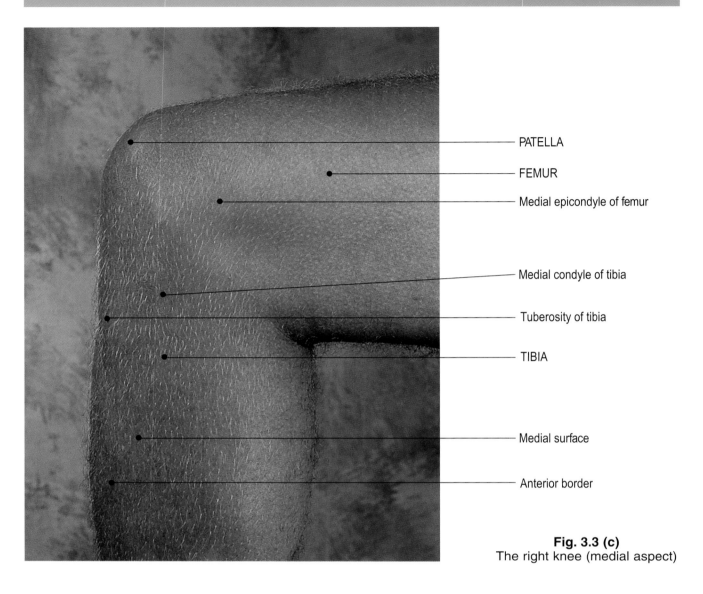

PATELLA

FEMUR

Medial epicondyle of femur

Medial condyle of tibia

Tuberosity of tibia

TIBIA

Medial surface

Anterior border

Fig. 3.3 (c)
The right knee (medial aspect)

Medial aspect

On the medial side of this region the large, elongated medial condyle of the femur sits on top of the flattened plateau of the medial tibial condyle. The centre of the medial surface of the femoral condyle is marked by a tubercle termed the medial epicondyle. Vertically above this is the medial supracondylar line marked at its lower end by the adductor tubercle.

Below the femoral condyle the flattened medial tibial condyle continues downwards as the medial surface of the tibial shaft, bounded in front by its anterior border marked at its upper end by the tibial tuberosity.

Palpation

The medial surface of the femoral condyle is readily palpable, with the epicondyle projecting from its mid point (Fig. 3.3). Approximately 2 cm proximal to the medial epicondyle the adductor tubercle is just palpable, being hidden to a certain extent by the attachment of the tendinous part of the adductor magnus. This tubercle represents the most distal part of the medial supracondylar ridge, little of which can be palpated.

The medial tibial condyle (Fig. 3.3c, d) is also easily palpable below the femoral condyle. It appears to be larger than the lateral, and can be traced around the medial side, becoming continuous

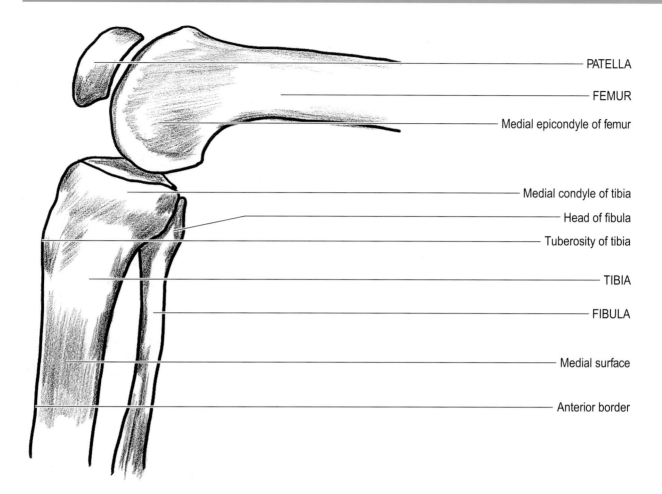

PATELLA

FEMUR

Medial epicondyle of femur

Medial condyle of tibia

Head of fibula

Tuberosity of tibia

TIBIA

FIBULA

Medial surface

Anterior border

Fig. 3.3 (d)
Bones of the right knee (medial aspect)

below with the medial surface of the shaft of the tibia and its anterior border (the shin), the whole of which is subcutaneous and palpable as far as the medial malleolus.

Palpation on movement

With the model standing and the knee extended place the fingers of one hand on the medial condyle of the femur and the fingers of the other hand on the medial border of the patella. If the model now flexes the knee the patella will be observed sliding downwards and backwards on

the femoral condyle until it lies inferiorly. Return the knee to the extended position. Now move the fingers from the patella and place them on the upper part of the medial surface of the medial condyle of the tibia, close to the joint line. If the knee is flexed again the tibial condyle will be observed moving backwards and upwards on to the posterior aspect of the femoral condyle. As in the case of the lateral condyles, in this position the anterior part of the tibial condyle appears to part from the femoral condyle due to the smaller articular surface at the posterior part of the femoral condyle.

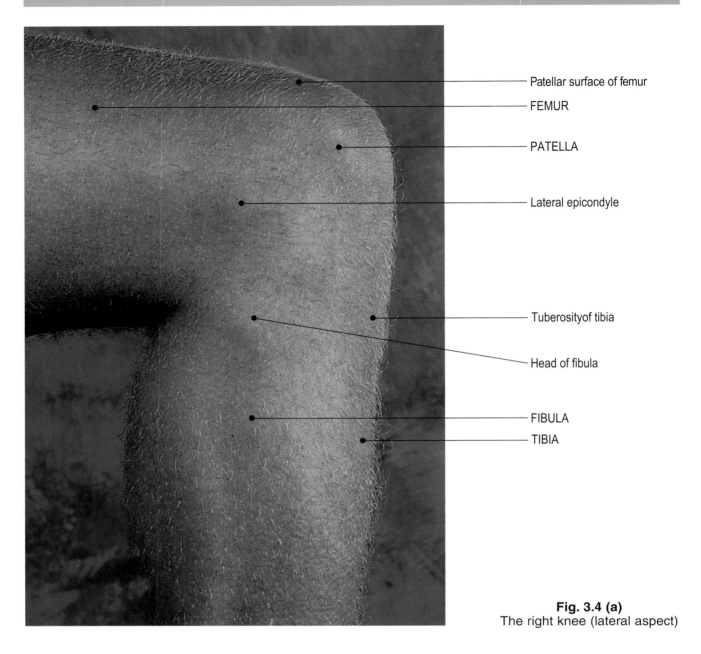

Patellar surface of femur

FEMUR

PATELLA

Lateral epicondyle

Tuberosityof tibia

Head of fibula

FIBULA
TIBIA

Fig. 3.4 (a)
The right knee (lateral aspect)

Lateral aspect

On the lateral side of this region the stout lateral condyle of the femur sits on top of the plateau of the lateral condyle of the tibia. Posteriorly, the two condyles are close together; however anteriorly, they diverge into a small hollow which is bounded at the front by the lower section of the patella and the ligamentum patellae. The head of the fibula lies below and posterior to the knee joint.

Palpation

With the model standing, the flat lateral surface of the lateral femoral condyle can readily be palpated, lying posterior to the lateral border of the

patella. It is marked by a tubercle at its centre (the lateral epicondyle). Running your fingers upwards from this lateral epicondyle the lateral supra-condylar ridge may be just palpable running verti-cally upwards. This is difficult to palpate as the iliotibial tract tends to follow the same line.

Approximately 2 cm below the lateral epicondyle the lower border of the lateral femoral condyle and the upper border of the lateral tibial condyle can be palpated running horizontally and diverging anteriorly. Finally, approximately 1 cm below this rim, the head of the fibula can be palpated, with its styloid process projecting upwards, and the narrower neck just below (Fig. 3.4). The remainder

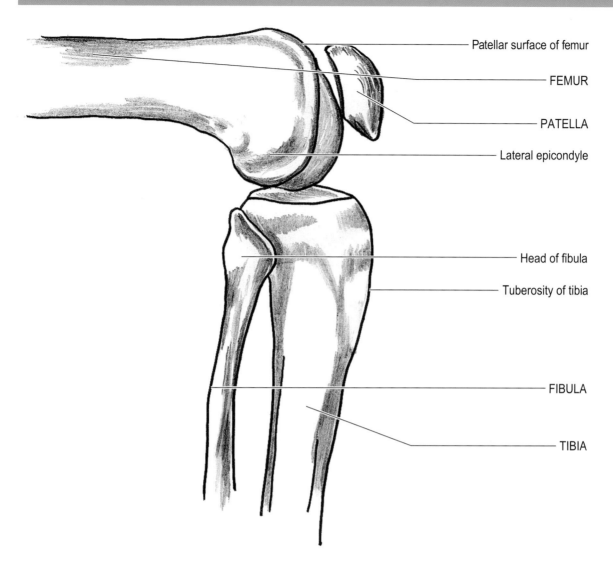

Patellar surface of femur

FEMUR

PATELLA

Lateral epicondyle

Head of fibula

Tuberosity of tibia

FIBULA

TIBIA

Fig. 3.4 (b)
Bones of the right knee (lateral
aspect)

of the upper end of the shaft of the fibula is sur-rounded by muscles and is therefore not palpable. The head can easily be located by running the palm of the hand up the lateral aspect of the leg.

Palpation on movement

With the model's knee fully extended, place your fingers of one hand on the lateral side of the patella and the fingers of the other hand on the lateral surface of the femoral condyle. If the model now flexes the knee the patella will be observed sliding downwards and backwards under the condyle, finally ending up inferiorly. Return the knee back to the extended position. Now remove the fingers from the patella and place them on the lateral condyle of the tibia close to the knee joint. If the model flexes the knee again the tibia will be observed gliding backwards and upwards on to the posterior surface of the femoral condyles. At this position the anterior part of the tibial condyle appears to part from the femoral condyle. This is due to the posterior surface of the femoral condyle being smaller than that of the tibia.

The head of the fibula moves with the tibia.

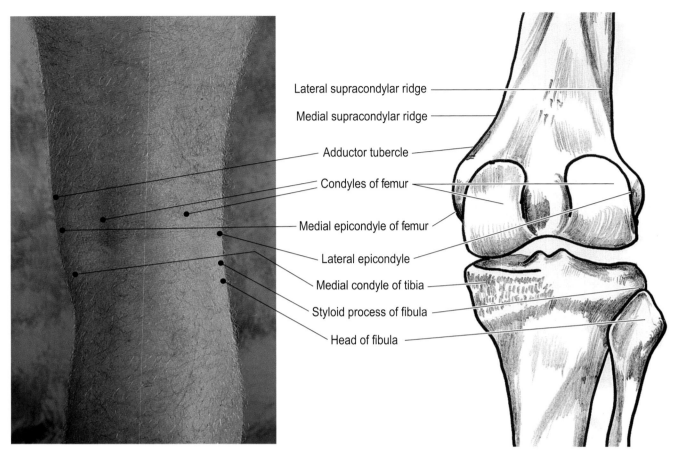

Lateral supracondylar ridge

Medial supracondylar ridge

Adductor tubercle

Condyles of femur

Medial epicondyle of femur

Lateral epicondyle

Medial condyle of tibia

Styloid process of fibula

Head of fibula

Fig. 3.4 (c), (d)
The right knee region (posterior aspect)

Posterior aspect

Virtually no bony features can be palpated on the posterior aspect of the knee, either when it is flexed or extended. The posterior aspect of the sides of each **femoral condyle** and the medial surfaces of the tibia soon become hidden by the fascia and muscles at the back of the knee. The **head of the fibula** (Fig. 3.4), however, can easily be palpated on the lateral side of the popliteal fossa, with the tendon of biceps femoris attaching to its upper section. Palpation from this aspect must be approached with care, as the common peroneal nerve passes down the back of the head of the fibula *en route* to its passage around the lateral side of the neck.

When the knee is extended and the quadriceps femoris is relaxed, the patella can easily be moved from side to side, producing a knocking effect as it crosses either side of the grooved patellar surface of the femur. This manoeuvre, an accessory movement, exposes a strip of the patellar surface of the femur, on the side away from the direction of the movement. If held to one side, the articular surface of the patella on that side can also be palpated for approximately 1 cm on its posterior surface.

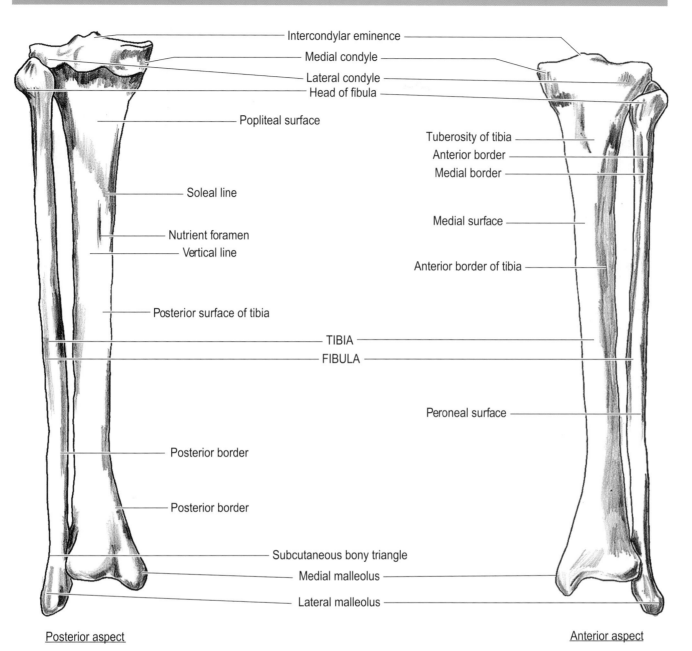

Intercondylar eminence

Medial condyle

Lateral condyle

Head of fibula

Popliteal surface

Tuberosity of tibia

Anterior border

Medial border

Medial surface

Anterior border of tibia

Soleal line

Nutrient foramen

Vertical line

Posterior surface of tibia

TIBIA

FIBULA

Peroneal surface

Posterior border

Posterior border

Subcutaneous bony triangle

Medial malleolus

Lateral malleolus

Posterior aspect

Anterior aspect

Fig. 3.4 (e), (f)
The tibia and fibula

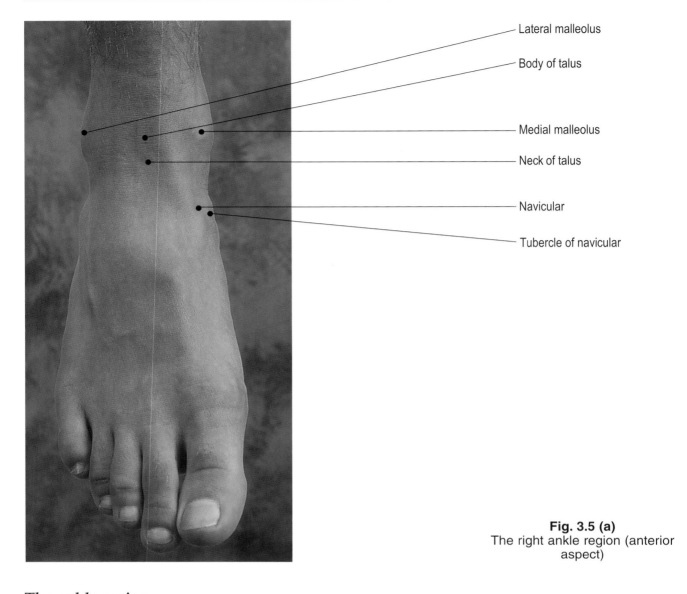

Lateral malleolus

Body of talus

Medial malleolus

Neck of talus

Navicular

Tubercle of navicular

Fig. 3.5 (a)
The right ankle region (anterior aspect)

The ankle region

There are four bones taking part in the formation of this area: the lower ends of the tibia and fibula, the talus and the calcaneus.

The lower end of the tibia

From its narrowest cross-section, two-thirds of the way down the shaft, the bone expands to form part of the mortice for the formation of the ankle joint. Its medial side presents a large projection downwards, termed the medial malleolus. On its lateral side there is an elongated triangular area for the attachment of an extremely strong interosseous ligament which binds the two bones together. Its under surface and the lateral side of the malleolus are smooth for articulation with the talus in the ankle joint.

The lower end of the fibula

The slender shaft of the fibula expands below to form the pointed lateral malleolus, which forms

the lateral section of the mortice of the ankle joint. It is flattened from side to side, having a smooth articular surface on its medial side and a roughened surface on its lateral, subcutaneous side.

The talus

This bone is formed of a body, a neck and a head. The body is narrower at the back and wider anteriorly. It is pulley-shaped superiorly and slightly concave inferiorly. It has smooth, articular surfaces on its superior, inferior, lateral and the upper part of its medial surfaces.

The neck passes forwards and medially to expand into the head, which articulates with the posterior surface of the navicular.

The calcaneus (see page 138)

At the ankle the muscles of the leg have become tendinous and thus the bones are easier to palpate and identify between and deep to the tendons and retinacula.

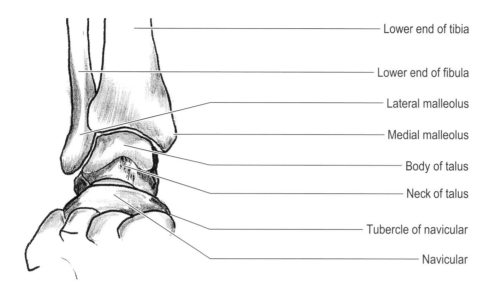

- Lower end of tibia
- Lower end of fibula
- Lateral malleolus
- Medial malleolus
- Body of talus
- Neck of talus
- Tubercle of navicular
- Navicular

Fig. 3.5 (b)
Bones of the right ankle region
(anterior aspect)

Palpation

Anterior aspect. Placing the hands on the subcutaneous medial surface of the tibia, trace down to the medial malleolus. The anterior border of the tibia (shin) appears to form the anterior part of the malleolus, which is clearly defined (Fig. 3.5a,b). It has an anterior border and tip which can be palpated, and a posterior border which is partially hidden by tendons and the flexor retinaculum. The anterior border of the malleolus [*malleolus* (L) = a small hammer] continues upwards and laterally under the extensor tendons and extensor retinacula, marking the line of the ankle joint.

On the lateral side of the ankle the lateral malleolus of the fibula is the most outstanding feature (Figs 3.4e, f, 3.5). From its tip, which lies at a lower level than that of the medial malleolus, both the anterior and posterior borders can be traced upwards, encompassing the large prominence of the malleolus. Just above the level of the ankle joint, at approximately 2.5 cm, the fibula narrows to a triangular subcutaneous lateral surface. The shaft can be traced upwards for approximately 15 cm, where it becomes hidden by muscle, the peroneus tertius anteriorly and the peroneus brevis and tendon of peroneus longus posteriorly.

With your right hand over the front of the ankle region, place your index finger on the lateral, and your thumb on the medial, malleolus of the subject's left ankle. Draw your finger and thumb forward into a small hollow on either side. Between your thumb and finger you will feel the head of the talus. Immediately anterior you can palpate the narrow gap of the talonavicular joint and posterior part of the navicular with its prominent **tubercle**, medially. If the foot is plantar flexed, the neck of the talus [*talus* (L) = the ankle bone] can also be palpated, and deep beneath the tip of your index finger, just lateral to the head of the talus, you will feel the anterior section of the upper surface of the calcaneus [*calx* (L) = a heel] and the origin of extensor digitorum brevis.

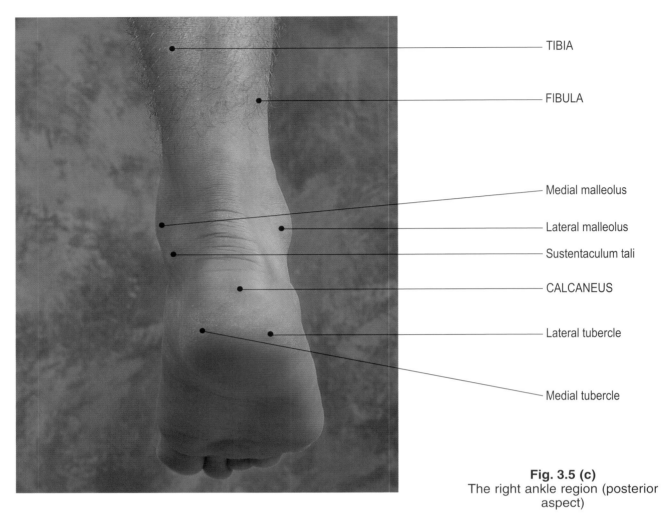

TIBIA

FIBULA

Medial malleolus

Lateral malleolus

Sustentaculum tali

CALCANEUS

Lateral tubercle

Medial tubercle

Fig. 3.5 (c)
The right ankle region (posterior aspect)

Posterior aspect. From the posterior aspect very little of the talus can be seen as the body has narrowed down to just two tubercles and a groove running downwards and medially. The mortice of the ankle joint (see page 136) is formed by the two malleoli and the inferior border of the tibia. Both the malleoli are marked posteriorly by a fossa for the attachment of ligaments.

The calcaneus

This is the largest of the tarsal bones and is situated below the talus and behind the navicular and cuboid. It is oblong in shape, projecting forwards and backwards beyond the talus. The backward projection forms the heel. It has six surfaces: an anterior, which is smooth, a superior, marked by a smooth articular surface centrally, and a medial, which is fairly smooth and converted into a hollow by the projection medially from its upper section by the sustentaculum tali. The lateral surface is roughened, presenting two tubercles, and the posterior surface is rounded and roughened across its centre for the attachment of the tendo-calcaneus. Its inferior surface is slightly concave downwards and is roughened for the attachment of muscles and fascia. It presents three broad, rounded tubercles. The medial and lateral lie

posterior, almost on the junction with the posterior surface, and the anterior lies central, approximately 1 cm from its anterior border.

Palpation

Place your hands at the tip of the medial malleolus. Move your fingers 1 cm down from this tip and you will feel the horizontal ridge of the sustentaculum tali. It runs for approximately 2–3 cm and is clearer anteriorly and posteriorly. If the foot is everted the sustentaculum tali becomes more prominent. At the anterior end of this ridge there is a small gap before encountering the tubercle of the navicular. This gap is spanned by the 'spring ligament'.

Because the tendocalcaneus lies almost 2 cm clear of the ankle joint, few bony features can be identified posteriorly. On close examination of the posterior borders of the lateral and medial malleoli, a small depression can be palpated, the malleolar fossa. Tracing superiorly, the posterior border of the lateral malleolus forms the posterior border of the triangular area referred to above. The posterior surface of the medial malleolus is continuous with the posterior border of the medial surface of the tibia (Fig. 3.5c, d).

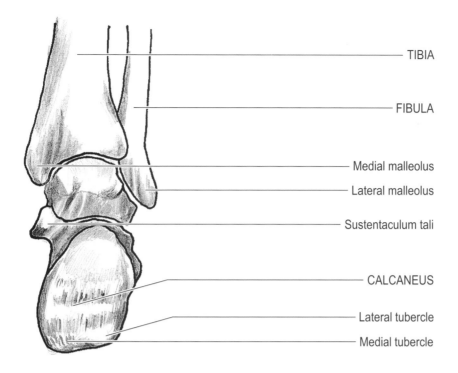

TIBIA

FIBULA

Medial malleolus

Lateral malleolus

Sustentaculum tali

CALCANEUS

Lateral tubercle

Medial tubercle

Fig. 3.5 (d)
Bones of the right ankle region
(posterior aspect)

Palpation on movement

Anterior. With the model lying, stand facing the lateral side of the model's right ankle region. With your left hand grip the two malleoli with your fingers on the medial and your thumb on the lateral. With your right hand grip the anterior part of the body and neck of the talus with your fingers in the hollow just anterior to the medial malleolus and your thumb in the hollow just anterior to the lateral malleolus. Both sets of fingers and both sets of thumbs should be close to each other.

Starting from the fully plantarflexed position, if the model now dorsiflexes the foot you will feel the anterior part of the body disappearing into the gap between the two malleoli. In fact, the fingers of your right hand will now be gripping the neck and head of the talus. At this point the ankle is in its close-packed position and no side-to-side movement is possible. When the model fully plantarflexes from the dorsiflexed position the head and neck of the talus will move forwards and downwards and the anterior section of the body will reappear from within the mortice. At this point the head and neck of the talus can be rocked from side to side. This is an accessory movement.

Medial. With the ankle returned to the mid position, adopt the same position with your hands but now move the fingers of your right hand to just below the tip of the medial malleolus. Here you will find the horizontal rim of the sustentaculum tali. If the model now rhythmically plantar- and dorsiflexes the ankle, you will feel the sustentaculum tali moving forwards and backwards, describing a shallow arc around the medial malleolus.

Lateral. Similarly, if the left hand remains in its original position and your right thumb is placed on the two tubercles below the lateral malleolus, movement forwards and backwards around the malleolus can be observed when plantar- and dorsiflexion is performed.

Posterior. With the model and yourself in the same position, keep your left hand gripping the two malleoli, place your right hand under the heel with the fingers resting on the posterior aspect of the calcaneus either side of the tendocalcaneus. As the model moves into dorsi- and plantarflexion, the calcaneus will be observed moving forwards and backwards away and towards the posterior part of the tibia. It is worth noting that when it passes downwards it is nearly impossible to move from side to side. This is due to the anterior part of the talus moving into the mortice of the ankle joint.

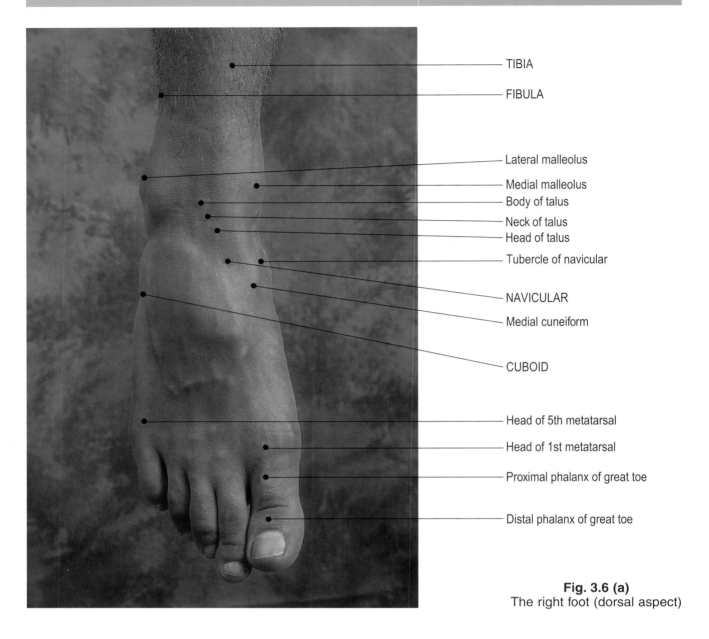

TIBIA

FIBULA

Lateral malleolus

Medial malleolus

Body of talus

Neck of talus

Head of talus

Tubercle of navicular

NAVICULAR

Medial cuneiform

CUBOID

Head of 5th metatarsal

Head of 1st metatarsal

Proximal phalanx of great toe

Distal phalanx of great toe

Fig. 3.6 (a)
The right foot (dorsal aspect)

The foot

There are three main groups of bones forming the skeleton of the foot. Posteriorly is the tarsus, comprising large irregular bones, while anteriorly are the phalanges, miniature long bones forming the toes. Between these two groups are the metatarsals, which are also miniature long bones, linking them together (Fig. 3.6).

The calcaneus forms the heel and is the largest and most posterior of the group of tarsal bones. In front and to the lateral side is the cuboid [*kubgides* (Gk) = cube shape]. Sitting on the middle section of the upper surface of the calcaneus is the body of the talus, with its neck and head passing forwards and medially, superomedially to the cuboid. The navicular lies in front of the head of the talus with the three cuneiform [*cuneus* (L) = a wedge] bones interposed between the anterior surface of the navicular and the three medial metatarsal bones.

The two lateral metatarsals lie anterior to the cuboid.

Dorsal aspect

From the medial and lateral malleoli run your index finger and thumb forwards, as before, until the head of the talus is gripped between them. The upper part of the talocalcaneonavicular joint can be palpated. The roughened dorsal surface of the navicular can be traced medially to its large tuberosity which projects downwards and medially, being approximately 2.5 cm downwards and forwards from the tip of the medial malleolus (Figs 3.5a, b, and 3.6). Immediately distal to the navicular the medial cuneiform can also be palpated, projecting downwards. The dorsal surfaces of the middle and lateral cuneiforms can be identified on the dorsum of the foot, lying lateral to

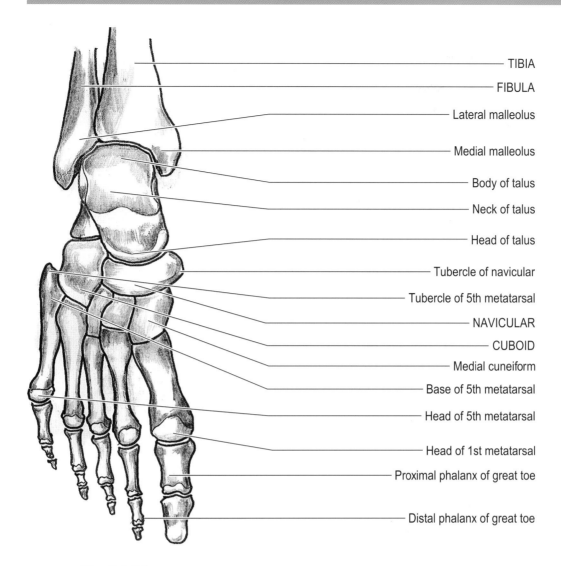

TIBIA

FIBULA

Lateral malleolus

Medial malleolus

Body of talus

Neck of talus

Head of talus

Tubercle of navicular

Tubercle of 5th metatarsal

NAVICULAR

CUBOID

Medial cuneiform

Base of 5th metatarsal

Head of 5th metatarsal

Head of 1st metatarsal

Proximal phalanx of great toe

Distal phalanx of great toe

Fig. 3.6 (b)
Bones of the right foot (dorsal
aspect)

the medial cuneiform. The base, shaft and head of the first metatarsal are clearly identifiable, being much stouter than those of the other four. In some individuals the head projects medially, carrying the base of the toe with it. This causes inflammation of the bursa on its medial side, often accompanied by pain and swelling. Such medial deviation of the metatarsal head commonly progresses to a condition termed 'hallux valgus'.

Carefully running the pads of your fingers over the dorsum of the foot, the base, shaft and head of each of the remaining metatarsals can be palpated. The base of the second metatarsal is traced further proximally than the others to the middle cuneiform, the third to the lateral cuneiform and the fourth and fifth to the cuboid (Fig. 3.6). The base of the fifth metatarsal is more expanded than

the rest and has, projecting proximally, a tubercle or styloid process on its lateral side. The base is easily located by tracing backwards along the shaft of the fifth metatarsal. The large lateral projection is elongated proximally and overlies the lateral side of the cuboid.

The lateral side of the calcaneus is marked by the peroneal tubercle 1 cm below and just anterior to the tip of the lateral malleolus. This tubercle is elongated downwards and forwards and if the foot is everted, two tendons appear to pull clear. The one above the tubercle is peroneus brevis, the one below is peroneus longus. This tubercle must not be confused with that of the calcaneofibular ligament which can be found with careful palpation just below and posterior to the tip of the lateral malleolus.

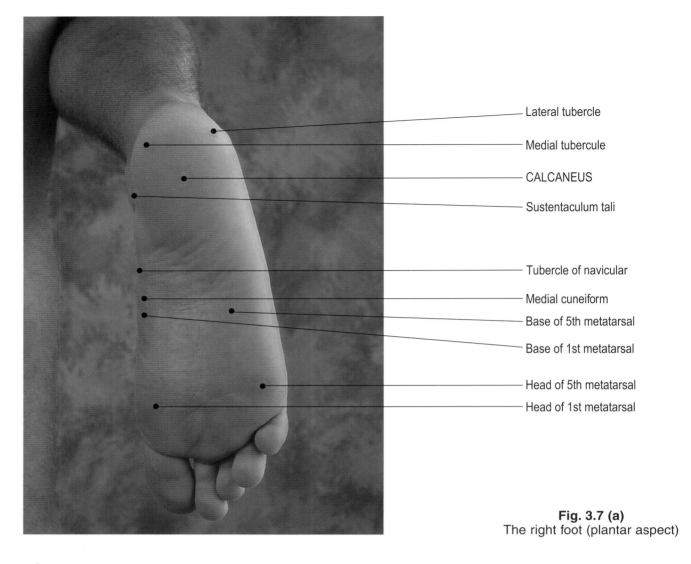

Lateral tubercle

Medial tubercule

CALCANEUS

Sustentaculum tali

Tubercle of navicular

Medial cuneiform

Base of 5th metatarsal

Base of 1st metatarsal

Head of 5th metatarsal

Head of 1st metatarsal

Fig. 3.7 (a)
The right foot (plantar aspect)

Plantar aspect

As in the palm of the hand, very few bony points are palpable in this region due to the presence of overlying muscles, as well as a dense and thick layer of plantar fascia, termed the 'plantar aponeurosis'.

The heel is the most posterior and inferior aspect of the calcaneus, on either side of which are two large broad tubercles (medial and lateral) which give attachment to the more superficial of the plantar muscles. On the posterior aspect of the heel there is often a horizontal raised area to which the tendocalcaneus attaches. The tendon and its attachment are usually quite clear (see Fig. 3.22b). Below this the posterior surface of the calcaneus is covered with a pad of tough fibrous tissue and fat.

Below and in front of the tip of the lateral malleolus, the calcaneus is marked by an elongated tubercle (the peroneal tubercle), which has the tendons of peroneus brevis above and peroneus longus below.

Immediately below the tip of the medial malleolus, a horizontal ridge can be felt – the sustentaculum tali – which is slightly hidden by the tendon of flexor digitorum longus. The inferior surface of

the navicular tuberosity can be palpated on the medial side of the foot 3 cm anteroinferior to the tip of the medial malleolus. On the lateral side of the foot, the base of the fifth metatarsal and its tubercle are covered by the plantar fascia and muscles. The heads of the metatarsals are relatively easy to find (Fig. 3.7). Those of the first and fifth metatarsals lie deep to a pad of harder skin at the broadest part of the foot on the medial and lateral side, respectively. The heads of the second, third and fourth metatarsals are less easy to palpate, lying on a well-formed anterior metatarsal arch; normally they can be palpated with little difficulty when the arch is flat. If the toe is grasped between the finger and thumb of one hand and passively extended, the metatarsal head can readily be felt on the plantar surface proximal to the base of the toe. If, however, the toe is flexed at the metatarsophalangeal joint, the metatarsal head appears on the dorsum of the foot, as the knuckles would in the hand.

The base of the proximal phalanx can be identified just beyond the corresponding metatarsal head. The heads of the proximal phalanges,

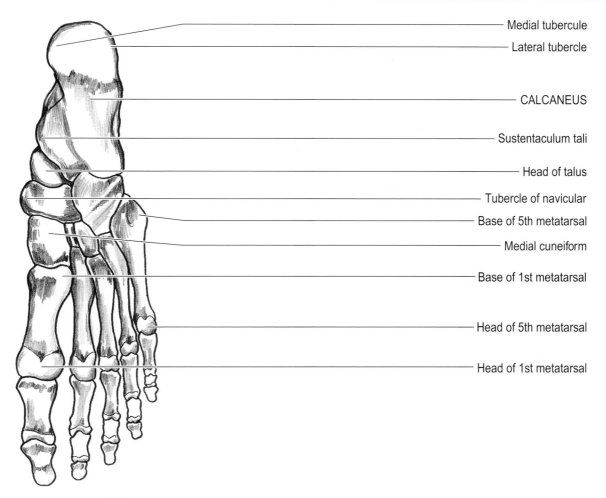

Medial tubercule

Lateral tubercle

CALCANEUS

Sustentaculum tali

Head of talus

Tubercle of navicular

Base of 5th metatarsal

Medial cuneiform

Base of 1st metatarsal

Head of 5th metatarsal

Head of 1st metatarsal

Fig. 3.7 (b)
Bones of the right foot (plantar
aspect)

particularly those of the second, third and fourth, are often flexed and project forwards on their dorsum, being covered by hard skin and a bursa which often swells and becomes inflamed and may lead, if not corrected, to a condition known as 'hammer toes'. If the toes are extended at the proximal interphalangeal joint, the small bicondylar head can be identified (Fig. 3.7).

Palpation on movement

Take up the same position and the same hand holds as for palpation on movement, anterior aspect (page 139). If the model now plantarflexes the ankle and then moves the foot into adduction and abduction, the head of the talus can be observed moving from side to side. Remember, this will not occur in dorsiflexion due to the close-packed nature of the ankle joint.

Now move your hands down so that the head of the talus is gripped in the left hand and the right fingers come into contact with the tubercle of the navicular and the thumb grips around the base of the fifth metatarsal. As the model everts the foot, the tubercle will descend and the metatarsal rises. As the model inverts the foot, the tubercle will rise and the metatarsal will descend. The navicular is rotating around an axis running through the neck and head of the talus.

If the hands are now moved down to the base of the great toe and the left hand grips the first metatarsal just proximal to the head and the right hand grips the proximal phalanx, when the model extends the toe, the head becomes quite clear with the phalanx moving towards the dorsum of the head. When the toe is flexed, the phalanx can be palpated moving downwards around the head. This movement can be observed in all the metatarsophalangeal joints, but to a lesser extent.

A similar movement can be felt in the interphalangeal joints with the head of the phalanx becoming quite palpable when the toes are flexed.

SELF ASSESSMENT

Page 124

1. Which three bones form the pelvic girdle?

2. Describe what is meant by 'The true pelvis'.

3. Explain the term 'false pelvis'.

4. By what Latin name is the hip bone known?

5. List the three components of the hip bone.

6. Where are the three bones united?

7. What forms the upper boundary of the ilium?

8. What structures form the boundaries of the obturator foramen?

9. Which three bony processes form the upper end of the femur?

10. Explain why this area is difficult to palpate.

11. The lower boundary of the waist is limited by which bony landmarks?

Page 125

12. Where is the anterior superior iliac spine located?

13. What lies at the posterior end of the iliac crest?

14. Describe the shape of the iliac crest from above.

15. What lies 5 cm posterior to the ASIS on the lateral side of the crest of the ilium?

16. Which structure attaches to this process?

17. Approximately, how far apart are the two anterior superior iliac spines?

18. Name the bony process which lies approximately 2 cm below the anterior superior iliac spine just above the acetabulum.

19. Name the rim of bone palpable at the lower, central part of the abdomen and approximately 4 cm above the genitalia.

20. What can be palpated centrally on this rim?

Please complete the labels below.

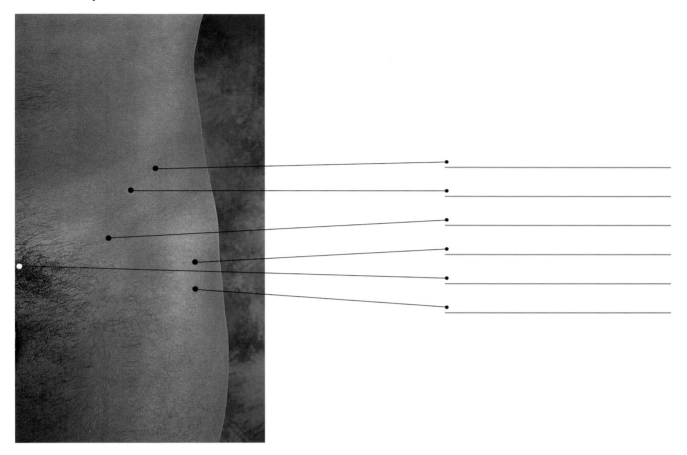

Fig. 3.1 (a) The left hip region (anterior aspect)

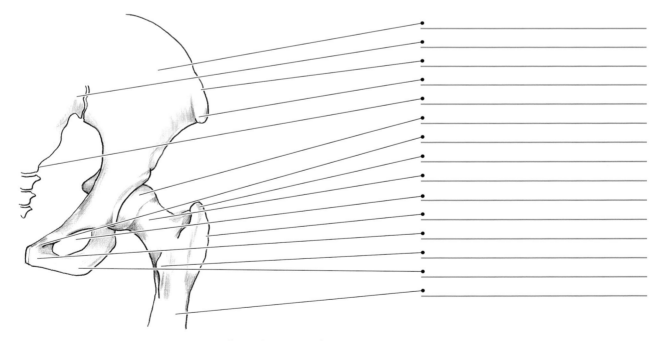

Fig. 3.1 (b) Bones of the left hip region (anterior aspect)

21. List the bones and the processes which comprise this rim.

_____

22. About 10 cm below the iliac crest, laterally, a large bony process is palpable. What is it called?

_____

Page 126

23. Name the process which lies approximately 2.5 cm below the posterior superior iliac spine.

_____

24. What notch does the posterior border partially form below this point?

_____

25. Which bone forms the medial boundary of this notch?

_____

26. Name the bony process at the lower end of the sacrum.

_____

27. How far above the line of the posterior superior iliac spines does the upper border of the sacrum reach?

_____

28. Which bony processes lie centrally down the posterior aspect of the sacrum?

_____

29. What name is given to the line of tubercles which lie just lateral to the mid line of the sacrum?

_____

30. Explain why this area is difficult to palpate.

_____

31. What lies at the lower end of the ischium?

_____

32. How is this structure made easier to palpate?

_____

Page 127

33. What partially covers the two tuberosities, posteriorly?

_____

34. The tuberosities give attachment to which muscle tendon?

_____

35. What may occur in these bursii if they are put under pressure for a period of time?

_____

36. If the lumbar spine is arched and the abdomen dropped forward, in which direction does the pelvis rotate?

_____

37. Around which axis does this movement occur?

_____

38. Lateral tilting of the pelvis occurs around which axis?

_____

39. Name the muscle groups which produce this movement.

_____

40. Explain how one can produce forward and backward rotation of the pelvis.

_____

Please complete the labels below.

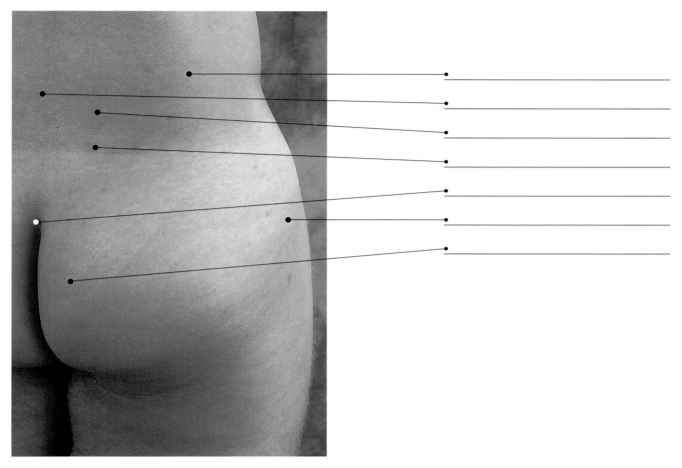

Fig. 3.2 (a) The right hip region (posterior aspect)

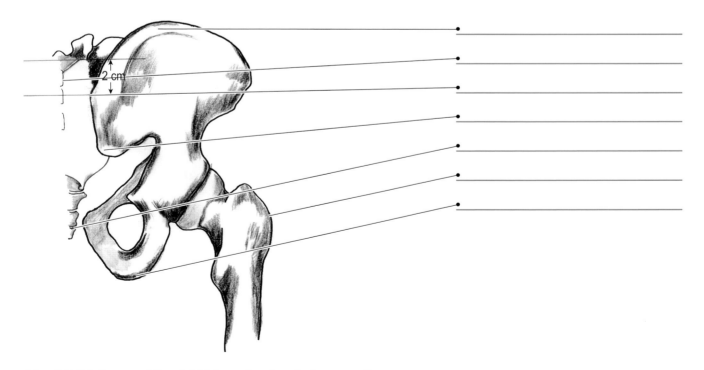

2 cm

Fig. 3.2 (b) Bones of the right hip region (posterior aspect)

Page 128

41. Which three bones take part in the knee joint?

42. What term is used to describe the posterior border of the femur?

43. Name the notch which lies posteriorly at the lower end of the femur.

44. Which is the stouter of the two femoral condyles?

45. From anterior to posterior, which is the longer condyle?

46. What type of cartilage covers the condyles inferiorly?

47. By what name is the triangular articular surface on the front of the two femoral condyles known?

48. Name the ridge above the two condyles, posteriorly.

49. What is the term used to describe the central raised area between the two condyles of the tibia?

50. What shape is the patella?

51. Which area of the patella is smooth and covered with articular cartilage?

52. With what does the upper end of the fibula articulate?

53. What bony prominence does its lower end form?

54. In which direction does the apex of the patella point?

Page 129

55. What attaches to the base of the patella?

56. The apex of the patella gives attachment to which ligament?

57. What structure covers the lower part of the tuberosity of the tibia?

58. Where may the two menisci be palpated?

Page 130

59. In which area is the medial epicondyle of the femur located?

60. Which tubercle lies just above the medial epicondyle?

61. Name the ridge which runs vertically up from this tubercle

Please complete the labels below.

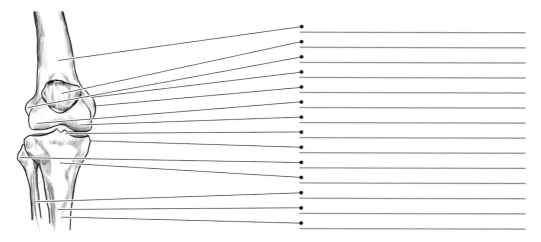

Fig. 3.3 (b) Bones of the right knee region (anterior aspect)

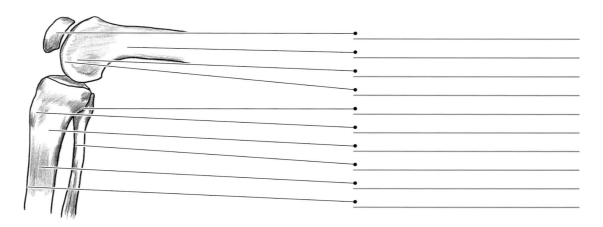

Fig. 3.3 (d) Bones of the right knee (medial aspect)

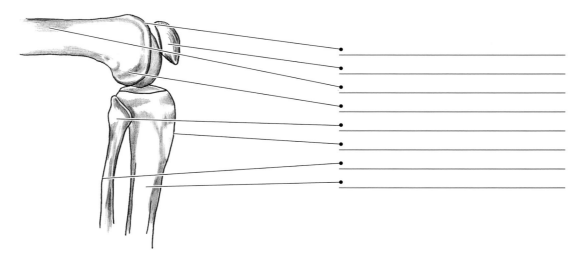

Fig. 3.4 (b) Bones of the right knee (lateral aspect)

62. The flattened medial condyle of the tibia continues downwards as what structure?

63. What structure bounds this surface anteriorly?

64. Of the following three structures, which is the easiest and which is the most difficult to palpate: the medial epicondyle of the femur, the adductor tubercle or the medial supracondylar ridge?

65. How far down the leg is the medial surface of the tibia palpable?

Page 131

66. What is the anterior border of the tibia commonly called?

67. Which tubercle projects laterally from the mid point of the lateral condyle of the femur?

68. How far below the knee joint is the head of the fibula situated?

69. What projects upwards from the head of the fibula?

Page 132

70. What structure lies below the lateral condyle of the femur?

71. Name the projection of bone which is palpable below the knee joint on the lateral side.

72. What marks the centre of the lateral surface of the lateral condyle of the femur?

73. Explain why it is difficult to palpate the lateral supracondylar ridge.

74. How far below the rim of the lateral condyle of the tibia can the head of the fibula be palpated?

Page 133

75. Explain why it is difficult to palpate the middle sections of the shaft of the fibula.

76. Describe how the head of the fibula may be easily palpated.

77. When the knee is being flexed, in which direction does the patella move?

78. With which part of the femoral condyle is the tibia in contact when the knee is in full flexion?

79. Describe the process which projects upwards from the head of the fibula.

Page 134

80. Which muscle attaches to the head of the fibula either side of this process?

Please complete the labels below.

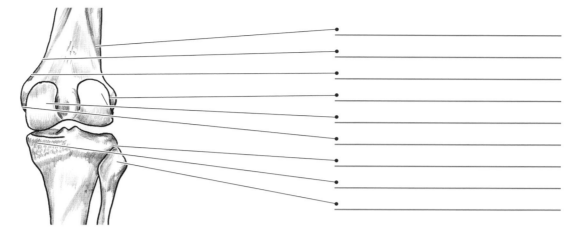

Fig. 3.4 (d) The right knee region (posterior aspect)

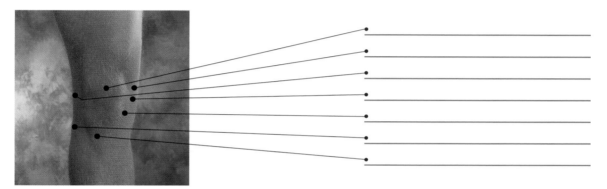

Fig. 3.3 (a) The right knee region (anterior aspect)

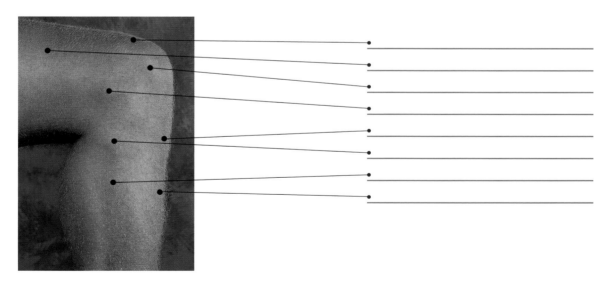

Fig. 3.4 (a) The right knee (lateral aspect)

81. Name a ligament which also attaches to the head of the fibula.

_____

82. Which nerve winds around the neck and back of the head of the fibula?

_____

SELF ASSESSMENT

Page 136

83. What bones take part in the ankle joint?

84. What is the name of the projection downwards at the lower end of the tibia?

85. With what bone does this projection articulate in the ankle joint?

86. List the bony components of the talus.

87. In which direction does the talar neck pass from the body?

88. With which bone does the head of the talus articulate anteriorly?

89. The tip of which malleolus projects the lowest?

90. Which joint can be palpated just anterior to the head of the talus?

91. Describe the posterior surface of the talus.

Page 138

92. Which bones form the mortice of the ankle joint?

93. What attaches to the fossa on the posterior border of the medial malleolus?

94. Name the largest tarsal bone.

95. What structure projects medially from the upper part of the medial surface of the calcaneus?

96. Where does the tendocalcaneus attach to the calcaneus?

97. List the three tubercles on the inferior surface of the calcaneus.

98. How far below the tip of the medial malleolus is the sustentaculum tali?

99. Describe a way in which the sustentaculum tali can be made more prominent.

100. What structure spans the gap between the anterior part of the sustentaculum tali and the navicular bone?

101. By what other name is this structure known?

Page 139

102. Describe what happens to the body of the talus on dorsiflexion of the ankle.

Please complete the labels below.

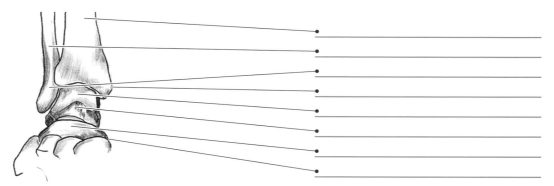

Fig. 3.5 (b) Bones of the right ankle region (anterior aspect)

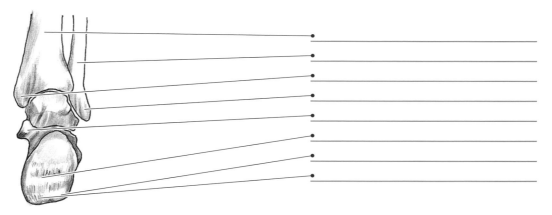

Fig. 3.5 (d) Bones of the right ankle region (posterior aspect)

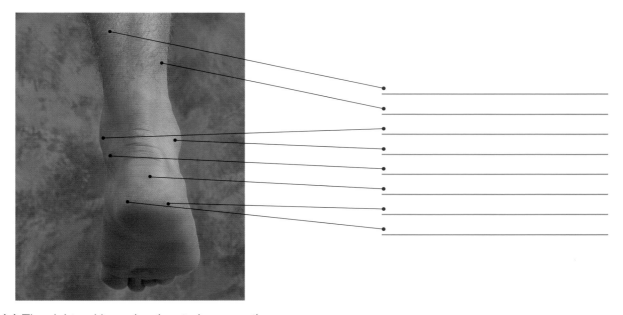

Fig. 3.5 (c) The right ankle region (posterior aspect)

103. How much side to side movement occurs at the ankle joint when it is dorsiflexed?

_____

104. What type of movement does the sustentaculum tali produce on plantar and dorsiflexion of the ankle joint?

_____

SELF ASSESSMENT

Page 140

105. How many groups of bones form the skeleton of the foot?

106. Name these groups, from posterior to anterior.

107. Which bones form the posterior group?

108. What structure projects downwards from the medial aspect of the navicular?

109. How far is this structure from the tip of the medial malleolus?

110. Which bones lie anterior to the navicula?

Page 141

111. In what ways does the first metatarsal bone differ from the other metatarsal bones?

112. Name the condition in which the head of the medial metatarsal projects more medially than normal.

113. Which metatarsal bones articulate with the cuboid bone?

114. List the identifying features of the fifth metatarsal.

115. Name the elongated tubercle, on the lateral surface of the calcaneus, anterior and below the tip of the lateral malleolus.

116. Which two tendons pass above and below this tubercle?

Page 142

117. Which is the upper of these two tendons?

118. Name the thick fascia under the plantar aspect of the foot.

119. What structure covers the posterior inferior aspect of the calcaneus?

120. Which tendon runs over the sustentaculum tali, medially?

121. Explain why the heads of the 2nd, 3rd and 4th metatarsals are more difficult to palpate from below.

122. Describe the deformity in the condition of 'hammer toes'. (fr)

123. Describe the head of the proximal phalanx.

124. On inversion and eversion, what movement occurs at the tubercle of the navicula?

Please complete the labels below.

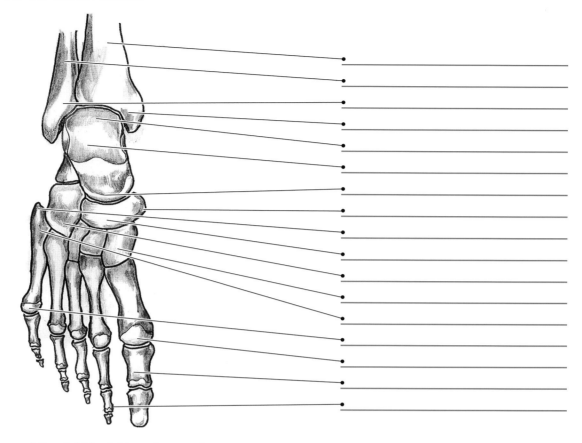

Fig. 3.6 (b) Bones of the right foot (dorsal aspect)

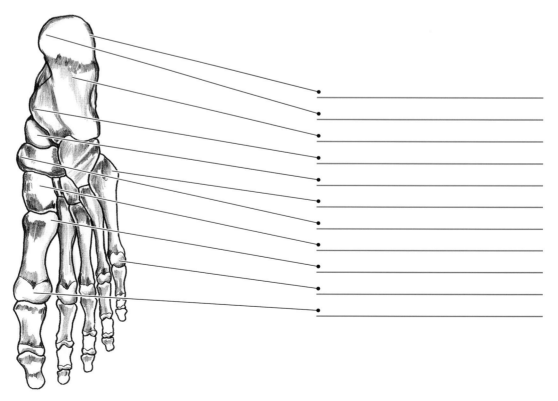

Fig. 3.7 (b) Bones of the right foot (plantar aspect)

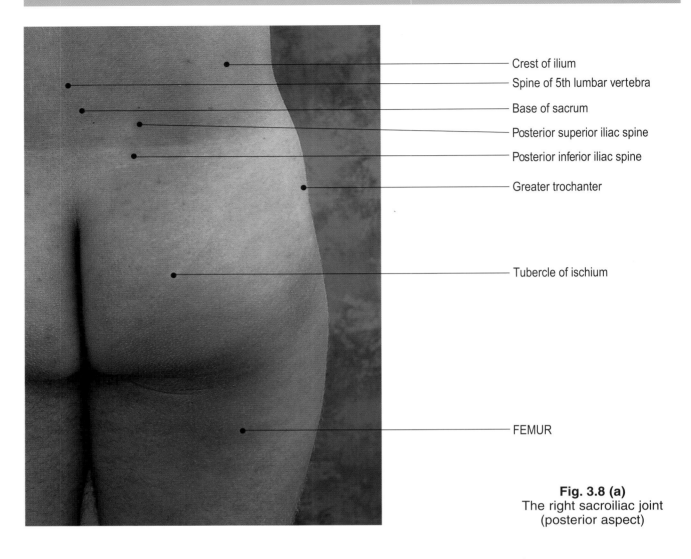

Crest of ilium
Spine of 5th lumbar vertebra
Base of sacrum
Posterior superior iliac spine
Posterior inferior iliac spine
Greater trochanter
Tubercle of ischium
FEMUR

Fig. 3.8 (a)
The right sacroiliac joint
(posterior aspect)

JOINTS

Although the joints of the lower limb are structurally similar to their counterparts in the upper limb, they tend to be more stable. Movement at the lower limb joints is more limited, with the weight transmitted across them being considerably more than in the upper limb. The sacroiliac joint and the pubic symphysis are really associated with the pelvis, but as this is the region from which the lower limb functions, they are included in this section.

The sacroiliac joint

Structure

This joint is situated deeply in the back of the pelvis and is formed by the auricular surface on the lateral side of the sacrum and the sacropelvic surface of the hip bone. It is a synovial joint surrounded by a capsule and lined with synovial membrane. The capsule is supported by anterior, posterior and interosseous ligaments and the joint is further supported by two accessory ligaments, the sacrotuberous and the sacrospinous.

Palpation and surface marking

This joint is set deeply at the back of the pelvis and is thus difficult to palpate. Nevertheless, certain landmarks can be identified, giving an accurate indication of its position (Fig. 3.8).

Find the posterior superior and inferior iliac spines, as outlined above (pages 126–127). The line of the joint can be marked by an oblique line passing downwards and medially at an angle of approximately 25° from a point 5 cm lateral to the spine of the fifth lumbar vertebra to a point just lateral to the posterior inferior iliac spine. The joint is, however, in a plane running forwards and laterally under the posterior part of the ilium, reaching as far forward as the apex of the greater sciatic notch (Fig. 3.9b).

Accessory movements

There is much controversy concerning the movements that may occur at this joint. The fact that it is a synovial joint with plane, although irregular, articular surfaces suggests that it is designed for movement. However, the irregularity of the articular surface, together with the presence of extremely strong, short interosseous ligaments,

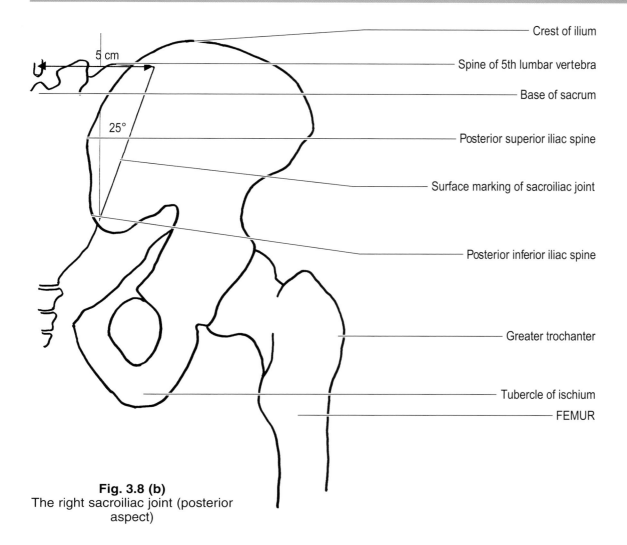

Crest of ilium

Spine of 5th lumbar vertebra

Base of sacrum

Posterior superior iliac spine

Surface marking of sacroiliac joint

Posterior inferior iliac spine

Greater trochanter

Tubercle of ischium

FEMUR

Fig. 3.8 (b)
The right sacroiliac joint (posterior
aspect)

means that in reality little movement is possible. In the young female, movement is often considerable, whereas in the elderly male, little or no movement is possible. The two joints on either side of the sacrum and the symphysis pubis anteriorly allow slight rotation and gapping movements to occur, which reduces the stresses imparted on the pelvis from the trunk and lower limbs.

Slight rotation of the sacrum forwards and backwards around a frontal axis running through its interosseous ligament may be regarded as normal physiological movement. It can, however, be aided by pressure placed alternately on the upper and lower aspects of its posterior surface, with the subject in prone lying, thereby rocking the sacrum between the ilia.

Rotation of the ilium can be enhanced by using the femur as a lever and localizing the movement of the joint with the other hand. With the subject lying on one side, stand behind the hip region and take the upper femur into extension; the other hand should be placed on the posterior aspect of the iliac crest. Considerable fixation of the rest of the pelvis can be achieved if the subject holds the alternate knee up to the chest. Flexion of the femur on the pelvis produces a backward rotation of the ilium on the sacrum, which can be enhanced by pressure applied from the front on the anterior superior iliac spine, and fixation by the subject extending the alternate lower limb.

With the subject supine, slight gapping of the posterior part of the sacroiliac joint can be achieved by rotating the pelvis and flexed lower limb to the side and applying a downward and inward pressure on the femur, towards the hip. During these movements, associated gapping and twisting occur at the pubic symphysis. For additional information consult the manipulation literature.

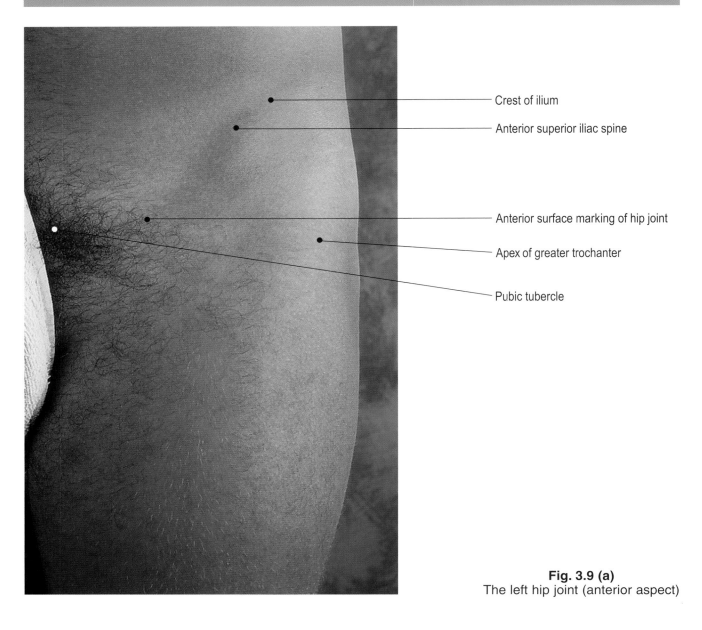

Crest of ilium

Anterior superior iliac spine

Anterior surface marking of hip joint

Apex of greater trochanter

Pubic tubercle

Fig. 3.9 (a)
The left hip joint (anterior aspect)

The hip joint [Fig. 3.9]

This is a large synovial ball-and-socket joint between the head of the femur and the acetabulum of the hip bone. It lies on the anterolateral aspect of the pelvis and affords a considerable amount of mobility to the lower limb. It is surrounded by a capsule which encloses a large part of the femoral neck, both lined with synovial membrane. The capsule is supported, externally, by the very powerful iliofemoral, ischiofemoral and pubo-femoral ligaments. In addition further support is afforded internally by the ligament of the head deep inside the joint and the acetabular labrum, which attaches to the rim of the acetabulum and transverse ligament, thus surrounding the head.

Surface marking

The joint lies in the groin some 1.5 cm below the mid point of the inguinal ligament, i.e. halfway between the **anterior superior iliac spine** and the **pubic tubercle** (pages 124–125). The acetabulum extends 4 cm vertically below this point deep to the head of the femur. Midway between the upper and lower limits, i.e. at the mid point of the joint, the acetabulum extends 2 cm either side of this vertical line (Fig. 3.9).

An alternative method of establishing the centre of the hip joint can be by tracing a line horizontally and medially from the upper border of the **greater trochanter** to a point below the mid point of the inguinal ligament. When viewed posteriorly, the hip joint centre lies 5 cm above and 3 cm lateral to the ischial tuberosity.

Palpation

Palpation of the joint from any aspect is, however, virtually impossible as it is covered by thick muscle crossing the joint, particularly posteriorly and laterally. Only if the hip is fully extended can

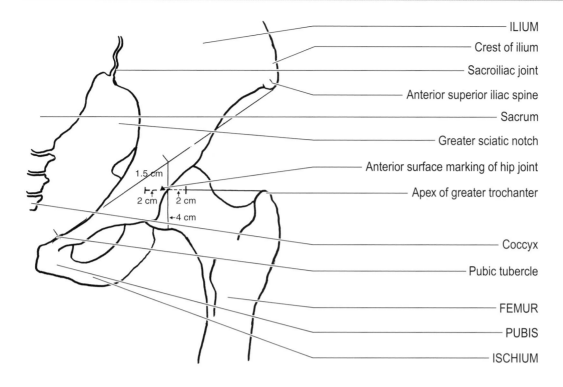

ILIUM
Crest of ilium
Sacroiliac joint
Anterior superior iliac spine
Sacrum
Greater sciatic notch
Anterior surface marking of hip joint
Apex of greater trochanter
Coccyx
Pubic tubercle
FEMUR
PUBIS
ISCHIUM

1.5 cm
2 cm 2 cm
4 cm

Fig. 3.9 (b)
Bones of the left hip joint (anterior
aspect)

movement be detected and then only anteriorly. If the fingers are placed on the anterior surface marking of the joint, with the subject standing, and the limb is then taken into approximately 15° of extension, the head of the femur can be palpated projecting forwards under the anterior covering of muscles (iliopsoas and pectineus).

Accessory movements

There is very little accessory movement at this joint. With the subject lying supine and the hip flexed approximately 30°, slight parting of the articular surfaces is possible. This is produced by applying strong traction to the femur.

Movements of flexion, extension and rotation of the hip, however, with the hands carefully controlling the movement from the lower end of the femur, can be a source of important information for the palpator. Quality and range of movement can be assessed and areas of 'grinding' and limitation can be located. Linked with the patient's symptoms and reactions, a much clearer picture of the problems involved can be visualized.

Combining the three components of movement, i.e. flexion/extension, abduction/adduction and medial/lateral rotation, can test the joint movement and function to extremes. Testing in these confined movements is often referred to as the 'quadrants' and for further information concerning these manoeuvres the manipulation and mobilization literature should be consulted (Maitland 1991). Fixation of proximal and distal joints in testing of the hip joint is essential, as compensatory movement is common in this area and can lead to incorrect diagnosis.

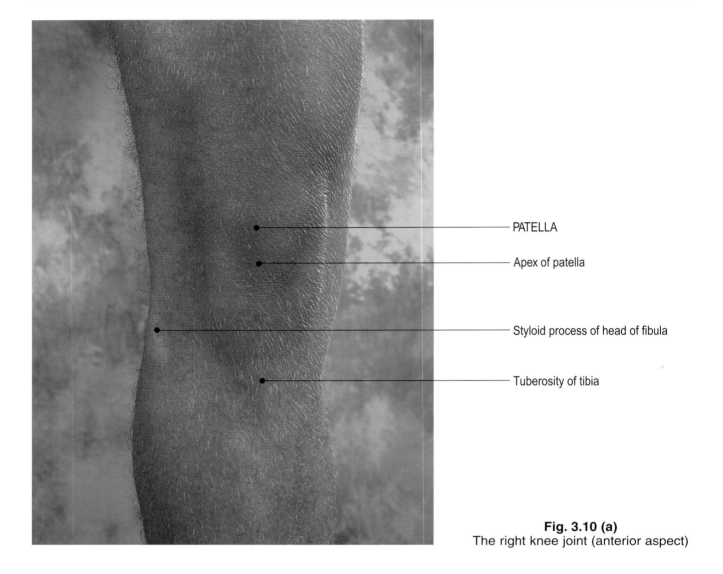

PATELLA

Apex of patella

Styloid process of head of fibula

Tuberosity of tibia

Fig. 3.10 (a)
The right knee joint (anterior aspect)

The knee joint [Fig. 3.10]

The knee joint is a synovial composite joint comprising the bicondylar section between the condyles of femur and tibia and the plane joint between the patella and the patellar surface of the femur. The joint functions as a modified hinge, with the main movements being flexion and extension. Rotation can be produced in the semiflexed position and in the final few degrees of full extension.

It is the largest joint in the human body and perhaps the most complex (see *Anatomy and Human Movement*, Palastanga, Field and Soames 1998).

The articular surfaces are covered with articular cartilage, but are not congruent. Those on the femur cover the superior, posterior, inferior and anterior surfaces of the large condyles, coming together anteriorly to form a triangular surface which is narrow at the top and is called the patellar surface. The articular surfaces of the tibia only cover the central section of the upper surface; its outer sections are covered by two crescentic-shaped menisci.

The joint is supported on its posterior, lateral and medial side by a fibrous capsule. Anteriorly

the capsule is formed by the lower section of the quadriceps femoris, the patella and the ligamentum patellae. The joint is lined by an extensive and complex synovial membrane and is supported by numerous ligaments, including the oblique popliteal, the tibial collateral, the fibula collateral externally and the anterior and posterior cruciate ligaments internally. It also relies heavily on the powerful surrounding muscles for its stability.

Anterior to the condylar section is the patello-femoral joint between the posterior surface of the patella and the patellar surface of the femur. This is a synovial plane joint, separate from the knee although it shares the same joint space and synovial membrane.

The knee joint appears at first sight to be a very unstable joint with the two rounded condyles of the femur sitting on top of the two flattened surfaces of the tibia. This, however, is not so. This joint rarely dislocates and even then only under extreme force, such as a car or aeroplane crash. It is, however, subject to many stresses and strains, particularly in sport.

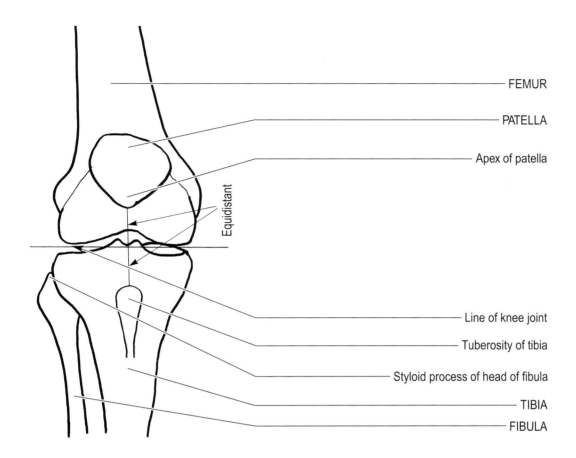

Fig. 3.10 (b)
The right knee joint (anterior aspect)

Surface marking

The joint lies on a line which bisects the ligamentum patellae horizontally (Fig. 3.10b,d), **halfway between the lower tip of the patella and the tibial tuberosity**. An alternative method of marking the joint is by drawing a line horizontally 1 cm above the tip of the styloid process of the fibula.

Palpation

With the fingers either side of the ligamentum patellae, two triangular depressions can be felt. These are bounded by the tibia below, the femur above and the ligamentum patellae centrally. At the apex of the depression, running horizontally, is the knee joint space; your fingers are now resting against the anterior aspect of the medial and lateral menisci. These can be observed moving forwards during rotation at the joint, the lateral meniscus on lateral rotation and the medial on medial rotation. Tracing the joint posteriorly, the space becomes narrower until just behind the mid point it becomes hidden by the medial collateral ligament medially and the lateral part of the joint capsule laterally. Posteriorly the joint is impossible to palpate due to the presence of muscle, tendon and fascial coverings, although the joint can be represented by a horizontal line drawn across the back of the popliteal fossa 1 cm above the tip of the styloid process of the head of the fibula (Fig. 3.10f).

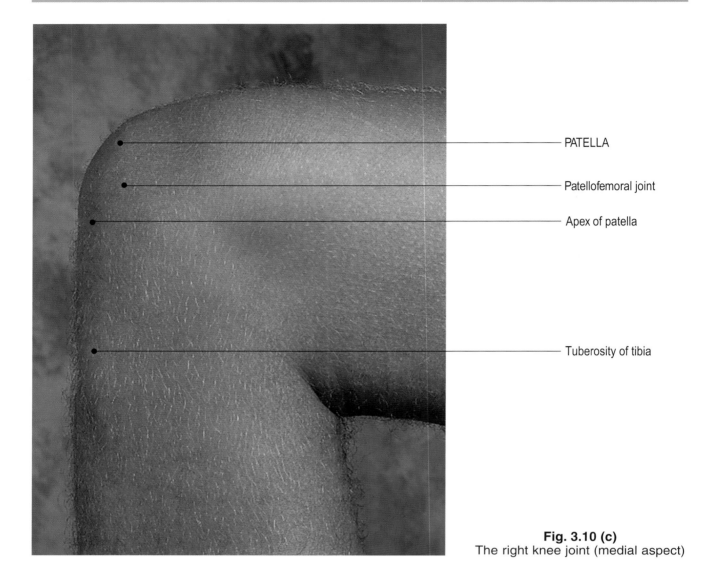

PATELLA

Patellofemoral joint

Apex of patella

Tuberosity of tibia

Fig. 3.10 (c)
The right knee joint (medial aspect)

Accessory movements

The knee joint becomes 'close packed' on full extension; therefore, accessory movements should only be performed avoiding the extreme of extension. With the subject lying supine, the knee flexed to 90° and the foot firmly fixed on the supporting surface (often achieved by the investigator sitting on the foot), the tibial condyles can be drawn forwards (anterior draw test), and pushed backwards, producing a gliding of the tibial condyles against the femoral condyles. There should be only a slight movement in either direction, forward movement of the tibia being limited by the anterior cruciate ligament and posterior movement being limited by the posterior cruciate ligament.

With the subject again lying supine with the knee flexed 15°, stabilize the under surface of the thigh with one hand and grasp the lower end of the leg just above the ankle with the other. A side-to-side movement can be produced. Distraction of the joint can also be achieved by pulling on the leg in the mid position, with the subject seated on a high plinth with the foot clear of the floor.

The patellofemoral joint lies deep to the patella, between it and the patellar surface of the femur, 1 cm deep to its anterior surface (Fig. 3.10c, d), sharing the same joint space as the bicondylar articulation. It is easily marked by tracing around the perimeter of bone. When the knee is in an extended and relaxed position, the patella can be moved from side to side across the patellar surface of the femur, resulting in a knocking effect. It can also be moved up and down as a gliding movement along the vertical groove of the femoral surface.

With the patella moved laterally, the medial edge of the patellar surface of the femur can be palpated, marked by a sharp ridge. In this position, the under surface of the lateral edge of the patella can also be palpated. Conversely, if the patella is moved medially, the lateral edge of the patellar surface of the femur and the medial under surface of the patella also become palpable.

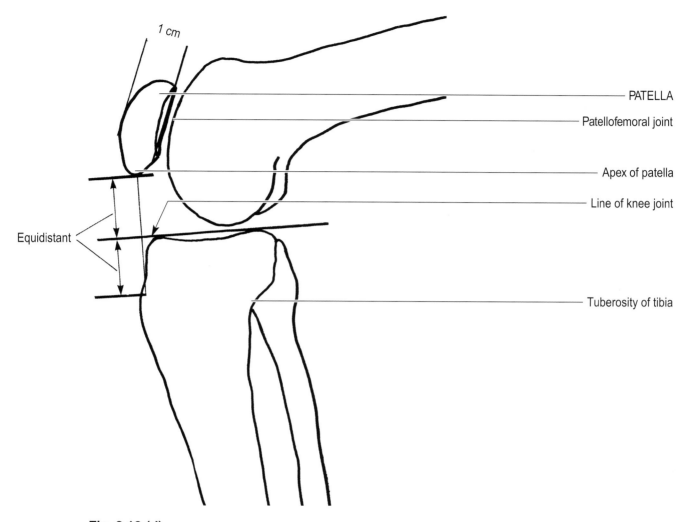

1 cm

PATELLA

Patellofemoral joint

Apex of patella

Line of knee joint

Tuberosity of tibia

Equidistant

Fig. 3.10 (d)
The right knee joint (medial aspect)

Functional anatomy

Little stress is applied to the structural components of the knee joint, on which it relies for its stability during normal activities, such as walking, running, jumping, swimming, etc. However, enormous tension is applied to these components during sporting activities where the lower limbs are used for varied directional propulsion and kicking. Lateral or medial forces applied to the knee, particularly when the knee is in its extended 'close-packed' position may cause strains, partial tears or even complete ruptures to medial or lateral ligaments. Violent over-extension of the knee may rupture the anterior cruciate ligament, and the posterior cruciate ligament may rupture when enormous force is applied to the anterior aspect of the proximal end of the tibia. When the knee is over-rotated in a flexed position the menisci, especially the medial, sometimes get trapped between the rolling condyle of the femur on the tibia, producing a tear in the meniscus.

In addition to all the ligamentous problems, the very powerful muscle surrounding the joint, on which stability is also dependent, may be partially torn or even completely ruptured. On a violent extension force such as kicking a stationary object, or falling from a height on to the feet, the quadriceps femoris tendon may rupture causing complete dysfunction of the joint.

When one considers all the fractures that may occur through direct or indirect violence to the bones of the joint and the degeneration due to age and all the stresses applied by virtually the whole body weight being transferred through the joint during movement, it is hardly surprising that the knee joints are a source of much pain and suffering, for many, in their senior years.

(For detailed study of structure, stability, function, dysfunction, remedies, etc., see *Anatomy and Human Movement*, Palastanga, Field and Soames 1998.)

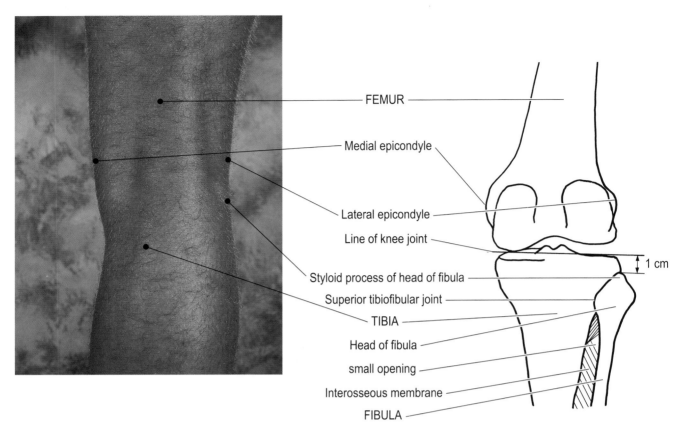

FEMUR

Medial epicondyle

Lateral epicondyle

Line of knee joint

1 cm

Styloid process of head of fibula

Superior tibiofibular joint

TIBIA

Head of fibula

small opening

Interosseous membrane

FIBULA

Fig. 3.10 (e), (f)
The right knee joint (posterior aspect)

The tibiofibular union

The tibia and fibula are joined together by two joints, the superior tibiofibular joint and the inferior tibiofibular joint, and an interosseous membrane. They unite the bones so tightly that very little movement occurs between the two. The interosseous membrane is composed of strong fibrous tissue with its fibres passing downwards and laterally. There is a small opening above (see Fig. 3.10f), with an additional group of fibres passing in the opposite direction just below the superior tibiofibular joint.

The superior tibiofibular joint

This is a synovial joint, with its surfaces covered with articular cartilage and it is surrounded by a capsule lined with synovial membrane. The capsule is supported by the anterior and posterior tibiofibular ligaments.

Surface marking

This joint can be represented, both anteriorly and posteriorly, by a line 1.5 cm in length running downwards and slightly medially just medial to the head of the fibula (Fig. 3.11a,b).

Palpation

With the model in supine lying and the knee straight, stand on the right side just below the level of the knee. Place the index finger of your left hand on the styloid process of the head of the fibula. From that point your thumb can trace downwards and medially along the anterior aspect of the joint. Your middle finger is just behind the joint, and similarly to the thumb, can trace downwards and medially along the posterior joint line. This is a little more difficult to palpate as it is covered by the lateral head of gastrocnemius.

Accessory movements

Although the head of the fibula can be felt gliding up and down during dorsiflexion and plantar flexion of the ankle joint, accessory movement between the two bones is virtually impossible. With the subject lying supine and the ankle joint plantar flexed, direct pressure, applied by the thumb, on the head of the fibula can produce a slight backward gliding. Forward gliding can be achieved using the same technique but with the subject lying prone. Extreme care must be taken, when performing this procedure, to avoid the common peroneal nerve as it winds around the neck of the fibula.

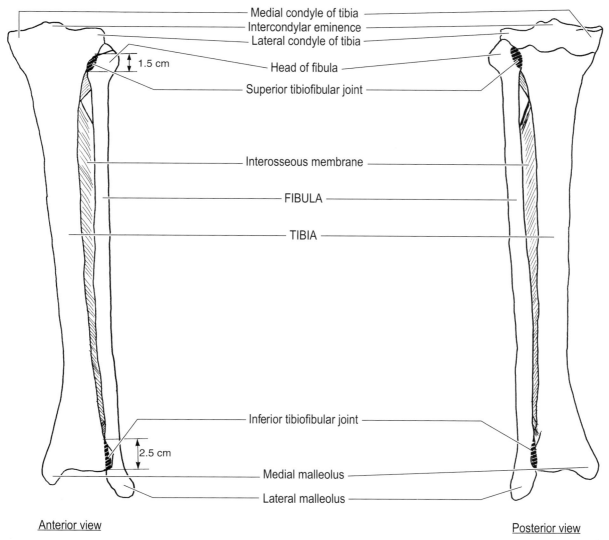

Fig. 3.11 (a), (b)
The superior and inferior tibiofibular joints and union of the left side

The inferior tibiofibular joint

This joint is a fibrous syndesmosis [*syndesmos* (Gk) = a band] between the lower lateral rough triangular surface on the tibia and a similar surface on the lower medial side of the fibula. The surfaces are bound together by a very strong interosseous ligament which is a continuation downwards of the interosseous membrane. The joint is further supported by an anterior, posterior and transverse tibiofibular ligament, the latter forming part of the socket of the ankle joint.

Surface marking

This joint can be represented by a vertical line 2.5 cm long running superiorly from the line of the ankle joint (see page 166) on the medial side of the **lateral malleolus**.

Palpation

Again it is difficult to palpate, except for its upper edge, as it is mostly covered by the superior extensor retinaculum and extensor digitorum longus tendons. Posteriorly, little can be palpated owing to the presence of the tendocalcaneus.

Accessory movements

Accessory movement of the inferior tibiofibular joint is not possible, except when diastasis (a parting of the inferior tibiofibular joint) has occurred. It is unwise to increase the unwanted movement in this injury, as this leads to even further instability tif the ankle joint.

The fibrous interosseous ligament between the two bones holds the two bones together and is referred to by some as a fibrous syndesmosis.

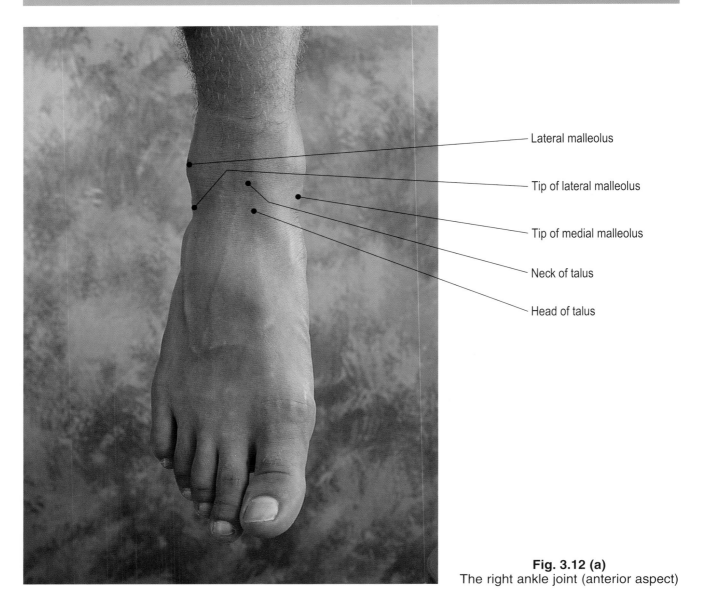

Lateral malleolus

Tip of lateral malleolus

Tip of medial malleolus

Neck of talus

Head of talus

Fig. 3.12 (a)
The right ankle joint (anterior aspect)

The ankle joint [Fig. 3.12]

The ankle joint is a synovial hinge joint involving the distal ends of the tibia and fibula proximally and the body of the talus distally. The weight-bearing surfaces are the trochlear surfaces of the tibia and talus. The stabilizing surfaces are those of the medial and lateral malleoli, which grip the body of the talus. The articular surfaces are composed of, above, the inferior surface of the tibia, the medial surface of the lateral malleolus and lateral surface of the medial malleolus, and, below, the superior, lateral and upper part of the medial surface of the talus. The surfaces are covered with articular cartilage. The joint is surrounded by a capsule lined with synovial membrane and is supported by very powerful lateral and medial (deltoid) ligaments. These two ligaments are delta-shaped, being narrower above and broader below. Above they are attached to the anterior and posterior borders, tip and fossae of each malleolus. Below, the medial attaches to the navicular, calcaneonavicular 'spring' ligament, sustentaculum tali and medial tubercle of talus, with a deep section attaching to the medial surface of the talus. The lateral has three portions, the anterior and posterior attaching to the talus and the middle portion to the calcaneus. The transverse tibiofibular ligament which passes across the posterior of the ankle joint, forming part of its socket, attaches to both malleoli and the lower border of the tibia.

A horizontal line drawn across the anterior surface of the ankle 2 cm above the tip of the medial and 3 cm above that of the lateral malleolus marks the superior limit of the joint. It is continued down the medial side of the lateral malleolus and the lateral side of the medial malleolus to their tips which completes the joint line (Fig. 3.12b, d, f).

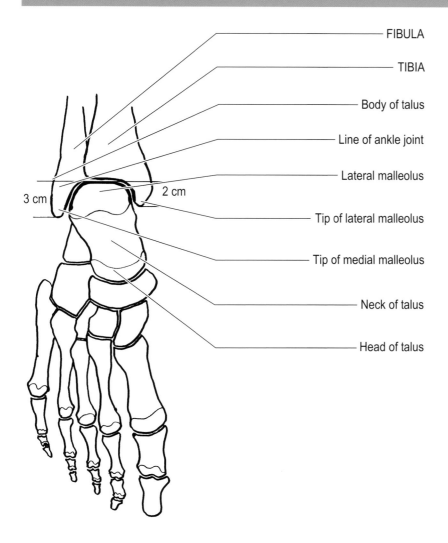

FIBULA

TIBIA

Body of talus

Line of ankle joint

Lateral malleolus

Tip of lateral malleolus

Tip of medial malleolus

Neck of talus

Head of talus

3 cm   2 cm

Fig. 3.12 (b)
The right ankle joint (anterior aspect)

Palpation

Careful palpation between the extensor tendons in the region of the horizontal part of the joint line reveals the lower border of the tibia. Medially the joint line can be traced on to the anterior border of the medial malleolus and down to the tip. It can be traced up the posterior border of the medial malleolus, above the malleolar fossa where the joint line is hidden by tissue which lies between the tendocalcaneus and the joint. Laterally the joint line can be palpated between the talus and lateral malleolus anteriorly, and can be traced down to the tip of the malleolus. As on the medial side, its posterior border can be traced upwards above the malleolar fossa until it too is lost under similar fascia. With the ankle plantarflexed, the body of the talus, i.e. its upper, lateral and medial surfaces, can be felt gliding forwards (Fig. 3.12c, d). Posteriorly the joint is hidden by tendons and fascia.

Accessory movements

The ankle joint allows the movements of dorsiflexion and plantarflexion. Side-to-side movement is limited by the presence of the two malleoli, there being no movement possible when the joint is dorsiflexed and 'close packed' as the body is gripped between the two malleoli. However, when the joint is plantarflexed, by gripping the foot with one hand and stabilizing the leg with the other, the narrower part of the body of the talus can be moved from side to side, as well as forwards and backwards.

Commonly the lateral (and less frequently the medial) malleolus is fractured by a lateromedial or mediolateral force. Unless the malleolus is replaced exactly, the talus is able to move sideways and the joint becomes less stable. The same mechanical problem will occur if the two bones are parted at the inferior tibiofibular joint (diastasis – see page 165).

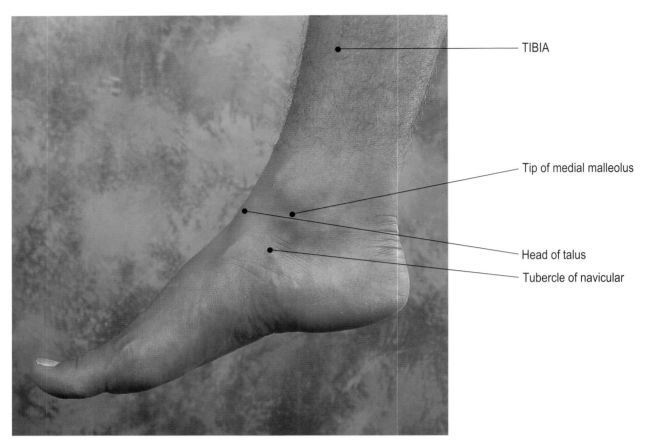

TIBIA

Tip of medial malleolus

Head of talus

Tubercle of navicular

Fig. 3.12 (c)
The right ankle joint (medial aspect)

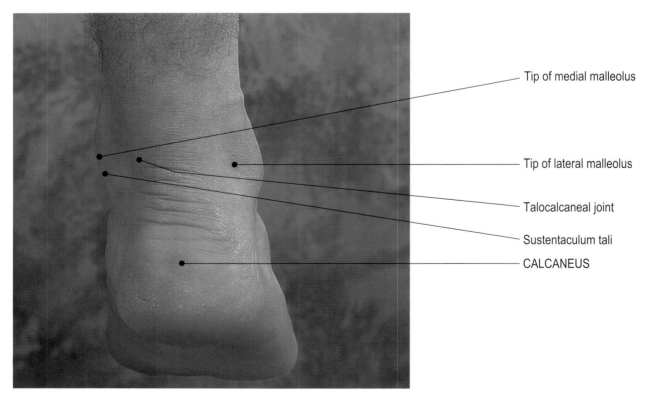

Tip of medial malleolus

Tip of lateral malleolus

Talocalcaneal joint

Sustentaculum tali

CALCANEUS

Fig. 3.12 (e)
The right ankle joint (posterior aspect)

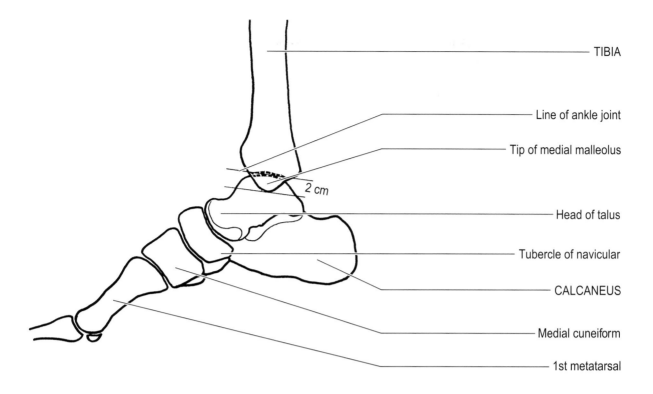

Fig. 3.12 (d)
The right ankle joint (medial aspect)

TIBIA

Line of ankle joint

Tip of medial malleolus

2 cm

Head of talus

Tubercle of navicular

CALCANEUS

Medial cuneiform

1st metatarsal

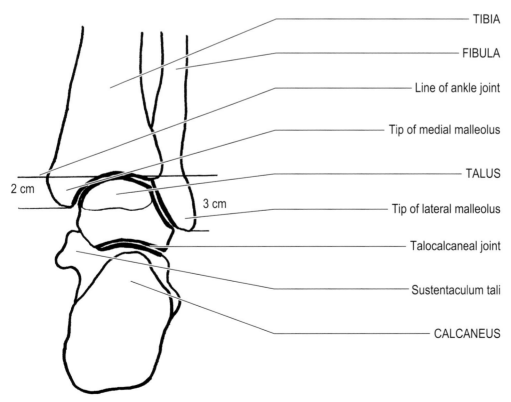

Fig. 3.12 (f)
The right ankle joint (posterior aspect)

TIBIA

FIBULA

Line of ankle joint

Tip of medial malleolus

TALUS

Tip of lateral malleolus

Talocalcaneal joint

Sustentaculum tali

CALCANEUS

2 cm

3 cm

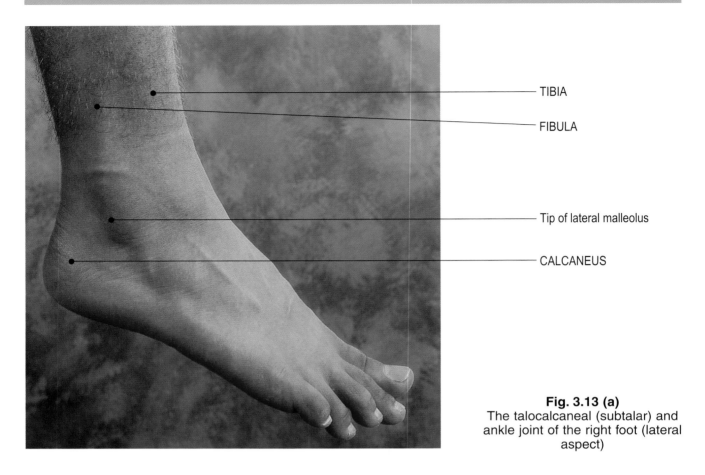

TIBIA

FIBULA

Tip of lateral malleolus

CALCANEUS

Fig. 3.13 (a)
The talocalcaneal (subtalar) and ankle joint of the right foot (lateral aspect)

The foot

The joints of the foot are divided into those between the tarsal bones (the intertarsal joints) and the tarsal and metatarsal bones (the tarso-metatarsal joints); between the metatarsal bases (the intermetatarsal joints); between the meta-tarsals and phalanges (the metatarsophalangeal joints) and those between the phalanges (the inter-phalangeal joints). Most of the joints are readily identifiable on the dorsum of the foot as they are only covered by thin fascia and the tendons of the long extensor muscles, whereas the plantar aspect of the foot is covered by numerous intrinsic muscles, in four layers, and very thick layers (up to 80) of plantar fascia.

The talocalcaneal (subtalar) joint [Fig. 3.13]

The talocalcaneal joint lies below the talus and is often referred to as the subtalar joint. The joint surfaces taking part in this joint are the inferior surface of the talus and the middle section of the superior surface of the calcaneus. Both surfaces are covered with articular cartilage and the joint is surrounded by a fibrous capsule lined with synovial membrane. The capsule is supported by medial, posterior, lateral and interosseous liga-ment. The interosseous ligament lies anterior to the joint and separates it from the talocalcaneo-navicular joint. There is also a short ligament which joins the neck of the talus to the sustentaculum tali at the lateral end of the sinus tarsi.

Surface marking

The joint is marked by a line running horizontally 1 cm below the tip of the lateral malleolus on the lateral side to a point 1.5 cm below the tip of the medial malleolus on the medial side (Fig. 3.13b).

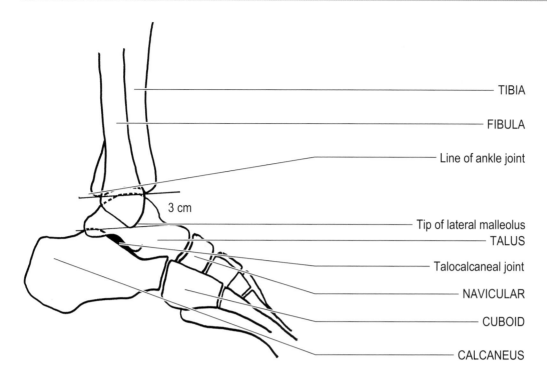

Fig. 3.13 (b)
The talocalcaneal (subtalar) and
ankle joint of the right foot (lateral
aspect)

Palpation

This is a very difficult joint to palpate due to the
fact that the medial and lateral malleoli and the
powerful ligaments tend to hide the joint. Find
the tip of the lateral malleolus and move forward
into the hollow. Below your finger you will feel the
sharp edge of the upper border of the calcaneus.
This is the anterior part of the lateral side of the
joint.

On the medial side find the tip of the medial
malleolus. Move down 2 cm and you will be able
to palpate a horizontal ridge. This is the medial
edge of the sustentaculum tali and its upper
border is the lower boundary of the subtalar joint.

Accessory movement

With the model in supine lying, stand to the
lateral side of the right foot (similar to the position
adopted for accessory movements of the ankle
joint). With your left hand grip the neck of the
talus with your finger on the medial side and
thumb laterally. With your right hand fit the
model's heel into your palm with your fingers
wrapping around the back of the calcaneus. The
calcaneus can now be made to glide very slightly
backwards and forwards. The calcaneus can also
be rocked from side to side producing a slight
gapping of the lateral and medial side of the joint
alternately.

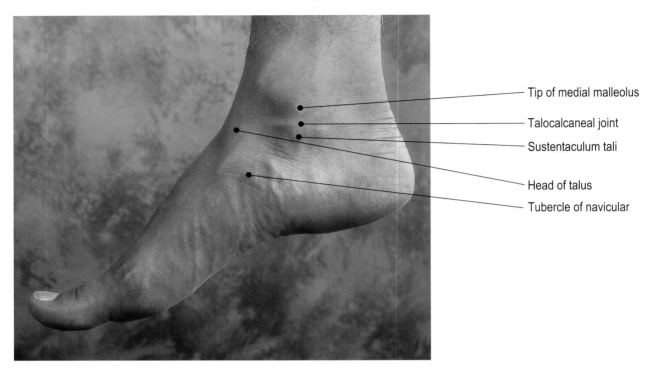

Fig. 3.13 (c)
The right talocalcaneal (subtalar) joint (medial aspect)

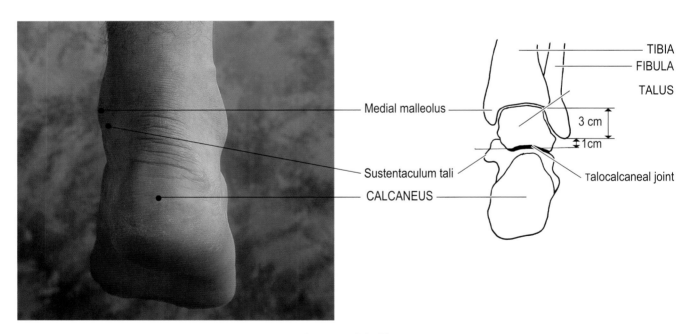

Fig. 3.13 (e), (f)
The talocalcaneal (subtalar) joint (posterior aspect)

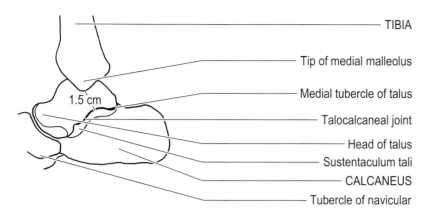

TIBIA

Tip of medial malleolus

Medial tubercle of talus

1.5 cm

Talocalcaneal joint

Head of talus

Sustentaculum tali

CALCANEUS

Tubercle of navicular

Fig. 3.13 (d)
The right talocalcaneal (subtalar) joint
(medial aspect)

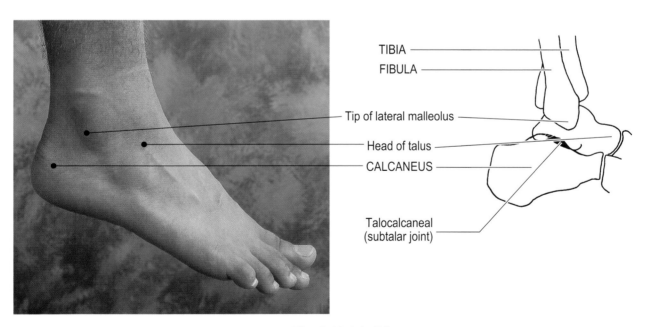

TIBIA

FIBULA

Tip of lateral malleolus

Head of talus

CALCANEUS

Talocalcaneal
(subtalar joint)

Fig. 3.13 (g), (h)
The talocalcaneal (subtalar) joint of the right foot (lateral aspect)

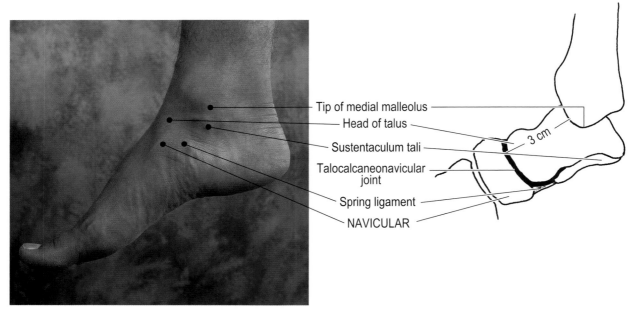

Fig. 3.14 (a), (b)
The talocalcaneonavicular joint of right foot (medial aspect)

The talocalcaneonavicular joint
[Fig. 3.14a–d]

This is a synovial, modified ball-and-socket joint between the head of the talus and a socket comprising the posterior surface of navicular, the superior surface of the sustentaculum tali of the calcaneus and the 'spring' ligament which joins the two (Fig. 3.14). It is surrounded by a capsule lined with synovial membrane and is supported by the talonavicular ligament dorsally, the medial band of the bifurcate ('Y'-shaped) ligament laterally, the tibionavicular part of the deltoid ligament medially and posteroinferiorly, under the neck, by the anterior section of the interosseous ligament in the sinus tarsi. The plantar calcaneonavicular (spring) ligament is a fibroelastic ligament forming part of the socket and lies below the head of the talus, having articular cartilage on its superior surface.

Surface marking

The surface marking of the joint can be represented by a line, convex distally, drawn transversely across the medial half of the dorsum of the foot at the level of the tubercle of the navicular.

As with nearly all the joints in the foot, palpation and identification is only possible on the dorsum. The plantar aspect is hidden deep to many layers of the plantar fascia, many short but powerful muscles and strong, dense ligaments.

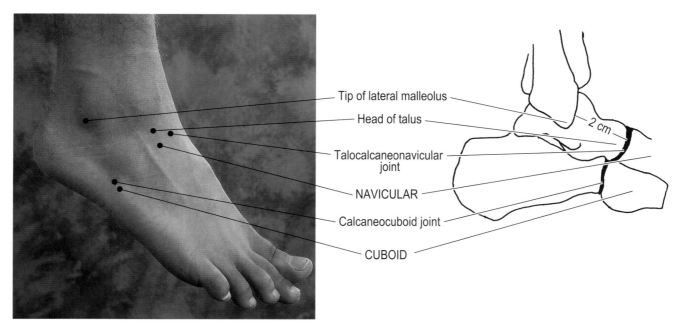

Fig. 3.14 (c), (d)
The talocalcaneonavicular and calcaneocuboid joints of right foot (lateral aspect)

Palpation

The tubercle of the navicular is situated 2.5 cm anteroinferior to the **tip of the medial malleolus** and is clearly palpable. As it projects slightly backwards, it is in line with the joint. The head of the talus can be traced down the proximal side of the tubercle to a small gap underneath, housing the 'spring' ligament. Posterior to the gap, the anterior section of the sustentaculum tali is palpable. If the foot is held in slight plantarflexion and the muscles relaxed, the joint can be traced across the dorsum of the foot almost to the mid point where the head of the talus and the navicular dip towards the bifurcate ligament. The tendons of tibialis anterior and extensor hallucis longus may have to be moved to the side to follow the line clearly.

Accessory movements

Stand lateral to the foot. With your proximal hand, stabilize the talus from the medial side with your fingers on the plantar and thumb on the dorsal aspect. With your distal hand, grasp the forefoot as far backwards as the navicular, again with your fingers on the plantar and thumb on the dorsal aspect. Slight up-and-down gliding can be obtained of the navicular on the head of the talus. Rotation of the forefoot on the head of the talus is also possible, but this is of course movement normally occurring during inversion and eversion.

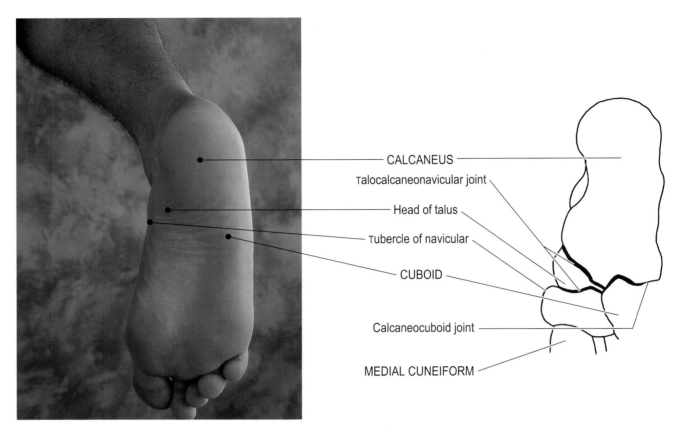

Fig. 3.14 (e), (f)
The talocalcaneonavicular and calcaneocuboid joint of right foot (plantar aspect)

The calcaneocuboid joint

This is a synovial, plane joint between the quadrilateral anterior surface of the calcaneus and the posterior surface of the cuboid. Both surfaces are covered with articular cartilage and the joint is surrounded by a capsule, lined with synovial membrane and supported by the lateral portion of the bifurcate ligament medially, by the dorsal calcaneocuboid ligament and by the plantar calcaneocuboid and long plantar ligaments.

Surface marking

The line of the joint is just proximal to the tubercle of the fifth metatarsal bone on the lateral and dorsal aspect of the base of the foot. It is slightly concave forwards.

Palpation

This joint is difficult to identify, although certain landmarks can be palpated. From the tip of the tubercle of the fifth metatarsal move dorsally 2 cm. Just proximal to your finger you will feel the anterior border of the superior surface of the calcaneus. This is 2 cm anterior to the tip of the lateral malleolus. The border can be traced medially until it dips towards the bifurcate ligament, and laterally to the anterior border of the lateral surface almost down to the tubercle.

Accessory movement

This plane synovial joint allows slight upward movement during eversion and slight downward movement during inversion accompanying the rotation of the navicular on the head of the talus. This movement is physiological and its loss would severely interfere with the functional movement of the foot. With the model in supine lying, stand to the right of the right foot. Stabilize the talus and calcaneus by gripping below the two malleoli with the fingers on the inside. With the right hand, grasp the cuboid with the thumb on the dorsum and the index and middle fingers underneath. Now move the cuboid up and down. Note, only slight movement will be present.

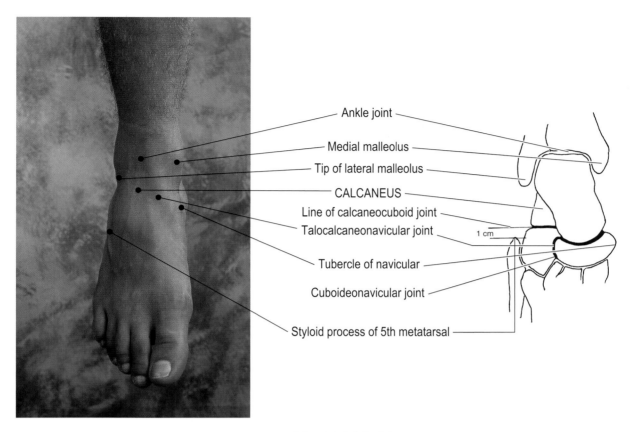

Fig. 3.14 (g), (h)
The midtarsal joint of the right foot (dorsal aspect)

The cuboideonavicular joint [Fig. 3.14h]

This joint between the navicular and the cuboid is normally a syndesmosis. The articular surfaces are joined entirely by a strong fibrous interosseous ligament and this is further supported by dorsal and plantar ligaments. Sometimes it is replaced by a small synovial joint which is surrounded by a capsule, lined by synovial membrane and supported by dorsal and plantar ligaments.

Surface marking

The joint is marked by a line 1 cm long running from back to front, 1 cm forward and 1 cm lateral to the lateral side of the head of the talus.

Palpation

The joint is impossible to palpate.

Accessory movements

As in all syndesmoses, there is usually a very minimal amount of movement, and as this restriction of movement is its function there is little point in trying to move the joint.

The midtarsal joint [Fig. 3.14g and h]

This is a composite articulation of the talocalcaneo-navicular joint medially and the **calcaneocuboid joint** laterally. The two proximal bones are firmly united by the interosseous ligament in the sinus tarsi and the two distal bones are firmly united by the cuboideonavicular syndesmosis. The two joints are therefore considered to move as one unit, particularly in inversion and eversion of the foot.

Surface marking

The joint line can be marked across the dorsum of the foot by a line from just proximal to the tuberosity of the navicular medially to a point 1 cm proximal to the tip of the tubercle of the fifth metatarsal laterally (Fig. 3.14g, h).

Palpation

As in the separate joints above.

Accessory movements

As in the separate joints above.

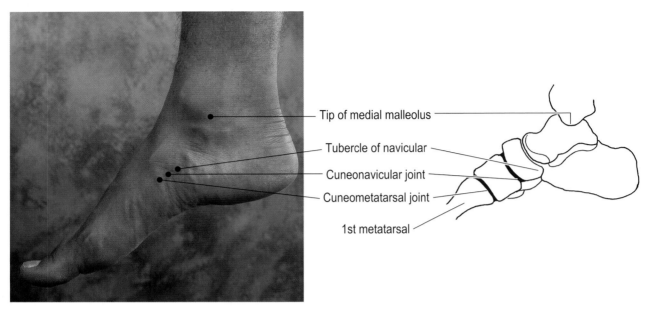

Fig. 3.14 (i), (j)
The cuneonavicular and cuneometatarsal joints of right foot (medial aspect)

The cuneonavicular and intercuneiform joints [Figs 3.14i,j and 3.15c,d]

The three cuneiform bones articulate proximally with the distal surface of the navicular by plane synovial joints. They are surrounded by a common capsule which is lined by synovial membrane and is supported by relatively weak dorsal and stronger plantar ligaments. The cuneiform bones are also bound together distally by interosseous ligaments.

Palpation

The cuneonavicular joint can be palpated on its medial and dorsal aspects just distal to the navicular tuberosity and, with care, can be traced across the foot between the extensor tendons, being slightly concave proximally (Fig. 3.14i, j).

The joints between the cuneiforms themselves, and between the lateral cuneiform and the cuboid, are extremely difficult to palpate, although the joint lines can be determined by following proximally from the first, second and third metatarsal bones (Fig. 3.15a, b).

Accessory movements

The joints between the navicular and the cuneiforms, as well as those between the cuneiforms themselves, are all plane synovial joints but as they also possess interosseous ligaments which bind the adjacent surfaces together, they possess very little movement. They can be moved passively by stabilizing the most proximal component with the fingers and thumb of one hand and gliding the distal component up and down with the other hand, the grip being similar to that used on the talocalcaneonavicular joint. Although only slight gliding is present at these joints, loss of this movement can lead to complete dysfunction of the foot.

The cuneocuboid joint is synovial but is also tightly bound together by an interosseous ligament, becoming, in part, a syndesmosis. Consequently, passive accessory movement between the two bones is virtually impossible.

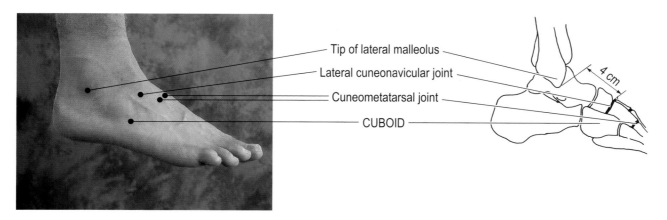

Fig. 3.15 (a), (b)
The cuneonavicular and cuneometatarsal joints of the right foot (lateral aspect)

The tarsometatarsal joints

The **tarsometatarsal joints** exist between the bases of the metatarsals and the cuneiform and cuboid bones. The first metatarsal articulates with the medial cuneiform bone, the second fits in between the medial and lateral cuneiforms with its base articulating with the middle, shorter, cuneiform, and the third metatarsal articulates with the lateral cuneiform. The fourth and fifth articulate with the cuboid. They are all plane synovial joints surrounded by a capsule which is lined with synovial membrane and supported by dorsal and plantar tarsometatarsal ligaments. There are also two or possibly three interosseous ligaments, two to the base of the second metatarsal as it fits into this mortice and the other between the lateral cuneiform to the fourth metatarsal.

Palpation and surface marking

The joint between the first metatarsal and the medial cuneiform can be palpated 2 cm distal to the navicular tuberosity. It can also be identified by following the first metatarsal proximally to where its base is marked by an expanded area. This line can be traced on to the dorsum of the foot, being crossed here by the tendon of extensor hallucis longus (Fig. 3.14i, j).

The joint between the second metatarsal and the middle cuneiform is extremely difficult to palpate as it is set more proximally between the medial and lateral cuneiforms. That between the third metatarsal and the lateral cuneiform, however, can be identified by following the line of the metatarsal to its base, which is slightly raised.

The same procedure will enable the joints between the fourth and fifth metatarsals and the cuboid to be identified. Its surface is marked by a line running laterally and proximally towards the tip of the tubercle on the fifth metatarsal (Figs 3.15a, b and 3.17a, b).

Accessory movements

With the model in supine lying, stand to the right of the right foot. With the cleft between your thumb and fingers of your left hand gripping the cuneiform bones and your right hand gripping the first metatarsal, movements up and down and even a little rotation can be obtained. There is a little movement obtained at these joints when the metatarsals are moved on each other (see Intermetatarsal joints, page 180).

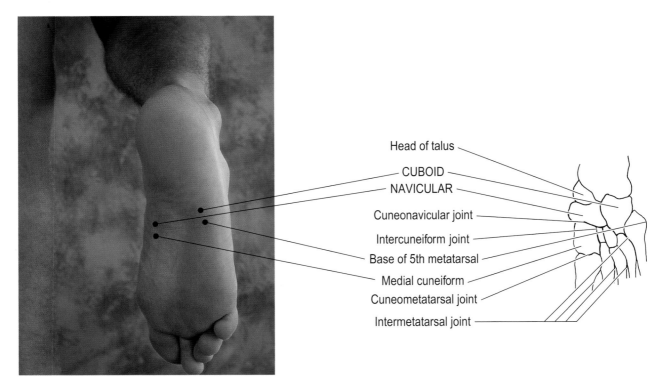

Fig. 3.15 (c), (d)
Joints of cuneiform bones and metatarsals of right foot, plantar aspect (not palpable)

The intermetatarsal joints [Fig. 3.15c–f]

These are four small synovial joints between the adjacent sides of the bases of the second to fifth metatarsal. They are surrounded by a capsule lined with synovial membrane and their joint space is continuous with that of the tarsometatarsal joints. The capsule is supported by a dorsal and plantar ligament and an interosseous ligament at its distal end. The base of the first metatarsal is connected to the base of the second by an interosseous ligament only.

Surface marking

From a line drawn across the dorsum of the foot from the base of the first metatarsal to the tubercle on the base of the fifth, the joints pass distally for 0.5 cm in line with the spaces between the second to fifth metatarsal.

Palpation

If a finger is placed between the metatarsals on the dorsum of the foot and drawn proximally, the space between them gradually narrows, with the bones eventually coming into contact with each other. These small plane joints run antero-posteriorly for approximately 0.5 cm, as far proximally as the line drawn across the dorsum of the foot from the base of the first metatarsal and the tubercle on the lateral side of the base of the fifth. That between the second and third metatarsals is slightly smaller due to the arrangement of the cuneiforms (Fig. 3.15e, f).

The interosseous ligament between the first and second metatarsals can be marked in a similar fashion.

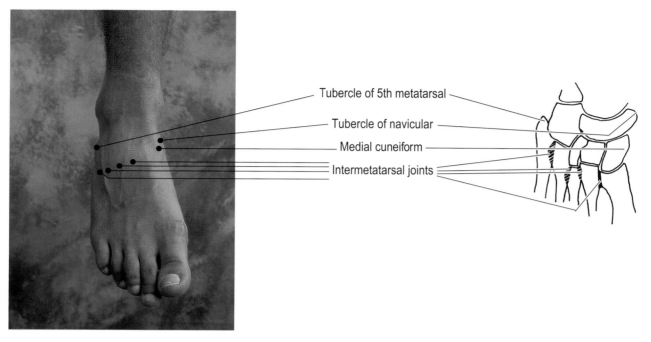

Fig. 3.15 (e), (f)
The intermetatarsal joints of right foot (dorsal aspect)

Accessory movements

Movement between the metatarsal bases and either the cuneiforms or the cuboid is virtually non-existent. Only slight movements can be produced, even when the metatarsals are used as levers. Obviously this also results in a slight gliding movement at the intermetatarsal joints. With the subject lying supine, grip one metatarsal head between the fingers and thumb of one hand and the adjacent head with the other hand, both thumbs being on the dorsum of the foot. Downward pressure on one metatarsal head, and upward pressure on the other, results in a small degree of movement. This small movement between the heads

creates an even smaller, but definite, movement between the bases. If the lateral metatarsal head is taken in one hand and the metatarsal of the great toe is taken in the other, a considerable forward and backward movement is achieved due to combined movement of all metatarsal bases.

Although there is no contact between the two metatarsal heads, they are joined to each other by the powerful deep transverse metatarsal ligament. Occasionally this may become shortened; movement of one metatarsal head against its neighbour will help to mobilize this region.

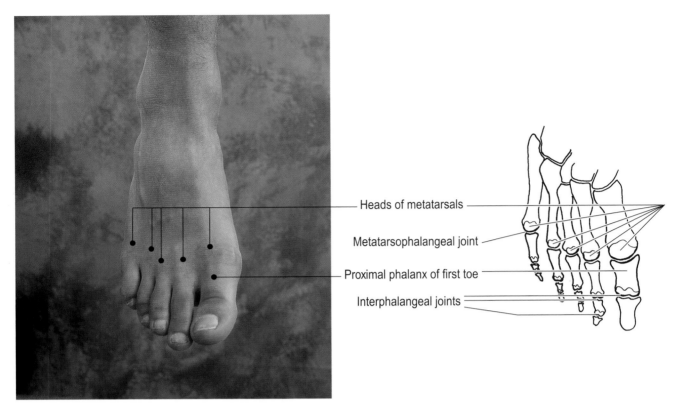

Fig. 3.16 (a), (b)
The metatarsophalangeal and interphalangeal joints of the right foot (dorsal aspect)

The metatarsophalangeal joints [Figs 3.16 and 3.17]

These joints exist between the smooth, rounded heads of the metatarsal bones and the shallow cavity on the base of the proximal phalange. They are synovial condyloid joints, surrounded by a fairly loose capsule which is lined with synovial membrane. The articular surface on the head of the metatarsal extends onto its dorsal, distal and particularly plantar surfaces. The capsule is supported by cord-like collateral and strong plantar ligaments. A deep transverse metatarsal ligament links all the plantar ligaments together, forming a strong link between the heads of the metatarsals while allowing some up-and-down movement to occur between them.

Surface marking

The metatarsophalangeal joints lie on a line drawn from just distal to the head of the first metatarsal to just distal to the head of the fifth metatarsal. The line is slightly convex forward at its centre.

Palpation

Grip the head of the first metatarsal between your fingers and thumb. Let them slide slightly forwards. The joint space can easily be identified on the medial and dorsal aspect just distal to the head. Although the under surface of the head is masked by a thick pad of fascia, the line of the joint can be traced with some difficulty.

If the lesser toes are strongly flexed, the heads of the metatarsals protrude on the dorsum of the foot. The joints can be palpated, with care, just beyond these heads. The tendons of extensor digitorum longus and brevis may have to be moved to the side. The joint of the fifth metatarsal can easily be palpated on its lateral side just beyond the head.

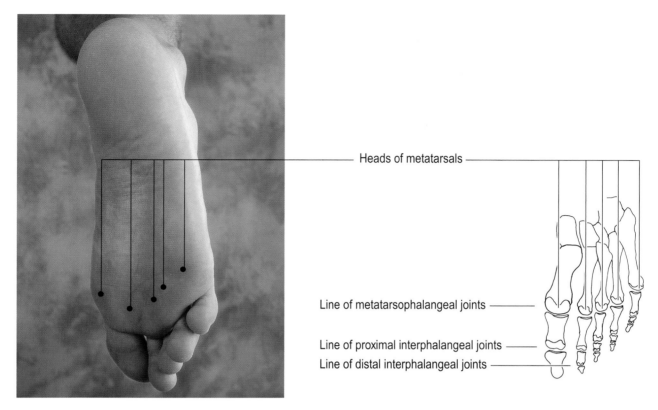

Fig. 3.16 (c), (d)
The metatarsophalangeal and interphalangeal joints of the right foot (plantar aspect)

With all the toes strongly extended, the joints can be identified from their plantar aspect but again they are partially masked by the thick fascia which covers them.

If the toes are rhythmically flexed and extended the proximal phalanges can be observed gliding over the heads of the metatarsals.

Accessory movements

Movement at the metatarsophalangeal joints is similar to that at the metacarpophalangeal joints of the hand, although a little more difficult to perform. These movements include rotation and a gliding of the proximal phalanx on the corresponding metatarsal head.

Grip the whole toe to be moved between the fingers and thumb of one hand, while stabilizing the remainder of the foot with the other. The toe can now be rotated about its long axis, and moved upwards, downwards and from side to side against the metatarsal head.

As in the case of many of the synovial joints with comparatively loose capsules, these joints can also be distracted, although not as much as the metacarpophalangeal joints of the hand and certainly not enough to cause the 'popping' sound that can be produced sometimes in the hand.

Stabilize the whole foot with one hand and grip the appropriate phalange with the fingers and thumb of the other. Now just apply a traction force on the phalange.

Although abduction and adduction is an active movement at these joints, it is often quite difficult to perform. This movement is easily obtainable, however, using the same technique as above and moving the phalange from side to side.

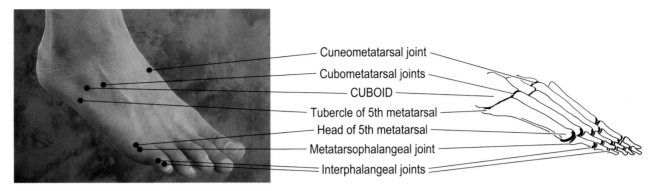

Fig. 3.17 (a), (b)
The metatarsophalangeal and interphalangeal joints of the right foot (lateral aspect)

The interphalangeal joints [Figs 3.16 and 3.17]

These joints exit between the proximal and middle, and middle and distal phalanges of each of the lesser toes. As there are only two phalanges in the great toe, there is only one interphalangeal joint. These joints are synovial hinge joints surrounded by a capsule which is lined with synovial membrane and supported by strong collateral and thick plantar ligaments. The plantar ligaments are composed of fibrocartilage and form part of the joint capsule.

At the distal end of each distal phalange the joint surface is replaced with the nail bed.

Palpation

On the second to fifth toes, the proximal interphalangeal joints are usually flexed so that the head of the proximal phalanx is easy to palpate. In many subjects it is marked by a small bursa on its dorsal aspect. These joints can be palpated as a faint, horizontal line just beyond this bicondylar head, particularly if the middle phalanx is gripped between the finger and thumb and gently moved forwards and backwards. The joint is difficult to palpate on its plantar aspect. The distal interphalangeal joint is usually hyperextended and, although the joint itself is difficult to feel, the movement available clearly marks its line, particularly when palpated from the plantar aspect (Figs 3.16c, d and 3.17).

The interphalangeal joint of the great toe can be palpated just beyond the head of the proximal phalanx, particularly when the toe is flexed, and again can be emphasized by moving the distal phalanx forwards and backwards in a similar fashion to the lesser toes (Fig. 3.16c, d).

Accessory movements

The interphalangeal joints are hinge joints. However, with the joint in slight flexion some side-to-side rocking of the joint can be produced.

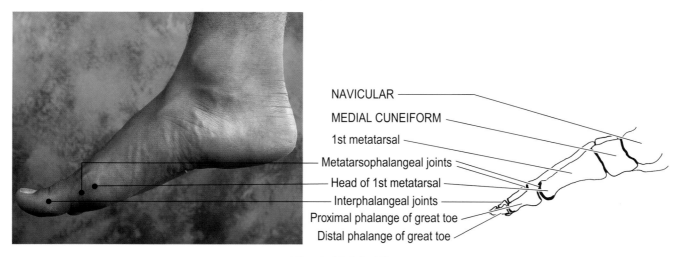

Fig. 3.17 (c), (d)
The metatarsophalangeal and interphalangeal joints of the right foot (medial aspect)

Grasp the proximal of the two phalanges between finger and thumb of one hand and the more distal in a similar grip with the other hand. The distal phalanx can now be moved from side to side.

The joints of the foot are generally more difficult to mark and palpate. They are, however, all important in the functions of the foot, especially locomotion. Stiffness of just one small joint may lead to severe pain and dysfunction. It is therefore important to be able to locate and mobilize all joints, noting the direction of their articular surfaces and the resultant shape of the part as a whole.

Most feet react favourably to fairly strong manipulative techniques being performed on them, and these combined with the correct strengthening and mobilizing exercises can improve function dramatically.

All the joints of the foot, including the ankle, contribute to the overall position and shape of the foot. This will vary considerably according to its function at the time, i.e. weight-bearing or non-weight-bearing, mobile or stationary. It is therefore important to examine the structure in as many varying positions as possible.

In the standing position, weight transference through the foot is worthy of close examination. Body weight is transmitted through the tibia to the talus and then via the longitudinal and transverse arches to the ground. The shape and position of the foot depend on where this downward force is applied to the arches and how the weight is distributed through the fore- and hind-foot to the ground. If the weight is applied too far to the medial side, the medial longitudinal arch becomes flattened, whereas if the weight is applied to the lateral side, the lateral longitudinal arch becomes flattened and the medial arch raised.

SELF ASSESSMENT

Page 156

1. Which surfaces take part in the sacroiliac joint?

2. Give the class and type of this joint.

3. Name the ligaments supporting the joint.

4. Which accessory ligaments support the joint?

5. What is the posterior surface marking of the sacroiliac joint?

6. How much movement is possible at this joint?

Page 157

7. Under normal circumstances, is the joint more mobile in young or elderly people?

8. Is the joint more mobile in males or females?

9. Why is it advantageous to have a slightly mobile pelvis?

10. Which movement is considered to be a normal physiological movement of the sacrum?

11. Describe the way in which a slight accessory movement of this joint may be produced.

Page 158

12. What class and type is the hip joint?

13. How extensive is the synovial membrane of the hip joint?

14. Name the ligaments which support the capsule.

15. Which internal ligaments help to support the hip joint?

16. Which ligament attaches to the rim of the acetabulum?

17. What is the anterior surface marking of the hip joint?

18. Give the posterior surface markings of the hip joint.

Page 159

19. Explain the technique for palpating this joint.

20. List the accessory movements which may be produced at the hip joint.

Please complete the labels below.

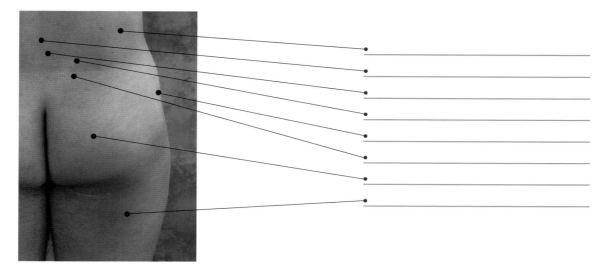

Fig. 3.8 (a) The right sacroiliac joint (posterior aspect)

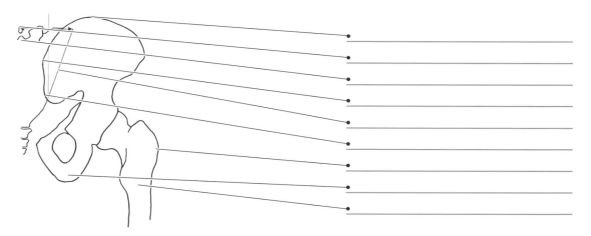

Fig. 3.8 (b) The right sacroiliac joint (posterior aspect)

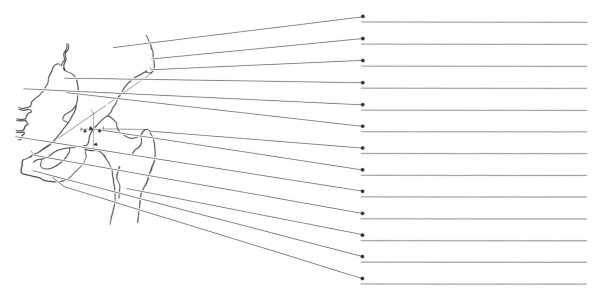

Fig. 3.9 (b) Bones of the left hip joint (anterior aspect)

SELF ASSESSMENT

Page 160

21. What is the class and type of the knee joint?

22. Which bones take part in this joint?

23. Describe the articular surfaces taking part in the knee joint.

24. List the movements that occur at this joint.

25. Describe the shape of the patella surface of the femur.

26. Which structures form the anterior part of the capsule?

27. Name the ligaments which support this joint externally.

28. Which internal ligaments support the joint?

29. Is this joint prone to dislocation?

Page 161

30. What is the surface marking of the knee joint?

31. Which structure can be palpated deep in the triangular spaces on either side of the ligamentum patellae?

32. Explain how slight movement of these structures can be produced.

33. Is it possible to palpate the knee joint from the posterior aspect?

34. What term is used to describe the position of the knee in full extension?

Page 162

35. Which accessory movements may be produced at the knee joint in the semiflexed position?

36. List the factors that limit these movements.

37. Which accessory movements can be produced at the patellofemoral joint when the knee is in full extension and the quadriceps muscles are relaxed?

Page 163

38. If violent force is applied to the anterior surface of the upper part of the tibia, which of the cruciate ligaments is put under stress?

39. Explain the mechanism by which the medial meniscus is usually damaged.

Please complete the labels below.

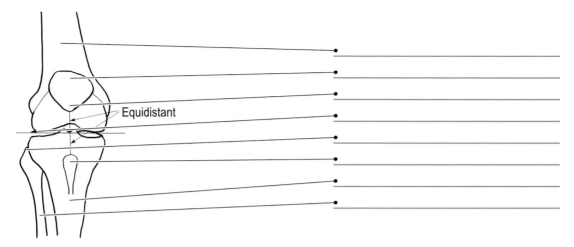

Fig. 3.10 (b) The right knee joint (anterior aspect)

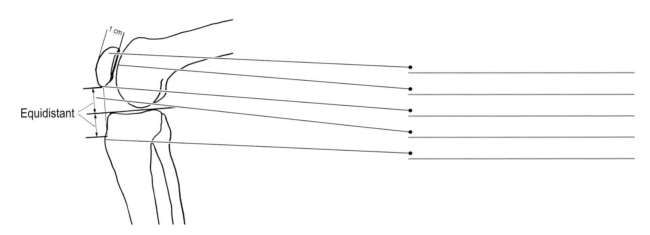

Fig. 3.10 (d) The right knee joint (medial aspect)

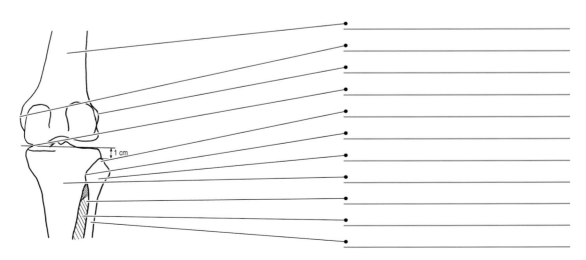

Fig. 3.10 (f) The right knee joint (posterior aspect)

SELF ASSESSMENT

Page 164

40. Name the joints which take place between the tibia and fibula.

41. What class and type is the superior tibiofibular joint?

42. Which ligaments support this joint?

43. What is the surface marking of the joint?

44. Which movement occurs at this joint during dorsiflexion and plantarflexion of the ankle joint?

45. Describe the accessory movements which can be performed at this joint.

Page 165

46. What is the class and type of the inferior tibiofibular joint?

47. What is the surface marking of this joint?

48. Name the very strong ligament which binds the two surfaces of the inferior joint together.

49. Which ligament of the inferior tibiofibular joint helps to form a socket for the ankle joint?

50. What structure binds the two shafts of the bones together?

51. In which direction do the fibres of this structure pass?

52. What term is used to describe the parting of the inferior tibiofibular joint caused by an injury? (fr)

Page 166

53. List the bones taking part in the ankle joint.

54. Describe the articular surfaces of these bones.

55. On which ligaments does the ankle joint depend for its stability?

56. Describe the extensive lower attachment of the ligament on the medial side of the joint.

57. What is the surface marking of the ankle joint?

Page 167

58. How much of this joint can be palpated?

59. Under what circumstances is the ankle joint described as 'close-packed'?

60. Which accessory movements can be produced at this joint and in what position?

Please complete the labels below.

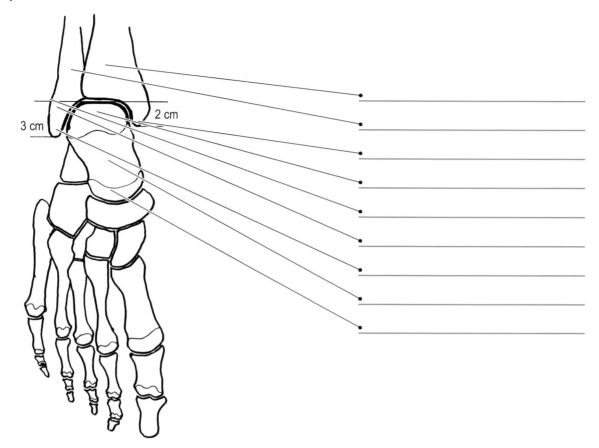

Fig. 3.12 (b) The right ankle joint (anterior aspect)

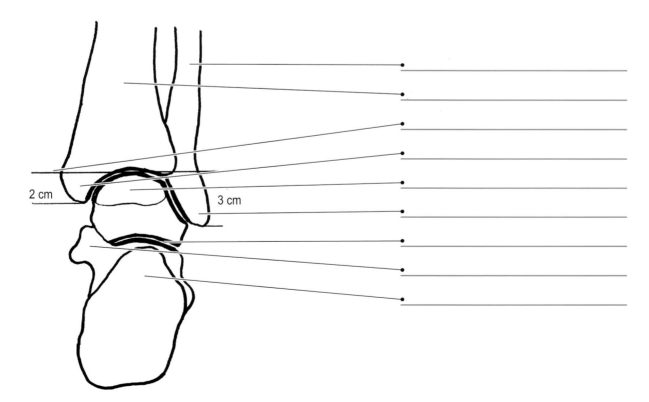

Fig. 3.12 (f) The right ankle joint (posterior aspect)

Page 170

61. List the different groups of joints in the foot.

62. Explain why it is difficult to palpate the joints of the foot from below.

63. Which surface of the talus takes part in the talocalcaneal joint?

64. Which surface of the calcaneus takes part in this joint?

65. On which ligaments does this joint rely for its support?

66. Describe the sinus tarsi.

67. What is the surface marking for the talocalcaneal joint?

68. Which surface of the sustentaculum tali is articular?

69. Name the bone which articulates with this surface.

Page 171

70. Which accessory movements may be produced at the talocalcaneal joint?

71. Describe the position of the hands used to obtain these movements.

Page 174

72. What is the class and type of the talocalcaneonavicular joint?

73. Which bony surfaces take part in this joint?

74. Name the ligaments which support the talocalcaneonavicular joint.

75. By what alternative name is the inferior ligament of this joint known?

76. What is the surface marking for the talocalcaneonavicular joint?

Page 175

77. How far, anteroinferiorly, is the tubercle of the navicular from the tip of the medial malleolus?

78. Which tendons may have to be moved aside to palpate the line of the joint?

79. Describe the accessory movements which can be produced at this joint.

Please complete the labels below.

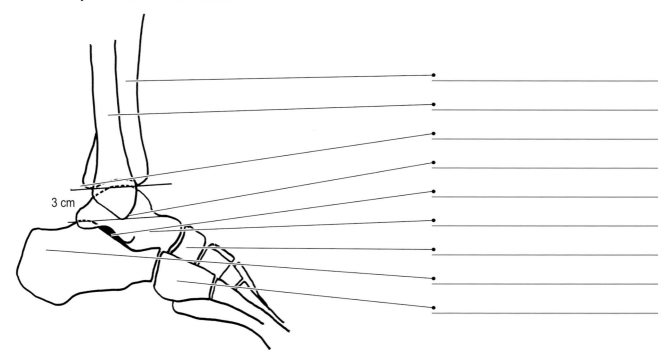

Fig. 3.13 (b) The talocalcaneal (subtalar) and ankle joint of the right foot (lateral aspect)

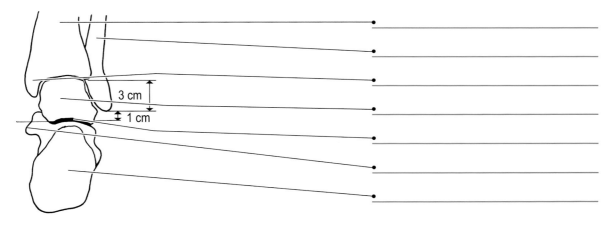

Fig. 3.13 (f) The talocalcaneal (subtalar) joint (posterior aspect)

Page 176

80. What is the classification and type the calcaneocuboid joint?

_____

81. Which surfaces take part in this joint?

_____

82. Which ligaments support this joint?

_____

83. What are the surface markings for the joint?

_____

Page 177

84. Give the classification of the cuboideonavicular joint.

_____

85. What is the surface marking of this joint?

_____

86. List the joints which are involved in the midtarsal articulation.

_____

87. What is the surface marking of this joint?

_____

Page 178

88. What class and type are the cuneonavicular and intercuneiform joints?

_____

89. Decribe how the cuneiform bones are bound together distally.

_____

90. With which structure do the three cuneiform bones articulate proximally.

_____

91. How much movement occurs between the cuneiform bones?

_____

Page 179

92. Which is the shortest of the three cuneiform bones?

_____

93. Which metatarsal bone articulates with all three cuneiform bones?

_____

94. With which bones do the 4th and 5th metatarsals articulate proximally?

_____

95. Name the ligaments supporting these joints.

_____

96. What is the surface marking of the tarsometatarsal joints?

_____

Please complete the labels below.

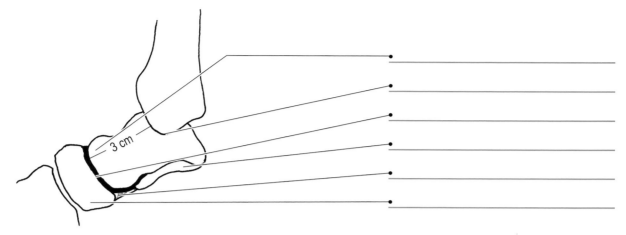

Fig. 3.14 (b) The talocalcaneonavicular joint of right foot (medial aspect)

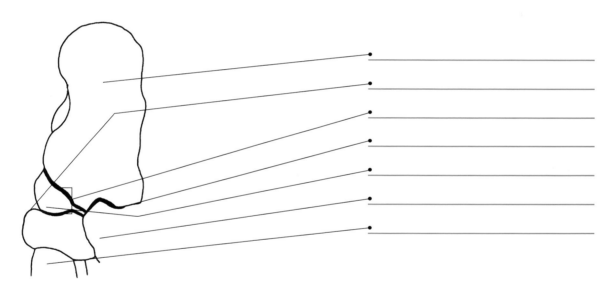

Fig. 3.14 (f) The talocalcaneonavicular and calcaneocuboid joint of right foot (plantar aspect)

Page 180

97. What is the classification and type of the intermetatarsal joints?

98. In which area are these joints located?

Page 181

99. Describe the way in which a limited amount of accessory movement can be produced at these joints.

100. What structure links the metatarsal heads together?

Page 182

101. What is the classification and type of the metatarsophalangeal joints?

102. Describe the articular surfaces taking part in these joints.

103. Name the ligaments which support these joints.

104. What are the surface markings of the metatarsophalangeal joints?

Page 183

105. Which accessory movements can be produced at these joints?

106. Name and describe a common deformity found at the first metatarsophalangeal joint. (fr)

Page 184

107. What is the classification and type of the interphalangeal joints?

108. Which ligaments support these joints?

109. Which accessory movements may be produced at these joints?

Page 185

110. Name and describe a common deformity found in the lesser toes. (fr)

111. Describe the way in which weight is distributed through the foot to the ground.

Please complete the labels below.

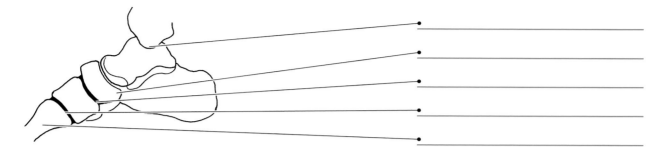

Fig. 3.14 (j) The cuneonavicular and cuneometatarsal joints of right foot (medial aspect)

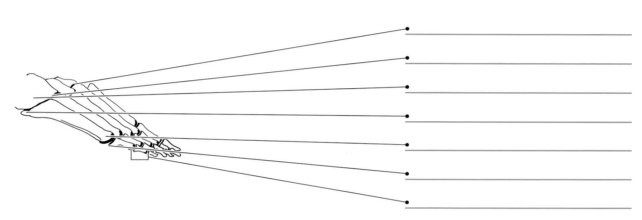

Fig. 3.17 (b) The metatarsophalangeal and interphalangeal joints of the right foot (lateral aspect)

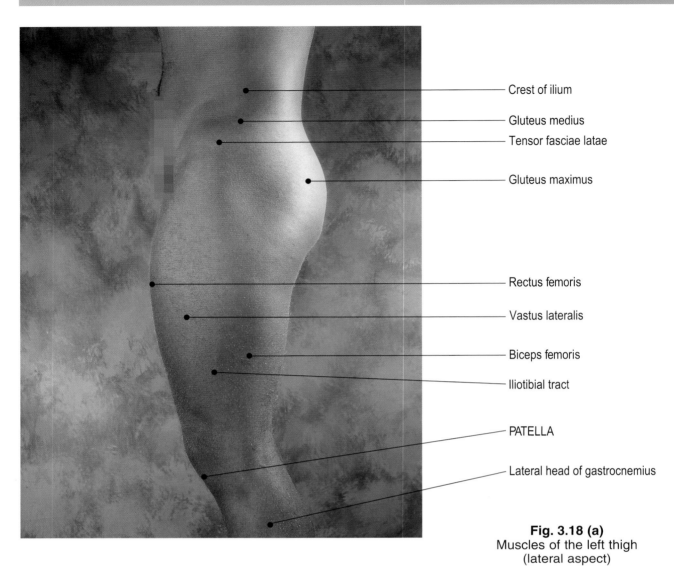

Crest of ilium

Gluteus medius

Tensor fasciae latae

Gluteus maximus

Rectus femoris

Vastus lateralis

Biceps femoris

Iliotibial tract

PATELLA

Lateral head of gastrocnemius

Fig. 3.18 (a)
Muscles of the left thigh
(lateral aspect)

MUSCLES

The lateral and anterior aspect of the hip

Gluteus medius, *gluteus minimus and tensor fasciae latae*

On the lateral aspect of the ilium, just anterior and deep to gluteus maximus, between the most lateral part of the iliac crest and the greater trochanter of the femur, gluteus medius can be located (Fig. 3.18a, b). It is covered by strong, thick fascia, but can, nevertheless, be felt contracting and relaxing when either, in standing, the weight is transferred from one leg to the other, the muscle preventing the pelvis dropping to the opposite side, or, in side lying, when the limb is raised and lowered. Anterior to gluteus medius, the bulk of gluteus minimus, covered by the tensor fasciae latae (Fig. 3.18a, b), is readily palpable between the anterior section of the iliac crest and the greater trochanter. The contraction of these two muscles is produced in lying or standing when the foot is medially rotated, as in the weight-bearing phase of walking when the lower limb is moving into

extension and medial rotation, just before the thrust phase produced by the gastrocnemius.

It is important to practise the palpation of these muscles, gluteus maximus, medius, minimus and tensor fasciae latae, in the subject or patient during ambulation. Much information can be gained from this region regarding the relationships of the bony structures and the power and timing of muscle contraction. As noted above, the gluteus medius should contract on the weight-bearing limb to prevent the pelvis dropping to the other side when the foot is raised from the ground. Therefore, the distance between the iliac crest and the greater trochanter of the femur, on the weight-bearing limb, should remain the same or even decrease slightly.

It is also worth noting, through palpation of these muscles, that as the weight-bearing limb

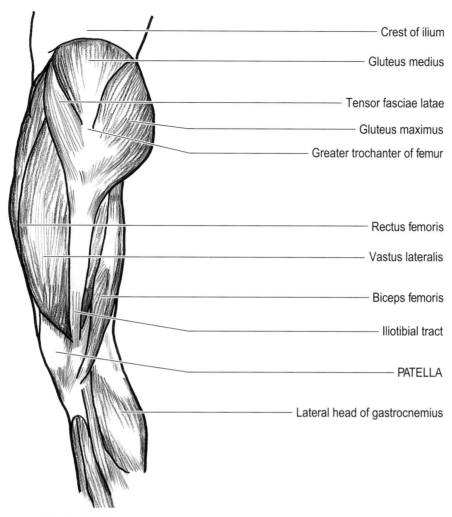

— Crest of ilium

— Gluteus medius

— Tensor fasciae latae

— Gluteus maximus

— Greater trochanter of femur

— Rectus femoris

— Vastus lateralis

— Biceps femoris

— Iliotibial tract

— PATELLA

Lateral head of gastrocnemius —

Fig. 3.18 (b)
Muscles of the left thigh
(lateral aspect)

moves from the flexed to the extended position, the muscles appear to contract in sequence from posterior to anterior. As the heel comes in contact with the ground, the limb is in lateral rotation and the posterior section of gluteus medius and possibly gluteus maximus are contracted. As the hip moves forwards over the foot, the middle of gluteus medius can be felt contracting, and as the limb moves into extension and medial rotation, the anterior section of gluteus medius, gluteus minimus and tensor fasciae latae are contracted. During this sequence, the pelvis will rotate around the weight-bearing hip joint towards the weight-bearing side. Finally, it is worth noting that immediately the limb is weight-bearing, the gluteus medius contracts.

Dysfunction of the hip joint may upset the precise *firing off* of these muscles.

Iliopsoas and pectineus

The front of the hip joint is crossed by iliopsoas and pectineus, the former being a broad tendon and the latter a quadrilateral muscle. Because they are both covered by several layers of fascia, as well as the femoral sheath and its contents, they are difficult to palpate (see Fig. 3.20a, b).

Palpation

With the subject lying supine and both the hip and knee supported and flexed to 90°, place your fingers on the anterior aspect of the hip joint 3.5 cm below the centre of the inguinal ligament. If the subject now gently flexes and extends the hip joint, the contraction of both iliopsoas laterally and pectineus medially can be palpated.

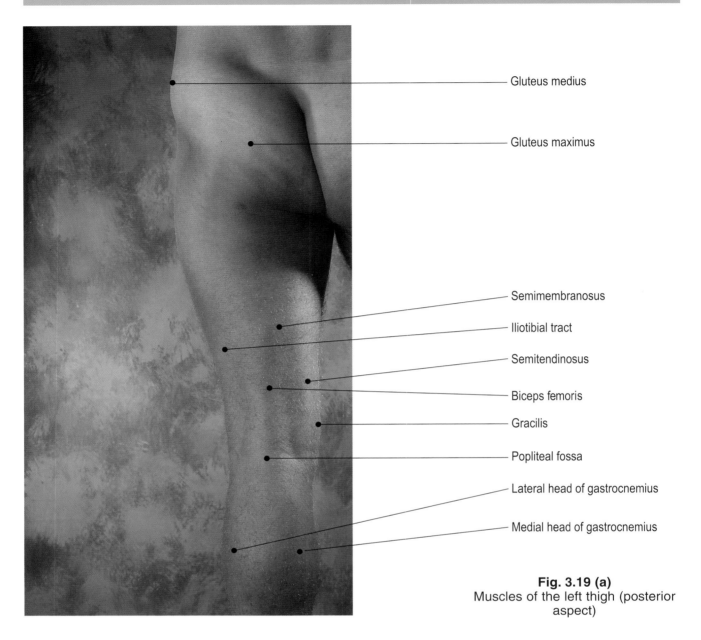

Gluteus medius

Gluteus maximus

Semimembranosus

Iliotibial tract

Semitendinosus

Biceps femoris

Gracilis

Popliteal fossa

Lateral head of gastrocnemius

Medial head of gastrocnemius

Fig. 3.19 (a)
Muscles of the left thigh (posterior aspect)

The posterior aspect of the hip and thigh

Gluteus maximus

The extremely well-developed muscles around the hip joint are the gluteal muscles, especially the gluteus maximus, which is important in maintaining the upright posture. It is a large and powerful muscle, giving the gluteal region its rounded shape.

Gluteus maximus (Figs 3.18 and 3.19) lies between the posterior part of the iliac crest superiorly, the anal cleft medially and the gluteal fold inferiorly. With care, its coarse fibres can be traced running downwards and laterally towards the greater trochanter of the femur. It is often possible, especially with the hip extended, to trace the more superficial fibres to their attachment into the fascia lata (iliotibial tract). The extent of the muscle is made clearer if the subject extends the hip when lying prone.

The hamstrings

Below the gluteal fold the hamstrings are evident. These powerful muscles cover the whole of the back of the thigh. Semitendinosus and semi-membranosus pass downwards and medially, with the biceps crossing to lie laterally as it passes down to the knee. The muscle bellies of the hamstrings separate approximately two-thirds of the way down the thigh, giving rise to their tendons – semitendinosus and semimembranosus medially and biceps femoris laterally (Fig. 3.19).

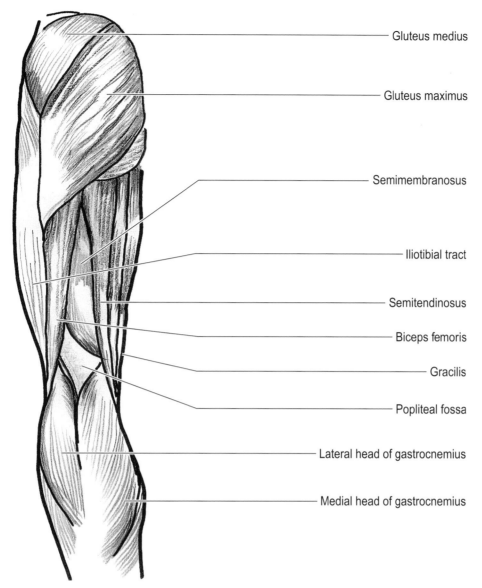

- Gluteus medius
- Gluteus maximus
- Semimembranosus
- Iliotibial tract
- Semitendinosus
- Biceps femoris
- Gracilis
- Popliteal fossa
- Lateral head of gastrocnemius
- Medial head of gastrocnemius

Fig. 3.19 (b)
Muscles of the left thigh (posterior aspect)

Palpation

With the subject lying prone and flexing the knee against resistance, the tendon of biceps femoris stands clear on the posterolateral side of the knee, and can be traced to its insertion to the head of the fibula. Proximally the superficial fusiform muscle belly can be followed towards the ischial tuberosity (Fig. 3.2). The deeper fibres of biceps femoris can be palpated on the medial side of the tendon in the upper part of the popliteal fossa. The tendon of semitendinosus can be observed, and palpated, on the posteromedial side of the knee joint as it passes downwards to its attachment on the medial surface of the tibial condyle and shaft. Proximally, its fusiform muscle belly joins that of biceps femoris near the gluteal fold. A slightly thinner tendon, lying anteromedial, can be identified. This is the tendon of gracilis whose muscle belly can be traced up the medial side of the thigh as far as the body of the pubis, particularly when the knee is flexed against resistance. Semimembranosus lies deep to semitendinosus just above the knee. It is difficult to palpate, even at its distal end, because it attaches, via a broad aponeurosis, to the posteromedial aspect of the medial condyle of the tibia.

With the knee supported in approximately 60° of flexion, press your fingertips and thumb into the space on either side of the semitendinosus tendon approximately 5 cm above the level of the knee joint. As the subject gently flexes and extends the knee, the muscle below can be felt contracting and then relaxing.

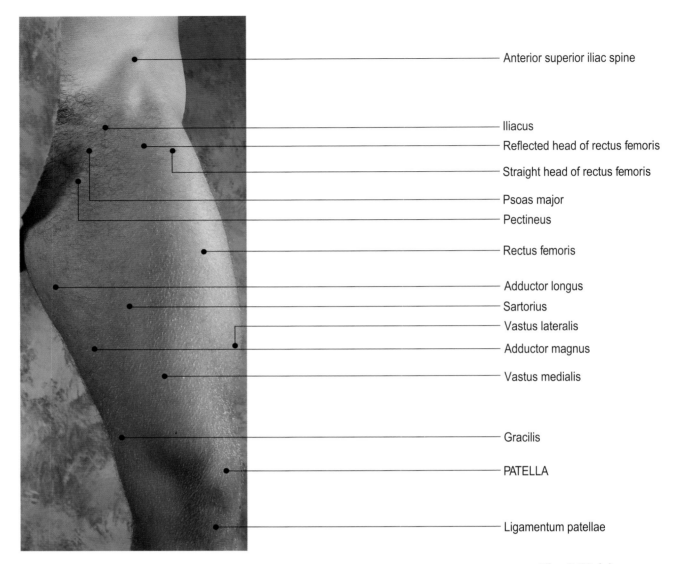

Anterior superior iliac spine

Iliacus

Reflected head of rectus femoris

Straight head of rectus femoris

Psoas major

Pectineus

Rectus femoris

Adductor longus

Sartorius

Vastus lateralis

Adductor magnus

Vastus medialis

Gracilis

PATELLA

Ligamentum patellae

Fig. 3.20 (a)
Muscles of the left thigh (medial aspect)

The anterior and medial aspects of the thigh

The adductors and quadriceps femoris

If the thigh is now adducted, the adductor group of muscles comes into action. The following can be palpated: the tendinous part of adductor magnus running down the medial aspect of the thigh from the ischial tuberosity to the adductor tubercle, adductor longus lying anteriorly and laterally with adductor brevis and the aponeurotic part of adductor magnus lying more posteriorly. However, it is difficult to identify the adductor muscles separately.

The great bulk of muscle on the front of the thigh is the quadriceps femoris, consisting of vastus medialis, vastus intermedius, vastus lateralis and rectus femoris. It extends from the anterior inferior iliac spine and above the acetabulum (the attachment of the rectus femoris) via the patella to the tibial tuberosity (Fig. 3.20).

Palpation

Three of the four bellies of quadriceps femoris can readily be palpated when the knee is extended against resistance. The belly of the vastus intermedius lies deep to the other three and is difficult to identify separately.

Rectus femoris passes straight down the front of the thigh from the anterior inferior iliac spine to the base of the patella. Its proximal and distal tendons can clearly be identified. Its belly appears as a fusiform shape on the front of the thigh.

The belly of vastus lateralis can be identified halfway down the lateral surface of the thigh, being flattened posteriorly by the fascia lata iliotibial tract (Fig. 3.18).

Vastus medialis can be identified on the medial side of the thigh just above the level of the patella. It varies considerably in size according to its use and is the first part of the quadriceps to show signs of weakness. Its lowest fibres can be traced

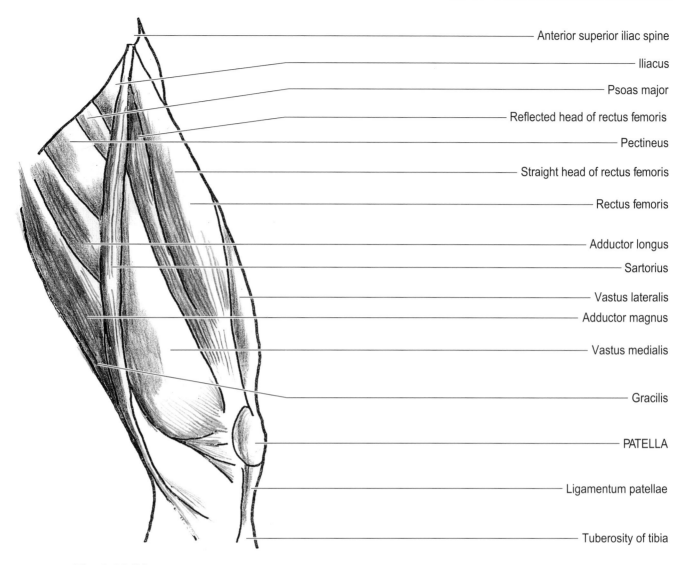

Anterior superior iliac spine

Iliacus

Psoas major

Reflected head of rectus femoris

Pectineus

Straight head of rectus femoris

Rectus femoris

Adductor longus

Sartorius

Vastus lateralis

Adductor magnus

Vastus medialis

Gracilis

PATELLA

Ligamentum patellae

Tuberosity of tibia

Fig. 3.20 (b)
Muscles of the left thigh (medial
aspect)

running almost horizontally and laterally to attach to the medial border of the patella.

The tendon of the quadriceps, particularly of rectus femoris and vastus intermedius, can be identified attaching to the upper border of the patella. There are often small depressions on its medial and lateral edges where it joins the expansion of vastus lateralis and vastus medialis. The patella is a sesamoid bone and lies within the tendon of quadriceps femoris, the ligamentum patellae being a continuation of the quadriceps tendon (Fig. 3.20). The ligamentum patellae joins the apex of the patella to the upper part of the tibial tuberosity. It is approximately 5 cm long and 2 cm wide, with its central point level with the knee joint (see pages 161 and 163). When the knee is fully extended, a strong tendon-like structure can be palpated lying lateral to the patella and running down to attach to the lateral tibial condyle

(Fig. 3.21a,b). This is the lower part of the iliotibial tract, and can be traced superiorly along the lateral side of the thigh to the ilium.

Sartorius

With the subject lying supine, resist the movement of flexion, lateral rotation, abduction of the hip and flexion of the knee by applying resistance to the heel. The long strap-like sartorius muscle can be observed and palpated, crossing the thigh from the anterior superior iliac spine above to the medial condyle of the tibia below (Fig. 3.20). Its upper third appears to stand away from the groin region. With the subject sitting with the knees extended, contraction of both muscles simultaneously produces the 'tailor sitting' position. Sartorius [*sartor* (L) = tailor] can be observed and palpated during this action.

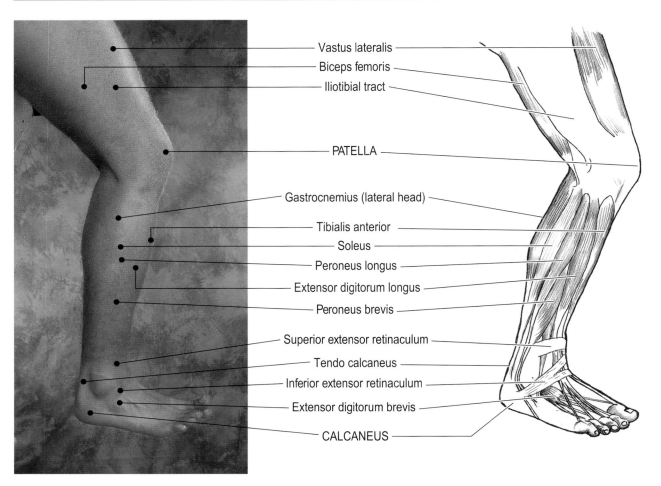

Fig. 3.21 (a), (b)
Muscles of the right leg (lateral aspect)

The anterior and lateral aspect of the leg and foot

The muscles in the anterior compartment of the leg are somewhat easier to identify than those in the corresponding aspect of the forearm. Even so, differentiation is easiest where the tendons pass over the front of the ankle joint. Consequently, palpation should begin here.

Tibialis anterior

With the subject lying supine and the foot dorsi-flexed, find the most medial tendon, that of tibialis anterior (Fig. 3.21). Although it lies deep to the superior and inferior extensor retinacula, it is clear to see and feel. Distally it can be traced to its insertion on the medial cuneiform and base of the first metatarsal. Proximally, the strong tendon gives way to a firm but narrow muscle which fills the space lateral to the anterior border of the tibia. The muscle is contained within strong fascia and becomes particularly hard on contraction. There is often a narrow space between the muscle and the tibia anteriorly.

Extensor hallucis longus

The tendon lying lateral to tibialis anterior at the ankle joint is that of extensor hallucis longus (Fig. 3.21c, d). It also stands clear of the joint and can be traced across the medial side of the foot to the great toe where, if the toe is extended, it can be followed to its insertion into the base of the distal phalanx. Proximally, the tendon is soon lost between the other muscles; however, if the line of the tendon is continued to the middle of the fibula, the muscle can be felt contracting deep to extensor digitorum longus.

Extensor digitorum longus

Lateral to the tendon of extensor hallucis longus lies the tendon of extensor digitorum longus (Fig. 3.21a–d). Immediately distal to the ankle it can be seen dividing into four separate tendons, which can be traced to the dorsal surface of the lateral four toes. Occasionally, when the toes are flexed at the metatarsophalangeal joint, the tendons can be felt and seen to 'bowstring' across the joint. Proximally, the tendon soon becomes muscular,

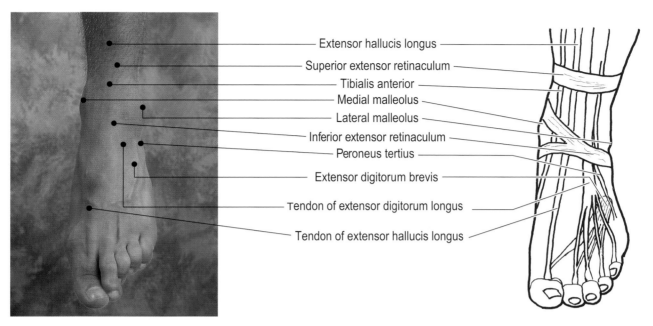

Fig. 3.21 (c), (d)
Tendons and muscles of the left foot (dorsal aspect)

extending superiorly as far as the superior tibio-fibular joint, lying between tibialis anterior medially and the fibula laterally.

Peroneus tertius

Although this small muscle is named as one of the peroneal muscles, peroneus tertius is considered to be part of the extensor digitorum longus, in fact its fifth tendon. This may be borne out as it does arise from the lower third of the fibula in line with, and does pass under, the superior extensor retinaculum and through the loop of the inferior retinaculum, with, and lateral to, the extensor digitorum longus. However, unlike the extensor digitorum longus, it does not insert into the digits but into the medial side of the dorsal surface of the base of the fifth metatarsal. In a small percentage of subjects the muscle is absent.

The tendon of the peroneus tertius is difficult to find, but is best located as it crosses the lateral part of the dorsum of the foot on its way to attach

to the medial side of the base of the fifth metatarsal (Fig. 3.21c, d).

Palpation

From the base of the fifth metatarsal, draw a line from its medial side towards the lower quarter of the shaft of the fibula. It is along this line that the tendon is most likely to be palpated, particularly when the foot is everted.

Extensor digitorum brevis

Extensor digitorum brevis presents as a large swelling some 2 cm anterior to the lateral malleolus on the dorsolateral aspect of the foot (Fig. 3.21). Four narrow tendons can be palpated, leaving its distal aspect passing towards the medial four toes. In the second, third and fourth toes the tendons join those of extensor digitorum longus, while in the great toe the tendon passes to the lateral side of the proximal phalanx.

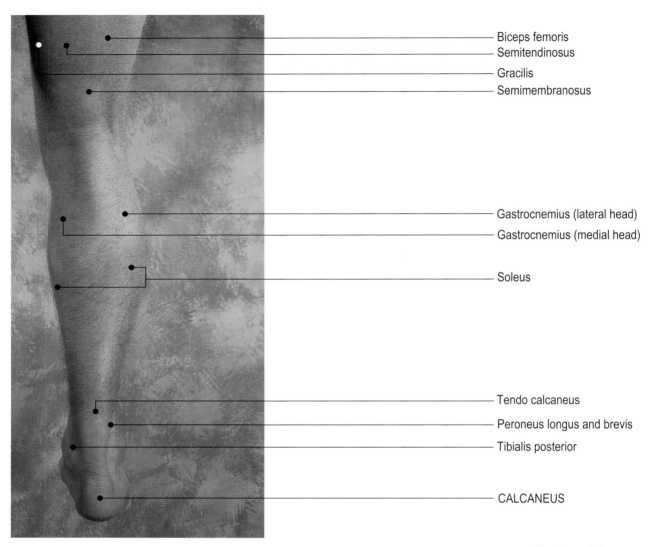

Biceps femoris
Semitendinosus
Gracilis
Semimembranosus

Gastrocnemius (lateral head)
Gastrocnemius (medial head)

Soleus

Tendo calcaneus
Peroneus longus and brevis
Tibialis posterior

CALCANEUS

Fig. 3.22 (a)
Muscles of the right leg and foot
(posterior aspect)

The posterior and plantar aspects of the leg and foot

Popliteus

Popliteus lies deep within the popliteal fossa high up on the posterolateral aspect of the knee joint. Its tendon, however, can be palpated as it passes below the lateral epicondyle of the femur. With the subject sitting and the knee flexed 90°, place the tips of your fingers on the lateral surface of the femoral condyle just below and in front of the lateral epicondyle. If medial rotation of the leg at the knee joint is now performed, the tendon of popliteus can be palpated as it runs forwards, in a groove, towards its femoral attachment.

Triceps surae (calf)

The posterior aspect of the leg is dominated by the beautifully shaped calf muscles gastrocnemius and soleus, the former being more superficial and the latter deep. Together they are attached distally by the tendo calcaneus to the posterior surface of the calcaneus. The two muscles, however, arise from different bones. The gastrocnemius from the femur, its medial head from the upper part of the medial condyle and the lateral head from just above the lateral epicondyle. The soleus, which is believed to derive its name from a flat fish, the sole, arises below the knee joint from the posterior surfaces of the tibia, fibula and interosseous membrane.

Plantaris, when present, passes lateral to medial, from the upper part of the lateral condyle of the femur downwards, between gastrocnemius and soleus to attach adjacent to the tendo calcaneus.

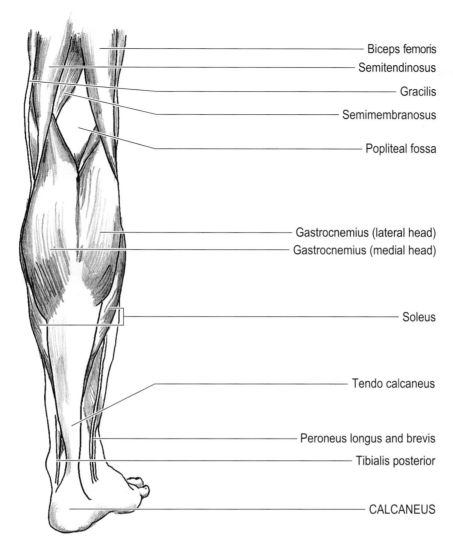

Biceps femoris
Semitendinosus
Gracilis
Semimembranosus
Popliteal fossa

Gastrocnemius (lateral head)
Gastrocnemius (medial head)

Soleus

Tendo calcaneus

Peroneus longus and brevis
Tibialis posterior

CALCANEUS

Fig. 3.22 (b)
Muscles of the right leg and foot
(posterior aspect)

Palpation

With the subject standing, begin at the posterior aspect of the heel, where the broad tendo calcaneus can easily be identified attaching to the calcaneus. Follow the tendon upwards for some 8 cm as it narrows to a width of approximately 1 cm, after which it rapidly widens into an aponeurosis about 8 cm wide. Here the muscle fibres of gastrocnemius can be palpated attaching to the superficial surface of the aponeurosis. Two large bellies, the medial and longer belly, stretch to the medial femoral condyle, and the lateral belly to the lateral femoral condyle (Fig. 3.22). The two bellies are separated by a faint vertical line which is easily palpable in a well-developed calf.

Soleus lies deep to gastrocnemius, its fibres contributing to the deep surface of the tendo calcaneus. Its upper attachment is to the posterior aspect of the tibia (soleal line) and to the head and shaft of the fibula. The muscle belly is broad and thick. As soleus is primarily a postural muscle,

preventing the tibia from tilting forwards in the standing position, it is easier to palpate when the subject is standing.

First locate the broad aponeurosis of the tendo calcaneus where it joins the muscle fibres of gastrocnemius, and run your fingers to the outer borders. Immediately adjacent is the muscle belly of soleus bulging either side and deep to the aponeurosis (Fig. 3.22). If the subject gently raises the heel, the muscle fibres of gastrocnemius can be felt contracting.

If the subject then fully flexes the knee and plantarflexes the foot, soleus can be felt contracting while gastrocnemius remains relaxed. This is because the upper (femoral) and lower (calcaneal) attachments of gastrocnemius are brought closer together, shortening the muscle and essentially preventing it from contracting. This is known as 'muscle insufficiency'.

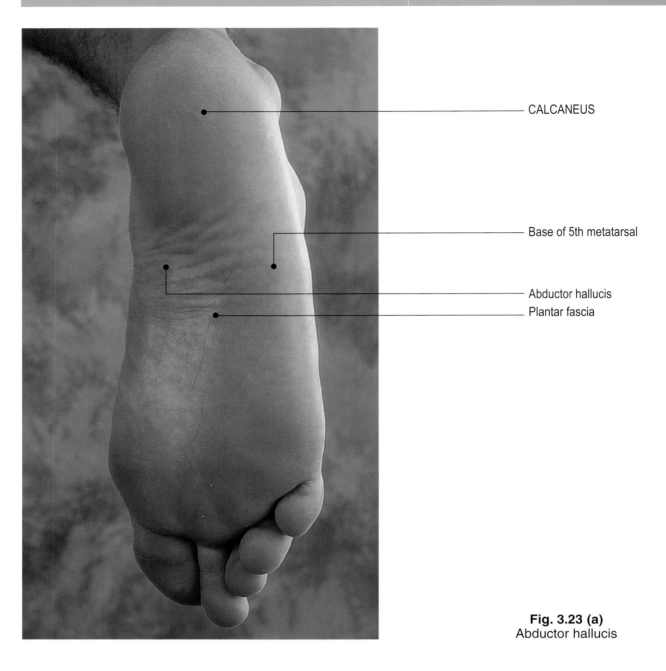

CALCANEUS

Base of 5th metatarsal

Abductor hallucis
Plantar fascia

Fig. 3.23 (a)
Abductor hallucis

Plantar muscles [Fig. 3.23]

The plantar surface of the foot is covered centrally by a thick dense layer of fascia known as the plantar aponeurosis. This is triangular in shape, being narrower posteriorly, where it attaches to the calcaneus, and broader anteriorly, where it splits to attach either side of the proximal phalanx of each toe. It gives the central portion of the plantar aspect a pale appearance, the heel, lateral border and under the metatarsal heads being darker and covered with harder skin for weight-bearing.

The plantar muscles are arranged in four layers deep to the plantar fascia, and are relatively easily recognized on dissection. The deepest muscles are the shortest, whereas those just deep to the plantar aponeurosis are the longest. All of these muscles except abductor hallucis are difficult to palpate due to the thickness and tension of the fascia.

Palpation

Only abductor hallucis is easily recognizable on the medial side of the foot. Some subjects may be able to abduct their great toe, in which case the belly of abductor hallucis can be palpated along the medial border of the foot. The broad fusiform-shaped muscle belly passes forwards from the medial tubercle of the calcaneus, continuing as a tendon to the medial side of the proximal phalange of the great toe.

If the subject is unable to abduct the great toe (really more of a party trick than anything else), shortening the foot while weight-bearing produces a powerful contraction of the muscle. This is most probably the muscle's main functional activity. The bulk of the muscle is palpated in its posterior section, with the relatively thick tendon distinct in its anterior half inserting into the medial side of

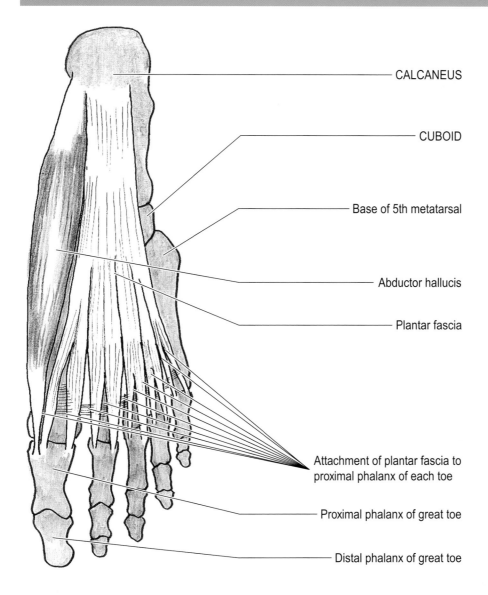

Fig. 3.23 (b)
Abductor hallux and plantar fascia of
the right foot (plantar aspect)

the base of the proximal phalanx of the great toe. If the toe is extended, the medial edge of the plantar fascia can be palpated as it is being stretched.

The use and type of footwear, if any, habitually worn, together with the activities and weight of the subject, will influence the structure and appearance of the foot. There is usually a thickening of the fascia and hardening of the skin over weight-bearing areas, these normally being over the heel, lateral border of the foot and heads of the metatarsals, particularly the first and fifth.

The amount of the sole of the foot which is in contact with the supporting surface is inversely proportional to the height of the plantar arches. The medial side of the foot is rarely in contact with the ground, except in subjects with extremely flat feet. Anteriorly, the metatarsal heads are normally in contact with the ground and may show a downward convexity, producing areas of hardened skin (callus), under the second, third and fourth metatarsal heads.

SELF ASSESSEMENT

Page 198

1. Describe the location of the gluteus medius.

2. In what area of the body can its contraction be felt?

3. What tissue covers the gluteus medius?

4. Give the attachments of this muscle proximally. (fr)

5. Where does it attach inferiorly? (fr).

6. In standing, which gluteus medius muscle contracts strongly when the left leg is raised from the floor?

7. Which two muscles lie anterior to the gluteus medius?

8. How can these two muscles be brought into action?

Page 199

9. When the weight-bearing lower limb is moving from flexion to extension, in which direction does the hip joint rotate?

10. How may dysfunction of the hip joint affect the surrounding muscles? (fr).

11. Which two muscles pass across the anterior aspect of the hip joint?

12. Explain why these two muscles are difficult to palpate.

13. Describe a technique whereby these muscles may be palpated.

14. Name one structure that lies in front of these muscles.

Page 200

15. In which area of the body is the gluteus maximus muscle located?

16. Name an important function of the gluteus maximus.

17. For which type of fibres is this muscle particularly noted?

18. In which direction do these fibres pass?

19. Where does the gluteus maximus muscle attach distally?

Please complete the labels below.

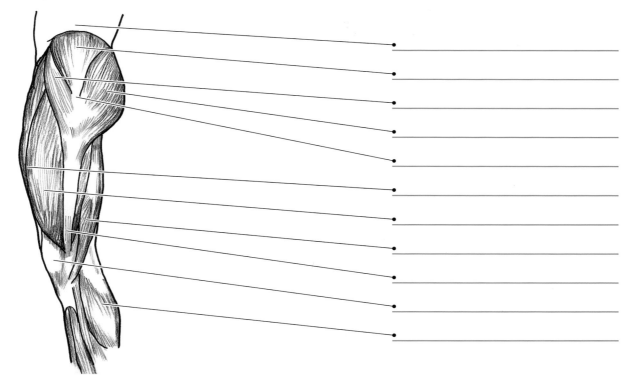

Fig. 3.18 (b) Muscles of the left thigh (lateral aspect)

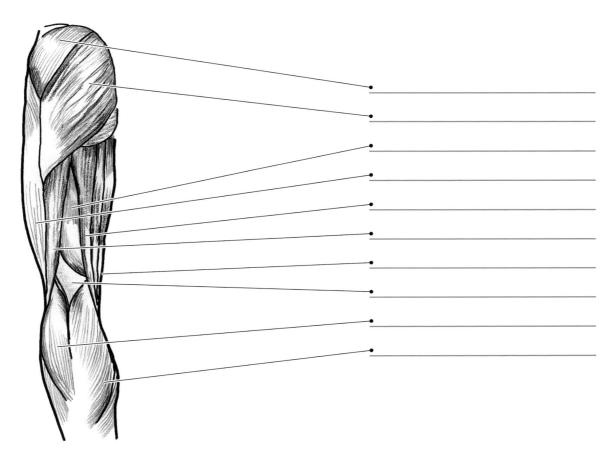

Fig. 3.19 (b) Muscles of the left thigh (posterior aspect)

20. Describe the way in which this muscle may be put into action.

21. In which area of the body are the hamstring muscles located?

22. List the muscles which comprise the hamstrings.

23. Which of these muscles pass downwards and medially?

24. Name the hamstring muscle which passes downwards and laterally.

25. How far down the thigh do the bellies of the hamstrings separate?

Page 201

26. Describe a technique for palpating these muscles.

27. Describe the distal attachment of the biceps femoris.

28. To what prominence of which bone do these muscles attach proximally?

29. In which area can the deeper fibres, from the short head, of the biceps femoris be palpated?

30. Describe where the tendon of the semitendinosus can be palpated.

31. Where does the tendon of the semitendinosus attach distally?

32. With which muscle does the semitendinosus blend proximally?

33. Name the muscle which has the thin tendon lying anteromedial to the tendon of semitendinosus.

34. Where does this thin muscle attach proximally?

35. Explain why the semimembranosus is difficult to palpate.

36. Where does semimembranosus attach distally?

37. What structure is given support by the fibrous lower attachment of semimembranosus? (fr)

38. Describe the way in which the semimembranosus can be palpated.

Please complete the labels below.

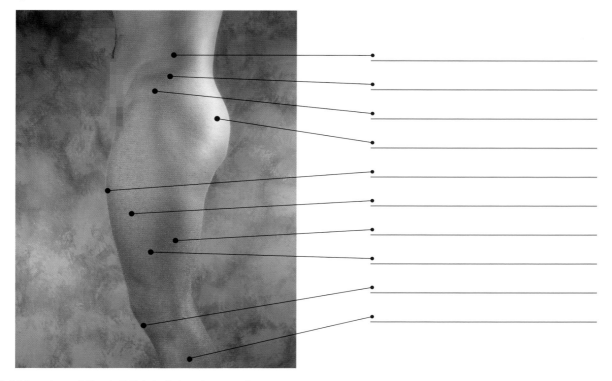

Fig. 3.18 (a) Muscles of the left thigh (lateral aspect)

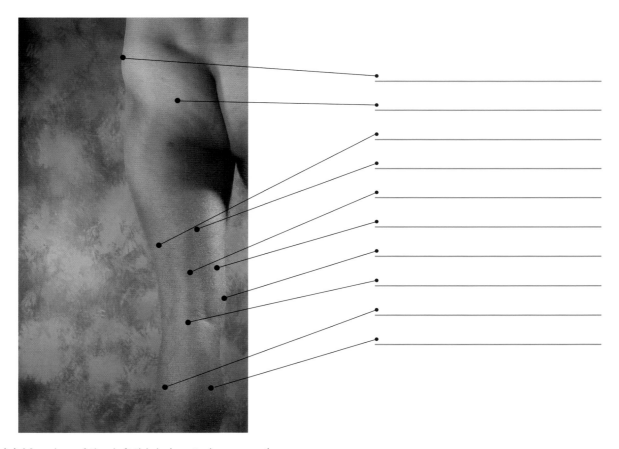

Fig. 3.19 (a) Muscles of the left thigh (posterior aspect)

Page 202

39. Which main muscle group is located on the medial aspect of the thigh?

40. List the muscles which comprise the medial group.

41. Where does the tendinous section of the largest muscle of the above group attach, distally?

42. What is the collective name of the main muscle group which forms the anterior aspect of the thigh?

43. From medial to lateral, list the muscles of the anterior group.

44. Where does the rectus femoris attach proximally?

45. What name is given to the section of the quadriceps tendon below the patella?

46. Where does this section of the quadriceps tendon attach distally?

47. Which three quadriceps muscles can be easily palpated?

48. Which structure flattens the lateral muscle of this group?

Page 203

49. Which is the lowest of the three quadriceps muscle bellies?

50. Following an injury, which of the quadriceps muscles usually atrophies first?

51. Name the two tendons which attach to the base of the patella.

52. What type of bone is the patella?

53. Under normal circumstances, how long is the ligamentum patellae?

54. Explain its relevance to the surface marking of the knee joint.

55. Name the tendon-like structure lying lateral to the patella when the knee is extended.

56. To what is this structure attached distally?

57. Where does the sartorius muscle attach proximally?

58. What is its attachment distally?

59. List the actions performed by the sartorius muscle.

60. Describe the position which results from its action.

61. What is the derivation of the name 'sartorius'?

Please complete the labels below.

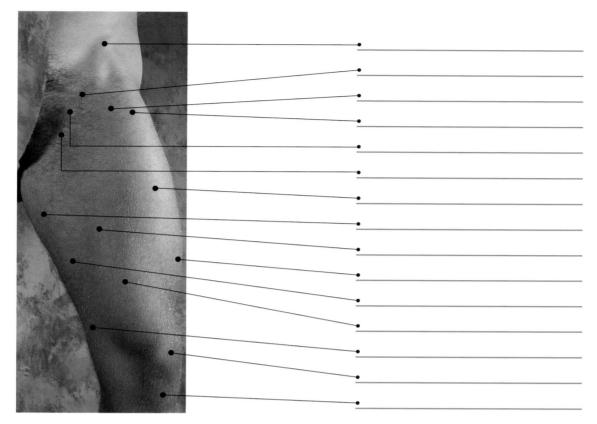

Fig. 3.20 (a) Muscles of the left thigh (medial aspect)

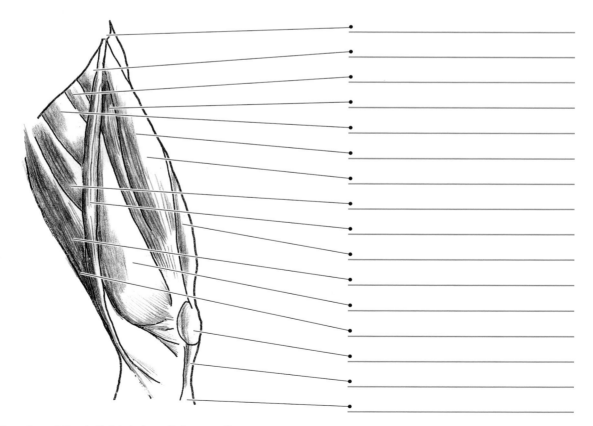

Fig. 3.20 (b) Muscles of the left thigh (medial aspect)

SELF ASSESSMENT

Page 204

62. List the muscles located in the anterior compartment of the leg.

63. Which is the most medial tendon, anteriorly, when the ankle joint is dorsiflexed?

64. Name the structure, beneath which this tendon passes, as it crosses the ankle joint.

65. Where does this muscle insert distally?

66. Which structure lies medial to the belly of this muscle?

67. Which tendon lies lateral to the above tendon?

68. What is the distal insertion of this tendon?

69. In which area can this muscle be felt contracting?

70. Which muscle tendon lies lateral to that of the extensor hallucis muscle?

71. Describe what happens to this tendon just below the level of the ankle joint.

Page 205

72. What is the peroneus tertius considered to be?

73. With which muscle does peroneus tertius pass through the loop of the extensor retinaculum?

74. Where does peroneus tertius insert distally?

75. What action is produced by this muscle?

76. Where is the extensor digitorum brevis muscle located?

77. Towards which four toes do the tendons pass?

78. Describe how these tendons differ in their insertion.

Page 206

79. Where in the body is the popliteus muscle situated?

80. Where can its tendon be located?

81. Describe how the popliteus muscle may be put into action.

Please complete the labels below.

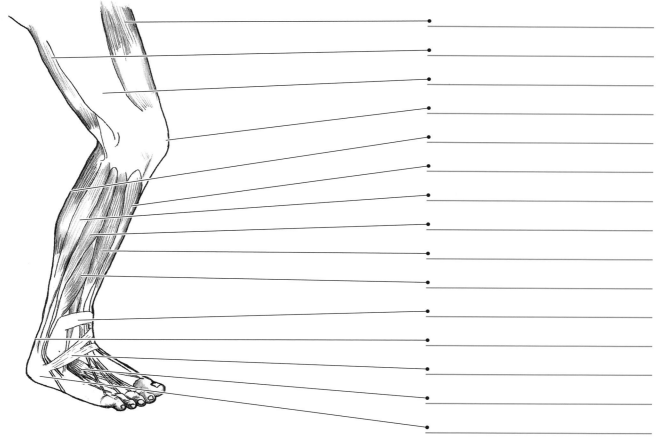

Fig. 3.21 (b) Muscles of the right leg (lateral aspect)

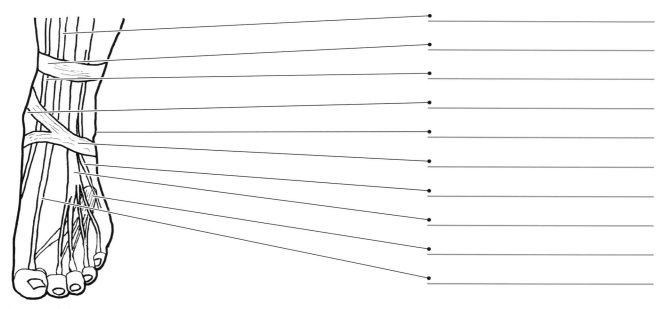

Fig. 3.21 (d) Tendons and muscles of the left foot (dorsal aspect)

82. By what other name is the calf muscle also known?

_____

83. List the muscles which comprise this group.

_____

84. Which muscle is more superficial than the others?

_____

85. Describe their attachment to the calcaneus.

86. Describe the attachment of the proximal end of the most superficial muscle.

87. What is the proximal attachment of the deepest of this muscle group?

88. Which muscle passes between the two?

89. Approximately, how long is the tendocalcanius?

90. How wide is it at its widest point?

91. Describe the muscular form of the most superficial muscle of the group.

Page 207

92. Under what conditions is it easiest to palpate the deepest muscle of this group?

93. In what area can the deepest muscle be palpated?

94. Describe a technique for putting the calf muscles into action.

95. Explain how a contraction of the deepest muscle can be obtained while achieving a simultaneous relaxation of the most superficial muscle.

Page 208

96. Which structure covers the central area of the plantar aspect of the foot?

97. Describe the shape of this structure.

98. Where does it attach posteriorly?

99. What is its anterior attachment?

100. Describe the general arrangement of the plantar muscles of the foot.

101. Which of these muscles is palpable?

102. In which area is this muscle palpated?

Page 209

103. Where does this muscle attach posteriorly?

104. What is its attachment anteriorly?

105. List the actions of this muscle.

Please complete the labels below.

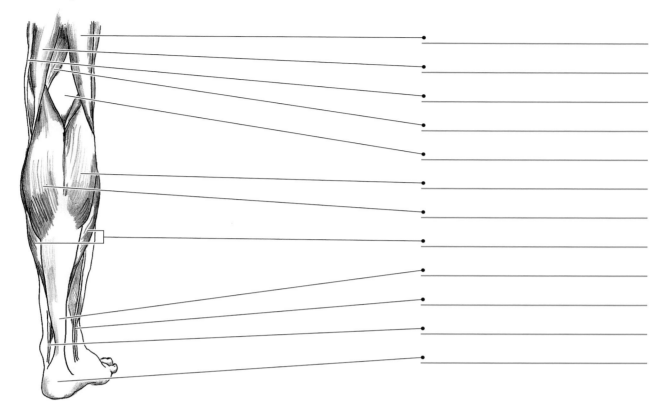

Fig. 3.22 (b) Muscles of the right leg and foot (posterior aspect)

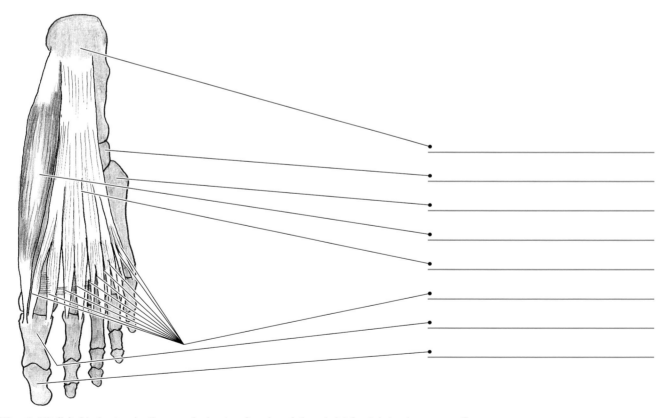

Fig. 3.23 (b) Abductor hallux and plantar fascia of the right foot (plantar aspect)

106. Under normal circumstances, in which area is the hardest skin of the plantar aspect of the foot located?

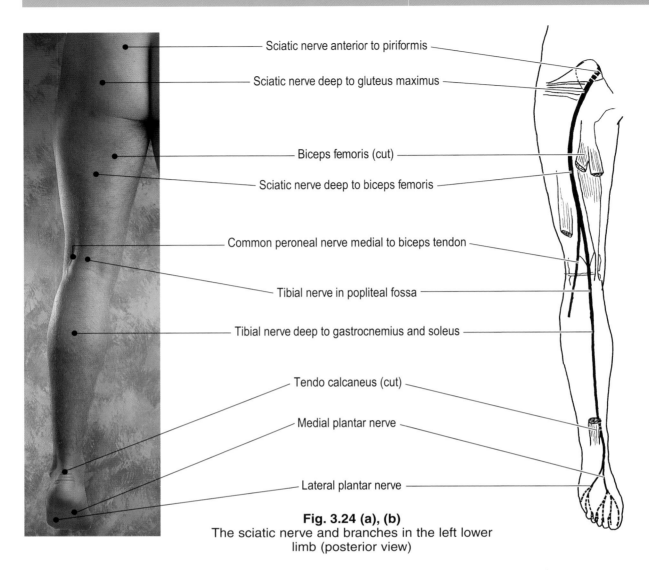

Sciatic nerve anterior to piriformis

Sciatic nerve deep to gluteus maximus

Biceps femoris (cut)

Sciatic nerve deep to biceps femoris

Common peroneal nerve medial to biceps tendon

Tibial nerve in popliteal fossa

Tibial nerve deep to gastrocnemius and soleus

Tendo calcaneus (cut)

Medial plantar nerve

Lateral plantar nerve

Fig. 3.24 (a), (b)
The sciatic nerve and branches in the left lower
limb (posterior view)

NERVES

The nerves of the lower limb are normally deep within the tissues and thus extremely difficult to palpate. Nevertheless, it is important to be aware of their location and to be able to palpate those that venture close to the surface.

The whole of the lower limb is supplied from the lumbar, sacral and coccygeal plexi. The lumbar plexus derives its fibres from T12, L1, L2, L3 and L4 roots. The sacral (lumbosacral) plexus derives its fibres from L4, L5, S1, S2, S3 and S4. The coccygeal (sacral) plexus derives its fibres from S4 and S5. These form a complex arrangement of nerves, most of which are not palpable, but nevertheless remain essential knowledge for the anatomist. The reader should refer to *Anatomy and Human Movement* (Palastanga, Field and Soames 1998) for further study.

Surface marking

The sciatic nerve derives its fibres from the anterior primary rami of L4 and L5 through the lumbosacral trunk, and S1, S2 and S3. It is formed in front of piriformis in the posterior part of the pelvis and emerges from the pelvis through the sciatic notch below piriformis and deep to the gluteus maximus. It is the largest peripheral nerve in the body. It runs vertically down the back of the thigh, deep to biceps femoris, having emerged from below piriformis approximately halfway between the greater trochanter of the femur and the ischial tuberosity. About two-thirds of the way down the thigh, it splits into its terminal branches – the tibial and common peroneal nerves (Fig. 3.24a–d). Although it is difficult to palpate the nerve directly, pressure applied over the area of its course can cause considerable discomfort to the subject.

The tibial nerve (Fig. 3.24a, b) continues through the popliteal fossa to enter the calf deep to gastrocnemius and soleus, to lie between superficial and deep groups of muscles. It is again difficult to palpate in this region, although an unpleasant sensation can be produced if excessive pressure is applied. In the lower third of the leg the tibial nerve becomes medial to the tendo calcaneus, and

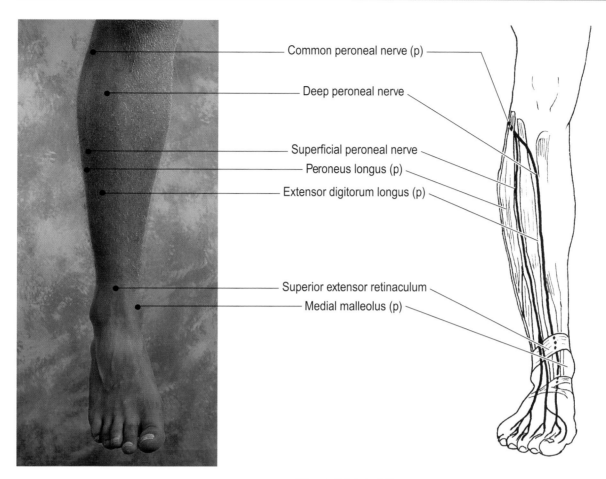

Fig. 3.24 (c), (d)
Branches of the common peroneal nerve of the right leg (anterior aspect) (p, palpable)

continues to the space behind the medial malleolus where it is palpable. It can be traced proximally into the leg, and distally into the foot, where it almost immediately divides into the medial and lateral plantar nerves. These terminal branches soon become too deep to be palpated.

The common peroneal nerve, the lateral terminal branch of the sciatic nerve, enters the popliteal fossa. It passes down the medial side of the tendon of biceps femoris where it can be palpated passing behind the head of the fibula to the neck (Fig. 3.24). It then winds anteriorly around the neck of the fibula, immediately splitting into superficial and deep branches.

Palpation

With the knee semiflexed, locate the tendon of biceps femoris as it passes down to the head of the fibula, posterolateral to the knee. Below the level of the knee joint the common peroneal nerve will be found just medial and deep to this tendon, passing behind the head of the fibula and winding

forwards around the neck of the fibula (Fig. 3.24). It is easier to palpate posteriorly but more difficult anteriorly as it becomes covered by peroneus longus and tibialis anterior.

The deep peroneal nerve lies deep within the anterior compartment of the leg and is impossible to palpate until it crosses the anterior aspect of the ankle joint between the tendons of extensor hallucis longus and extensor digitorum longus.

First find the anterior tibial pulse on the front of the ankle joint between extensor hallucis longus and extensor digitorum longus. The nerve runs just lateral to this, but it is difficult to find as it lies deep to the superior extensor retinaculum.

The superficial peroneal nerve can be palpated passing over the anterolateral aspect of the ankle, just medial to the anterior border of the lateral malleolus. It can be traced proximally for approximately 5 cm to where it emerges from between peroneus brevis and extensor digitorum longus. Distally it can be traced on to the lateral side of the dorsum of the foot, dividing into fine terminal cutaneous branches (Fig. 3.24c, d).

SELF ASSESSMENT

Page 220

1. List the three nerve plexi which supply the lower limb.

2. From which roots does the upper plexus derive its fibres?

3. Which roots give fibres to the middle of the three plexi?

4. From which roots does the lowest plexus derive its fibres?

5. The fibres of which roots comprise the sciatic nerve?

6. In front of which muscle is the sciatic nerve formed?

7. Describe the way in which the sciatic nerve emerges from the pelvis.

8. The sciatic nerve lies deep to which muscle as it emerges from the pelvis?

9. To which muscle does this nerve lie deep as it passes down the posterior aspect of the thigh?

10. Between which two bony landmarks does the sciatic nerve pass as it emerges from the sciatic notch?

11. In which area does the sciatic nerve divide into its two terminal branches?

12. The tibial nerve enters the calf deep to which two muscles?

13. On which side of the tendocalcaneus does the posterior tibial nerve emerge?

14. In which area is the posterior tibial nerve palpable around the ankle joint?

Page 221

15. Name the two branches of the posterior tibial nerve in the foot.

16. The common peroneal nerve lies medial to which muscle in the lower part of the thigh?

17. In which area around the knee joint can the common peroneal nerve be palpated?

18. Describe how the nerve passes to the anterior compartment of the leg.

19. Name the two branches into which the common peroneal nerve splits as it enters the anterior compartment of the leg.

20. Which nerve passes across the ankle between the extensor hallucis longus and the extensor digitorum longus?

21. Does this nerve lie deep or superficial to the superior extensor retinaculum?

Please complete the labels below.

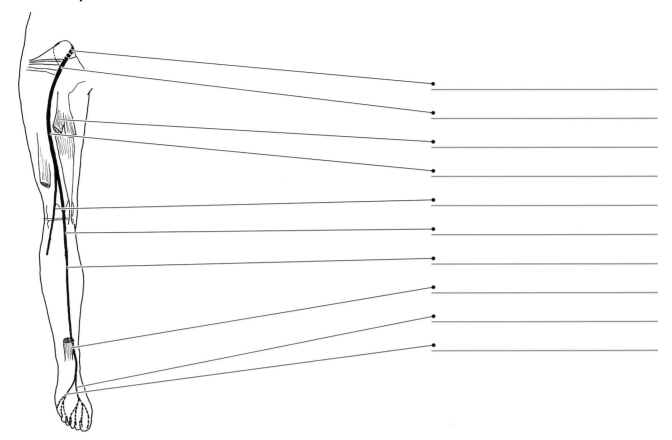

Fig. 3.24 (b) The sciatic nerve and branches in the left lower limb (posterior view)

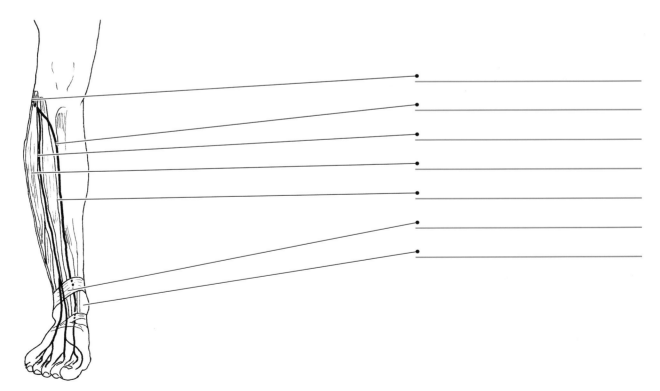

Fig. 3.24 (d) Branches of the common peroneal nerve of the right leg (anterior aspect) (p, palpable)

22. Which nerve can be palpated as it passes over the anterior aspect of the lateral malleolus?

_____

23. Describe what happens to this nerve as it passes onto the dorsum of the foot.

_____

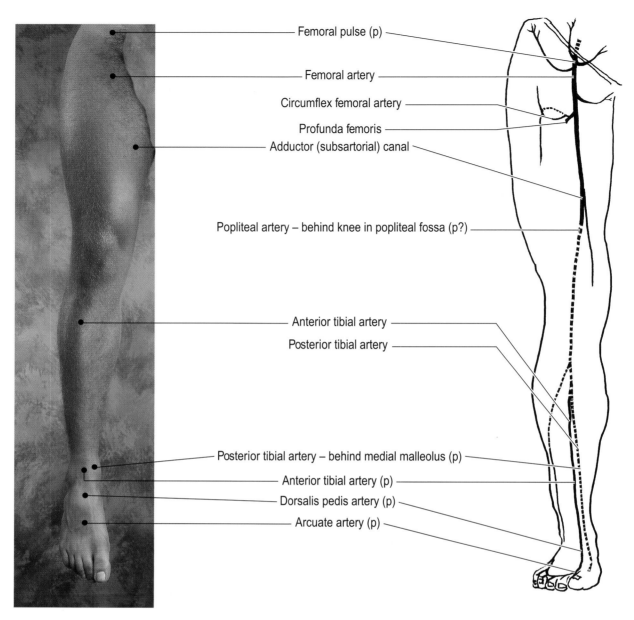

Femoral pulse (p)

Femoral artery

Circumflex femoral artery

Profunda femoris

Adductor (subsartorial) canal

Popliteal artery – behind knee in popliteal fossa (p?)

Anterior tibial artery

Posterior tibial artery

Posterior tibial artery – behind medial malleolus (p)

Anterior tibial artery (p)

Dorsalis pedis artery (p)

Arcuate artery (p)

Fig. 3.25 (a), (b)
The arteries of the right lower limb (anterior aspect) (p, palpable)

ARTERIES

As in the upper limb, most of the large arteries are located deep within the tissues and are normally difficult to palpate.

The pulsation of the femoral artery can be palpated in the groin just below the mid point (halfway between the anterior superior iliac spines and the pubic tubercle) of the inguinal ligament directly anterior to the head of the femur at the hip joint. Above, the vessel lies within the abdomen and below it is hidden by fascia as it lies in the femoral triangle on the proximal anteromedial aspect of the thigh. Just above the knee the femoral artery passes through the opening in adductor magnus (adductor hiatus) lying deep to the sartorius muscle in the adductor (subsartorial) canal to enter the popliteal fossa, becoming the

popliteal artery. This can be palpated with deep, sensitive pressure as it crosses the back of the knee joint. Its identification is facilitated if tension of the superficial tissues is reduced by bending the knee to about 45°. Success in palpation is largely dependent on the amount of fat within the fossa and, in reality, it is extremely difficult to find. This is, therefore, a good region in which to practise the careful use of the fingers in palpation of pulses.

As the popliteal artery enters the calf, it divides into the anterior and posterior tibial arteries. The anterior tibial artery passes over the main section of the interosseous membrane and below the most superior fibres (see pages 164 and 165), into the anterior compartment of the leg, deep to the anterior tibial muscles. The posterior tibial artery

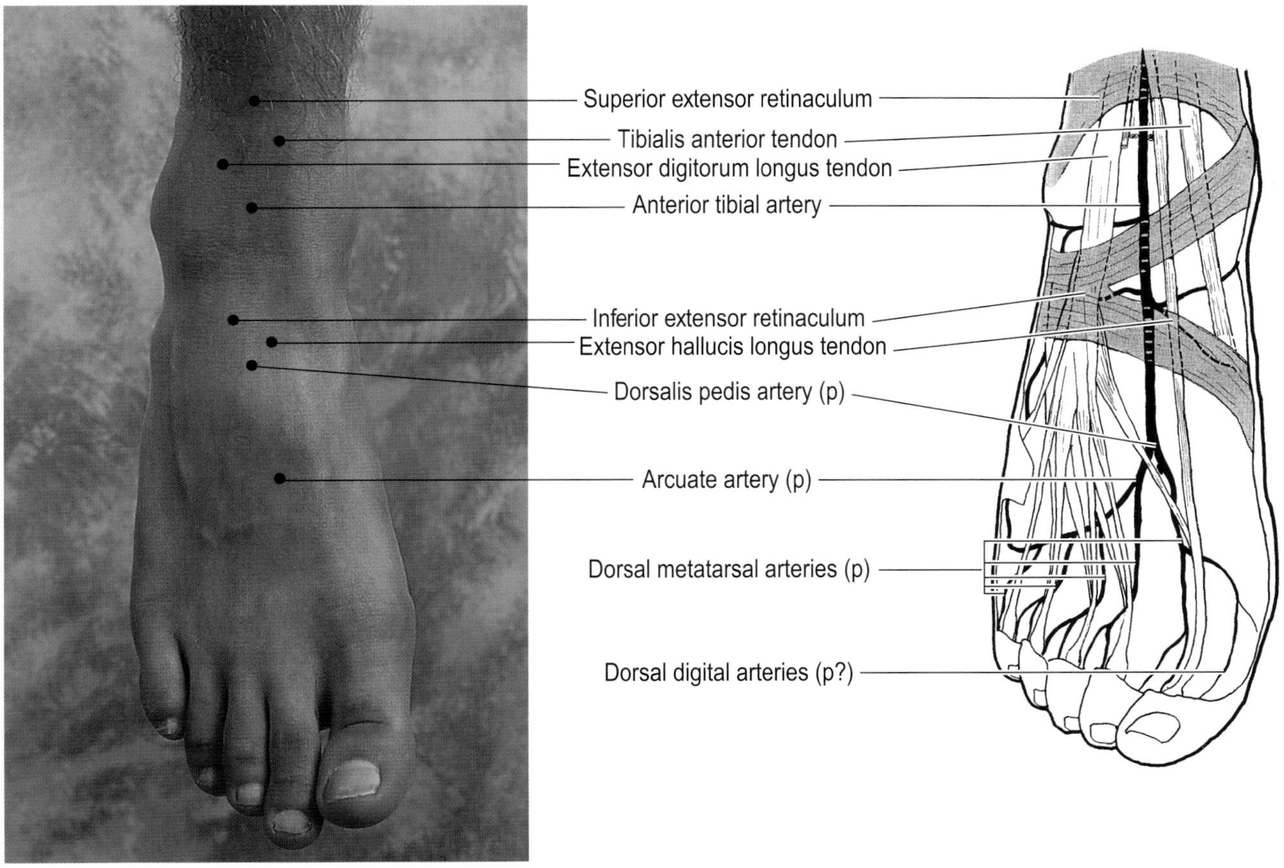

Fig. 3.25 (c), (d)
The arteries of the right foot (dorsal aspect) (p, palpable)

passes down the back of the leg deep to the gastrocnemius, soleus and plantaris (triceps surae).

The anterior tibial artery can be palpated as it crosses the anteromedial aspect of the ankle joint between the tendons of extensor hallucis longus and extensor digitorum longus where it lies medial to the deep branch of the common peroneal nerve. With careful palpation it can be traced down to the space between the first and second metatarsals where it passes into the plantar aspect of the foot between the two bones. Beyond the extensor retinaculum the artery is called the dorsalis pedis (Fig. 3.25a–d), and is commonly the point at which the arterial supply is checked. Care must be taken not to palpate too distally,

as the artery will have already passed through to the plantar aspect of the foot. In subjects with a good blood supply to the foot, the arcuate artery, a continuation of the dorsalis pedis on the dorsum of the metacarpals, can be palpated.

The posterior tibial artery crosses the ankle joint behind the medial malleolus between the tendons of flexor digitorum longus and flexor hallucis longus, medial to the posterior tibial nerve (Fig. 3.25a, b). Although it is quite clear as it crosses the ankle joint, it is difficult to trace into the medial side of the foot and the lower part of the leg.

It is important to practise finding these arterial pulses, as they give a good indication of the competence of the blood supply to the lower limb.

SELF ASSESSMENT

Page 224

1. In which area of the body may the pulsation of the femoral artery be palpated?

2. Name the gutter on the medial side of the thigh in which the artery lies.

3. Describe how the artery passes from the anterior to the posterior compartment of the thigh.

4. Through which canal does this artery pass?

5. Into which space does it pass on the posterior aspect of the knee?

6. What name is given to the artery in this space?

7. Name the muscle which lies deep to this artery.

8. List the branches into which this artery divides.

9. Describe how its anterior branch passes into the anterior compartment of the leg.

Page 225

10. Between which two tendons does the artery pass as it crosses the ankle joint?

11. Which nerve accompanies this artery?

12. Describe the course taken by the artery when it reaches the space between the first and second metatarsal bones.

13. By what name is the artery known at this point?

14. Name the artery which passes across the dorsum of the foot.

15. Describe the route of the posterior tibial artery in the posterior compartment of the leg.

16. Does the posterior tibial artery pass over or deep to the flexor retinaculum?

17. Between which tendons does this artery lie behind the ankle?

18. Which nerve accompanies this artery into the foot?

Please complete the labels below.

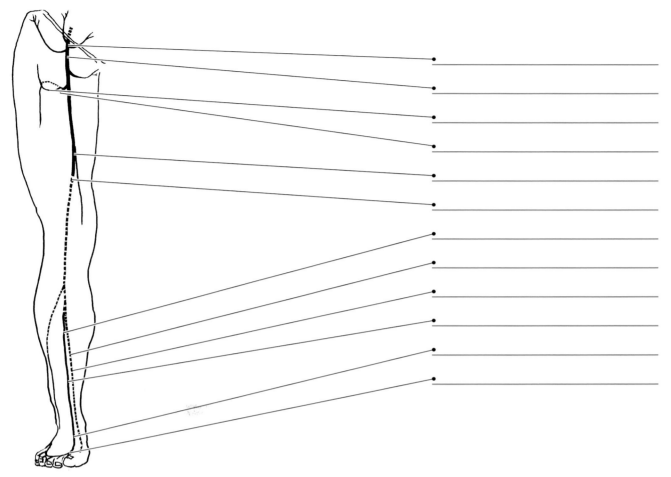

Fig. 3.25 (b) The arteries of the right lower limb (anterior aspect) (p, palpable)

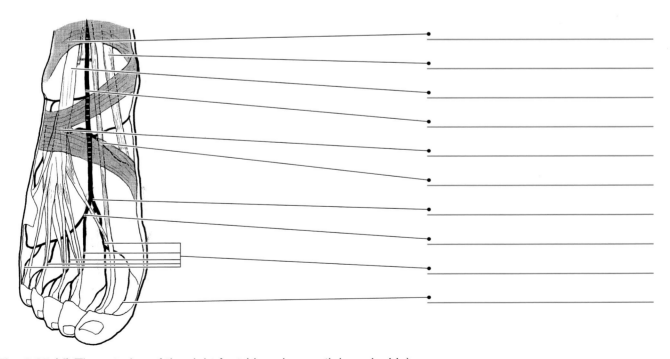

Fig. 3.25 (d) The arteries of the right foot (dorsal aspect) (p, palpable)

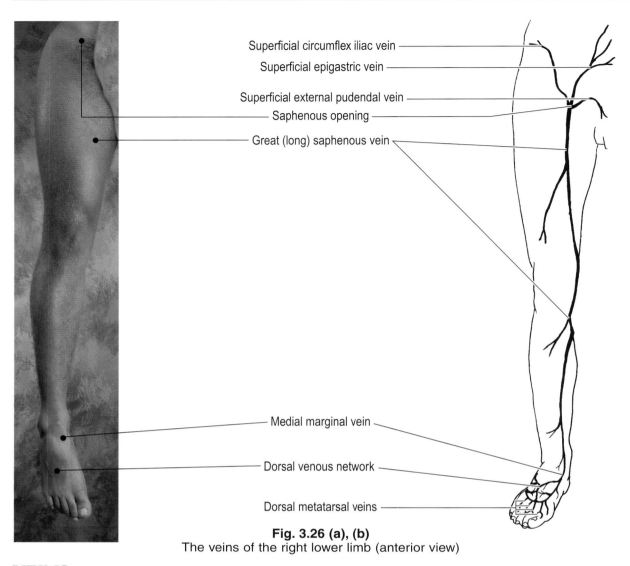

Superficial circumflex iliac vein

Superficial epigastric vein

Superficial external pudendal vein

Saphenous opening

Great (long) saphenous vein

Medial marginal vein

Dorsal venous network

Dorsal metatarsal veins

Fig. 3.26 (a), (b)
The veins of the right lower limb (anterior view)

VEINS

The arrangement of veins in the lower limb is similar to that in the upper limb (see pages 110 and 111), there being two main systems – deep, accompanying the arteries, and superficial, contained within the superficial fascia. All veins of the lower limb possess valves, which facilitate central venous return. The valves in the communicating vessels normally only permit blood to flow from the superficial to the deep system.

The deep veins

The smaller arteries are normally accompanied by two small veins (venae comitantes), one either side of the artery. The larger arteries are usually accompanied by a single large vein of approximately the same diameter as the artery. None of the deep veins can be palpated.

The superficial veins

In normal subjects most veins are difficult to see or palpate, except in the distal part of the leg and on the dorsum of the foot.

With the subject standing, the network of vessels on the dorsum of the foot appear blue and raised. They can be palpated with little difficulty. One vein on either side of the network appears to be slightly larger than the rest; these are termed marginal veins.

The great (long) saphenous vein

The great or long saphenous vein (Fig. 3.26a, b) begins on the medial side of the dorsal venous network as a continuation of the medial marginal vein. It passes proximally in front of the medial malleolus, along the medial side of the calf and crosses the knee joint just posterior to the medial condyles of both the tibia and femur. The vein then ascends on the medial side of the thigh to join the deep system (femoral vein) after passing through the saphenous opening which lies below the mid point of the inguinal ligament immediately medial to the pulsations of the femoral artery (see Fig. 3.25a, b).

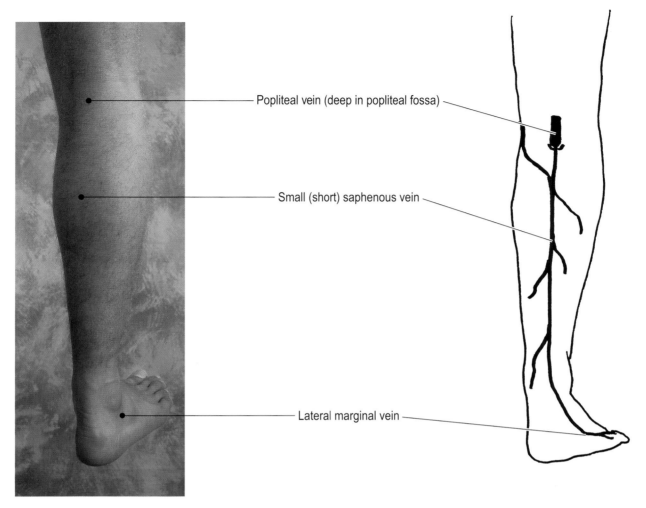

Popliteal vein (deep in popliteal fossa)

Small (short) saphenous vein

Lateral marginal vein

Fig. 3.26 (c), (d)
The veins of the right leg (posterior view)

Palpation

Only the lower part of the vein can normally be palpated as it lies deep within the superficial fascia. With the subject standing, find the medial marginal vein (the major vessel on the medial aspect of the dorsum of the foot). Brushing the skin surface with the fingertips, move up to the medial malleolus. Above this level the vein can be felt passing up the medial aspect of the calf. It can often be traced posteromedial to the knee, but soon disappears as it enters the thigh. In some individuals it can be seen in the thigh as a bluish line running upwards towards the mid point of the groin.

The small (short) saphenous vein

Beginning on the lateral side of the dorsal venous network as a continuation of the lateral marginal vein, the small or short saphenous vein passes behind the lateral malleolus and up the lateral side

of the tendo calcaneus to the posterior aspect of the calf. It pierces the deep fascia in the lower part of the popliteal fossa to join the deep popliteal vein (Fig. 3.26c, d).

Palpation

The lateral marginal vein is a little more difficult to recognize than the medial. It can be traced along the lateral side of the dorsum of the foot, but its continuation is difficult to palpate behind the lateral malleolus. That part between the lateral malleolus and the popliteal fossa is variable in its palpability; however, after a long period of standing it usually becomes quite visible and therefore easily palpable.

In some individuals, particularly the elderly, a network of vessels can be palpated on the medial side of the leg and thigh, which roughly follow the course of the great saphenous vein. Most of these join with the great saphenous vein along its length.

SELF ASSESSMENT

Page 228

1. Describe the general arrangement of the veins in the lower limb.

2. List the structures which facilitate central venous return.

3. In which direction do the communicating veins allow the blood to flow, superficial to deep or deep to superficial?

4. Name the two small veins that accompany small arteries.

5. In which areas in the lower limb are the veins most palpable or visible?

6. Name the two larger veins which run on either side of the foot.

7. Which vein drains the medial side of the foot and passes up the medial side of the lower limb?

8. Does this vein pass anterior or posterior to the medial malleolus?

9. Where does this vein cross the knee joint?

10. Which vein does it normally join in the upper part of the thigh?

11. Name the opening through which this vein passes from superficial to deep.

12. Where is this opening located?

13. Describe how this opening is formed. (fr).

14. Where can the long saphenous vein be palpated?

Page 229

15. Which vein passes up the lateral and posterior side of the leg?

16. Does this vein pass anterior or posterior to the lateral malleolus?

17. Lateral to which tendon does this vein lie?

18. Describe its arrangement in the popliteal fossa.

19. Describe a technique to facilitate the palpation of the majority of these veins.

Please complete the labels below.

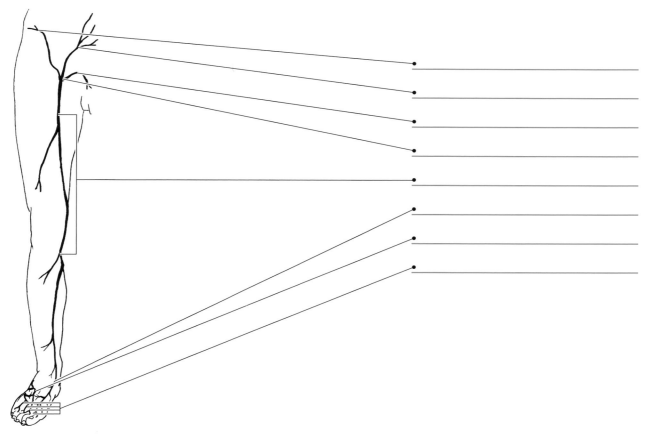

Fig. 3.26 (b) The veins of the right lower limb (anterior view)

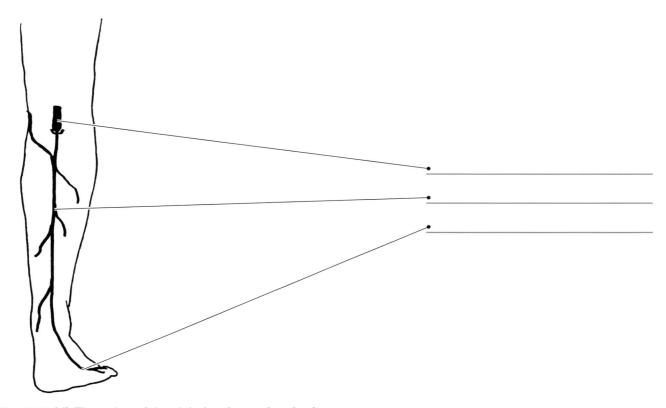

Fig. 3.26 (d) The veins of the right leg (posterior view)

The head and neck

Contents

At the end of this chapter you should be able to:

A. Find, recognize and name the constituent components of the external surface of the skull, noting their size and position.

B. Palpate many of the bony features, being able to relate one to another.

C. Locate, name and palpate the bony and cartilaginous structures at the front of the neck.

D. Recognize and palpate bony landmarks of the cervical spine.

E. Name all the joints of the skull recognizing the bones which form them.

F. Palpate and trace the lines of the sutures and joints of the skull and cervical spine, where possible, indicating their bony landmarks and surface markings.

G. Describe or carry out any accessory movements possible noting the ranges in which they are most evident.

H. Note the range of movement of the cervical spine and indicate the factors limiting the movement.

I. Give the class and type of each of the joints.

J. Name and demonstrate the action of all the muscles palpable in the head and neck.

K. Be able to draw the shape of the muscle on the surface and palpate its contraction.

L. Name all the main cutaneous nerves supplying the head and neck giving their distribution.

M. Name the main arteries of the head and neck giving their course and distribution.

N. Name the main veins of the head and neck noting their drainage areas and course.

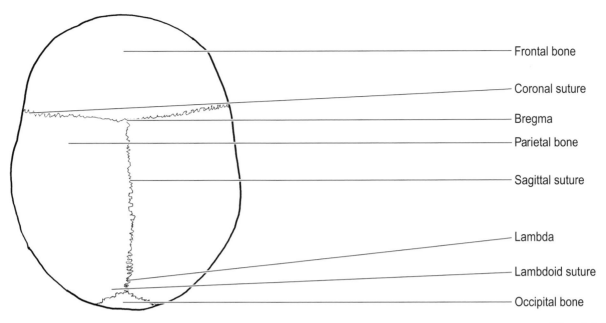

Fig. 4.1 (a)
The skull (superior aspect)

BONES

The skull

Superior aspect [Fig. 4.1a]

The skull, viewed from above, is shaped like a flattened egg. It is broader across the posterior dimension and narrower across the anterior dimension. Its length, from front to back, is normally almost twice its breadth from side to side.

It comprises the frontal, two parietal [*paries* (L) = a wall] and part of the occipital [*occipitum* (L) = the back of the head) bones. Viewed from above, the frontal bone makes up the anterior section, forming approximately one-third. The two parietal bones form most of the posterior two-thirds. The occipital bone fits into just the central posterior part of the skull.

The frontal bone joins the anterior borders of the two parietal bones at the coronal [*corona* (L) = crown] suture which runs transversely across the skull. The intersection of all three bones is known as 'bregma' [*brechein* (Gk) = to moisten, the most humid and delicate part of the infant's brain]. The two parietal bones join at the sagittal [*sagitta* (L) = an arrow, the direction in which an arrow would pass through the body) suture, which runs anteroposteriorly along the centre of the skull. The posterior borders of both parietal bones meet the anterior border of the squamous part of the occipital bone at the lambdoid [*lambda* = the Greek letter 'L'] sutures. The point at which all three bones meet is termed 'lambda'.

Palpation

The skull is covered, superiorly, by a fibromuscular sheet (aponeurosis) from the eyebrows anteriorly to the external occipital protuberance and the superior nuchal lines posteriorly. This is thick and adherent to the skin covering the skull but only attached to the pericranium by areola tissue. This gives it a certain amount of freedom to move over the skull. It is continuous laterally with the temporal and zygomatic fascia.

Due to this arrangement and the fact that there is normally a covering of hair, palpation of the bones, sutures and landmarks of the skull requires a slightly different technique if exact location is required. Use all the fingertips of both hands to locate and mark the structures, using a gentle forward and backward motion, moving the aponeurosis on the underlying bone.

Place your fingers anterior and posterior to the vertex of the skull. On pressing the tips in and moving them from side to side, the sagittal suture can be palpated, particularly posteriorly. Halfway between the vertex and the external occipital protuberance a hollow can be felt with two sutures running downwards and laterally in front of the occipital bone. This is the point 'lambda'. Moving approximately 5 cm forwards from the vertex there is another palpable slight hollow with the coronal suture running laterally to either side. This point is termed 'bregma'. In front of the coronal suture one can feel the frontal bone (forehead), sometimes with a central raised line where the two bones have fused.

Either side of the sagittal suture, behind the frontal bones and in front of the occipital bone, are the two large plates of the parietal bones.

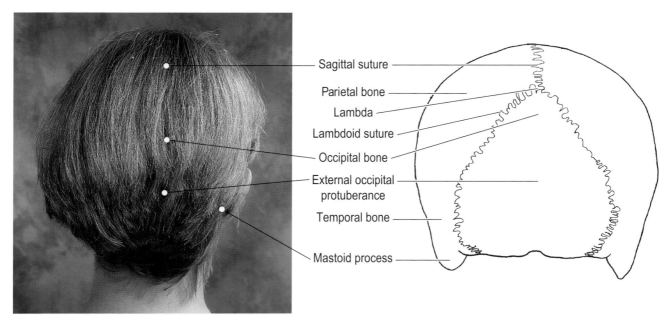

Fig. 4.1 (b), (c)
The skull (posterior aspect)

Posterior aspect [Fig. 4.1b and c]

The posteroinferior part of the skull consists mainly of the occipital bone. On either side it joins the temporal bones, each of which has a large downward-projecting prominence termed the mastoid [*mastos* (Gk) = a breast, *oeides* (Gk) = shape] process. Superiorly it joins the two parietal bones forming the vault of the skull. Its anterior portion forms the base of the skull, surrounding the foramen magnum and projecting forward as the basilar section.

Posteriorly, at its apex, the occipital bone fits between the two parietal bones at the point lambda (see previous page). Running downwards and laterally from this point, the two lambdoid sutures divide the occiput from the two parietal bones. The bone presents a large tuberosity, about 5 cm below the point lambda, termed the external occipital protuberance, with superior, middle and inferior nuchal lines radiating laterally. The external occipital protuberance varies considerably in its size, being very prominent in some and almost non-existent in others.

Palpation

The most prominent bony feature of the posterior aspect of the skull is the external occipital protuberance situated just below its centre. It varies in size and shape between individuals, being large and prominent in some and difficult to find in others. Radiating laterally and upwards from the external occipital protuberance are the two superior nuchal (believed to come from Arabic '*nugraph*' = the back of the neck) lines. These are palpable in their central section on most subjects, but are difficult to trace more than a few centimetres laterally. Approximately 5 cm above the external occipital protuberance the sagittal suture meets two occipitoparietal sutures. In the young child this is the region of the posterior fontanelle [*fons* (L) = small fountain or spring) which in the adult becomes the lambda. Inferiorly the occipital bone can be traced forwards under the skull, but is soon lost in the deep hollow at the level of the tubercle of the first cervical vertebra. Moving to either side, just behind the pinna of each ear, the mastoid process of the temporal bone can be palpated. It is pointed at its inferior aspect where sternocleidomastoid attaches.

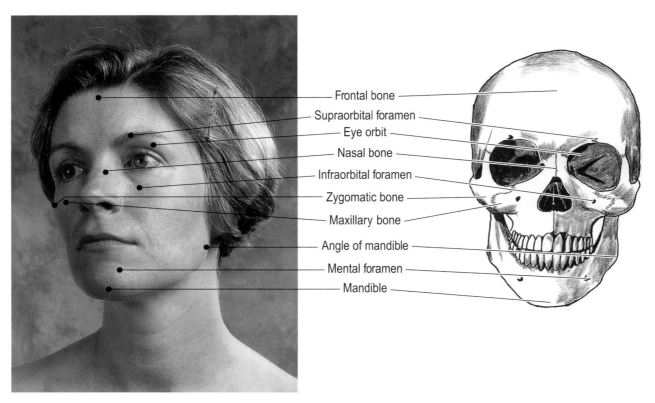

Fig. 4.2 (a), (b) The skull (anterior aspect)

Anterior aspect [Fig. 4.2a and b]

Each **eye orbit** is formed superiorly by the **frontal bone** (which forms the forehead), laterally by the **zygomatic bone**, medially by the **nasal bone** and inferiorly by the **maxilla**. The upper teeth are associated with the maxilla, while the lower teeth are located in the superior border of the **mandible**.

Palpation

Deep to the eyebrow the upper rim of the eye orbit can be palpated, being slightly notched at its centre where it is crossed by the supraorbital artery. The whole margin of the orbit is subcutaneous and can thus readily be palpated. The two nasal bones can be palpated centrally projecting forwards and continuing as a cartilage down to the centre of the nose. Below this can be palpated the upper part of the maxilla investing the upper teeth.

Lateral aspect [Fig. 4.2c and d]

The **temporal** [*tempus* (L) = time (pertaining to the passing of time and the greying of the temples)] **bone** forms the central area on the side of the skull. Posteriorly it articulates with the occipital bone, superiorly with the **parietal bone** and anteriorly, with the sphenoid [*sphen* (Gk) = a wedge] and zygomatic [*zygoma* (Gk) = a yoke or bar] bones.

The anterior section of the lateral aspect consists of the frontal bone and the maxilla, with the lateral part of the ethmoid [*ethmos* (Gk) = a sieve] just projecting between the sphenoid and frontal bones. Inferiorly the mandible [*mando* (L) = I chew] articulates by its **condyle** with the under surface of the temporal bone just anterior to the **external auditory meatus** [*meatus* (L) = a passage).

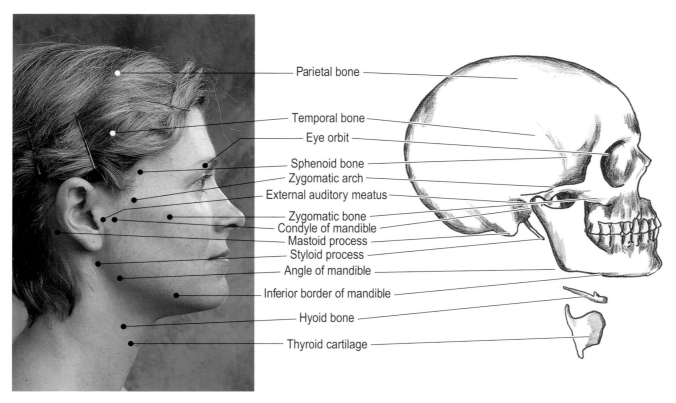

Fig. 4.2 (c), (d) The skull (lateral aspect)

Palpation

The external auditory meatus is an obvious landmark on the lateral side of the head. The little finger can be pressed deep into this opening to be surrounded by its bony walls. The pinna lies around three sides, while the tragus is the pointed area of soft tissue overlapping the meatus from the front. Running horizontally forwards just anterior to the tragus [*tragos* (Gk) and *tregus* (L) = a goat (possibly pertaining to the shape of a goat's beard)], a bony bridge can be palpated (the zygomatic arch). This forms the point of the cheek at the front where it joins the zygomatic bone (Fig. 4.2c, d). The arch is formed partly from the temporal and partly from the zygomatic bones.

Below the posterior part of the zygomatic arch anterior to the tragus a small tubercle can be palpated. This is the most lateral part of the condyle of the mandible. If the subject opens the mouth, this bony prominence can be felt, first rotating then moving forwards and downwards over the articular eminence of the temporal bone.

Some 7 cm directly below the condyle of the mandible, the angle of the mandible can be identified, being more prominent in men than in women as it is slightly everted. The inferior border of the mandible can be traced forward to a raised vertical line centrally at the front, where it joins the bone of the opposite side. A small tubercle (the mental tubercle) can be palpated on the inferior border either side of this line.

The anterior and lateral surfaces of the mandible are subcutaneous and can be traced posteriorly as far as the angle where it is hidden by the powerful muscles of mastication. The lower border is thickened all round, giving a concave appearance to the anterior surface. Below the zygomatic bone the maxilla can be palpated, with the teeth and gums easily identifiable through the flesh of the cheek and the upper lip.

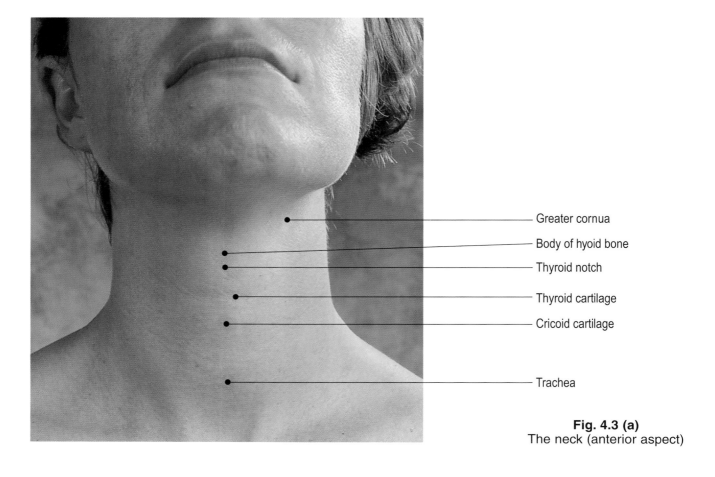

Greater cornua
Body of hyoid bone
Thyroid notch
Thyroid cartilage
Cricoid cartilage
Trachea

Fig. 4.3 (a)
The neck (anterior aspect)

The neck

Anterior aspect [Fig. 4.3a and b]

A series of midline structures run down the anterior aspect of the neck, being part of the respiratory tract. Just below the mandible is the small horseshoe-shaped hyoid bone [*hyoeides* (Gk) = U-shaped, i.e. shaped like the Greek letter upsilon]. Below, the thyroid [*thyreos* (Gk) = a shield] cartilage, formed from two cartilaginous plates fused at their anterior, but notched centrally above (the thyroid notch), projects slightly forward, particularly in the adult male, to form the 'Adam's apple'.

Behind the sternal notch lie the upper rings of the trachea [*trachys* (Gk) = uneven]. Interestingly, Aristotle mistakenly thought that this structure was an uneven surfaced artery. Between the upper ring and the thyroid cartilage lies the thicker and stronger signet-shaped ring of the cricoid cartilage [*krikos* (Gk) = a ring].

The larynx, formed mainly from the thyroid and cricoid cartilages, lies centrally at a level with the third to the sixth vertebral bodies and between the two sternomastoid muscles which are converging from above downwards.

The mandible, hyoid bone, thyroid and cricoid cartilages, and the upper part of the trachea, are all linked by muscle and ligaments and provide the tube for air to enter the lungs – 'the wind pipe'.

Palpation

It is quite unpleasant, and often frightening, to have these structures palpated by another person. It is therefore advisable to perform the palpation on yourself.

Place the fingers and thumb of one hand on either side of the mandible halfway along its inferior border (see page 237), and then slide your fingers and thumb down on to the sides of the throat. Some 3–5 cm below the mandible, the hyoid bone can be felt lying almost horizontal. It will appear as a horseshoe-shaped structure, rounded and thicker anteriorly and becoming pointed on

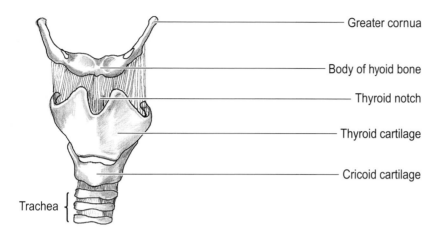

Greater cornua

Body of hyoid bone

Thyroid notch

Thyroid cartilage

Cricoid cartilage

Trachea

Fig. 4.3 (b)
Bones of the neck (anterior aspect)

either side posteriorly as it curves upwards slightly. This is the greater wing (*cornua*). Gentle pressure applied to either side will confirm its bony consistency.

Continue down the sides of the neck from the hyoid. After crossing a small space (felt as a depression), the broad flat lamina of the thyroid cartilage on either side is encountered. Each lamina is angled medially so that they meet in the midline anteriorly. A marked projection (the laryngeal prominence), more pronounced in men, will be found superiorly in the midline. This projection is commonly referred to as the 'Adam's apple'. If your finger is now placed on the antero-superior aspect of this prominence a small space can be palpated, concave upwards; this is the thyroid notch.

Trace down the sides of the thyroid cartilage for about 4 cm to a line just above the level of the medial ends of the clavicles. Here, after crossing another small space, a further ring-shaped structure will be palpated. This is the cricoid cartilage and it presents with a small tubercle at its centre.

Below the cricoid cartilage and deep in the suprasternal (jugular) notch, the cartilaginous rings of the upper part of the trachea can be palpated.

Each of the structures identified above can be taken between the finger and thumb of the same hand and carefully moved from side to side for a distance of about 1 cm. However, too much side movement can lead to tenderness in this part of the neck. During swallowing, each of the structures rises and then falls approximately 1 cm.

On either side of these central structures the sternocleidomastoid (sternomastoid) can be palpated, particularly if the supine subject tries to raise the head off a pillow. These muscles are widely spaced at the level of the hyoid bone but become much closer together as they approach the level of the clavicles.

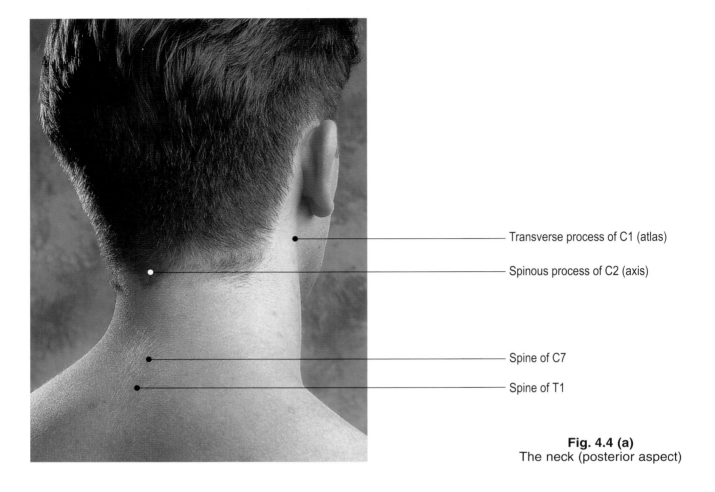

Transverse process of C1 (atlas)

Spinous process of C2 (axis)

Spine of C7

Spine of T1

Fig. 4.4 (a)
The neck (posterior aspect)

Posterior aspect [Fig. 4.4]

There are seven cervical vertebrae. Except for C1 (the atlas [derived from *atlao* (Gk) = I sustain]), C2 (the axis [*axis* (L) = a pivot or axle]) and C7, they all exhibit similar characteristics: small oval bodies, large vertebral canal, long laminae, a bifid spine and a broad transverse process with a foramen transversarium.

C1 does not possess a body, but has two lateral masses to support the weight of the head transferred via the occipital condyles. It has a posterior tubercle instead of a spine, and its transverse processes are wide and relatively pointed.

C2 has a tooth-like process projecting superiorly from its body, the dens or odontoid [*ódous* (Gk) = tooth) peg, a large prominent spine and small transverse processes. The seventh cervical vertebra is noted for its long non-bifid spine (vertebra prominens).

Palpation

Palpation of the neck is generally best carried out with the subject in the prone or supine position, achieving optimum relaxation. The natural curvature of the cervical spine is with the concavity backwards, thus adding to the difficulty of palpation.

With the subject lying prone, the forehead resting on the backs of the hands, the chin tucked in slightly and the neck straight, begin the palpation by finding the external occipital protuberance (see page 235), with the raised crescentic superior nuchal lines curving laterally. Running inferiorly and under the back of the skull from the protuberance, the external occipital crest can be palpated, ending at a deep hollow, which is level with the tubercle of the atlas (not palpable). The hollow is bounded below by the large prominence of the spine of the axis; this is approximately 3 cm below the external occipital protuberance. The spine

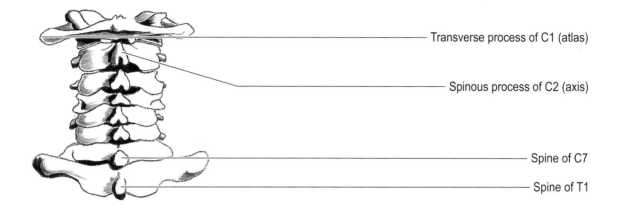

Transverse process of C1 (atlas)

Spinous process of C2 (axis)

Spine of C7

Spine of T1

Fig. 4.4 (b)
Bones of the neck (posterior aspect)

is easy to find and can be used for identification and location of other bony features.

Below, the spines of C3, 4 and 5 are closely packed together due to the curvature of the spine at this point. The spine of C3 lies close under the spine of C2 and is therefore difficult to palpate, the spine of C4 often being mistaken for that of C3.

Progress now to the lower part of the cervical spine, where two spinous processes can be felt projecting clearly. They are close together and rigid to the touch. The lower of the two is the spine of T1, that just above the spine of C7. The spine of C6 stands out clearly above that of C7 and can at times be mistaken for it. Differentiation between the spines of C6 and C7 can be carried out by asking the subject to extend the head and neck while keeping your finger on the spine of C6. It tends to move forward, causing it to disappear from beneath the palpating finger, while the spine of C7 remains stationary. Just above the spine of C6, that of C5 is identifiable, being very close to that of C4. It would be expected that flexion of the neck would improve identification. Unfortunately, except for the spines of C7 and T1, this is not the case as the tightening ligamentum nuchae hides the spines. The spines of C3, 4, 5 and 6, although difficult to identify separately, appear broad due to their bifid nature (Fig. 4.4).

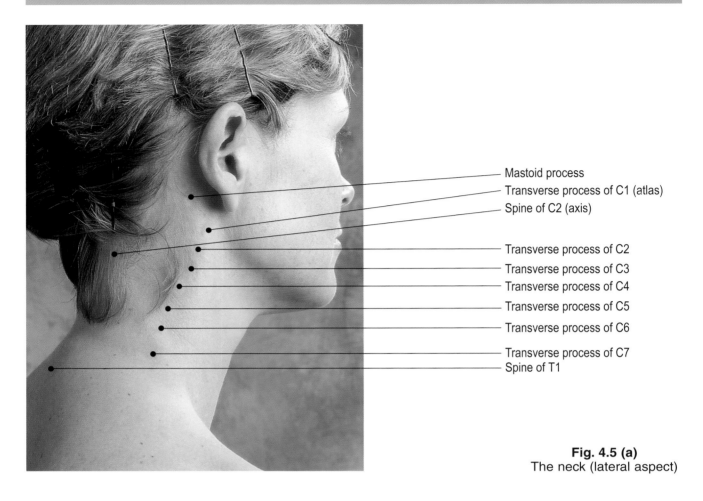

Mastoid process
Transverse process of C1 (atlas)
Spine of C2 (axis)

Transverse process of C2
Transverse process of C3
Transverse process of C4
Transverse process of C5
Transverse process of C6
Transverse process of C7
Spine of T1

Fig. 4.5 (a)
The neck (lateral aspect)

Lateral aspect [Fig. 4.5]

Although the transverse processes of the cervical vertebrae appear to project well out to the side, they are in fact quite difficult to palpate and identify. It is possible to palpate the tip of the transverse process of C1 between the angle of the mandible and the tip of the mastoid process. In some subjects the transverse process of C1 is not only palpable, but visible, as a small prominence. In others, it is difficult to identify even on deep palpation. This region can be quite tender if too much pressure is applied, and care must be taken to avoid the long and narrow styloid process just deep and anterior to the mastoid process.

The other transverse processes, with the exception of C2, present a double point laterally, the anterior and posterior tubercles, but owing to muscle attachments and fascial coverings they are not easy to distinguish. With the subject in prone lying, the line of the transverse processes can be identified from the back by easing the fingers into the side of the neck some 2 cm anterior to the tips of the spines. With care, the lower articular pillar of the vertebra above can be palpated immediately medial to each posterior tubercle. This is at the inferior limit of the facet (zygapophyseal) joint. Pressure on this tubercle will produce compression of the facet joint, whereas pressure just below the tubercle will produce an anterior movement of the lower articular pillar and slight gapping of the joint surfaces.

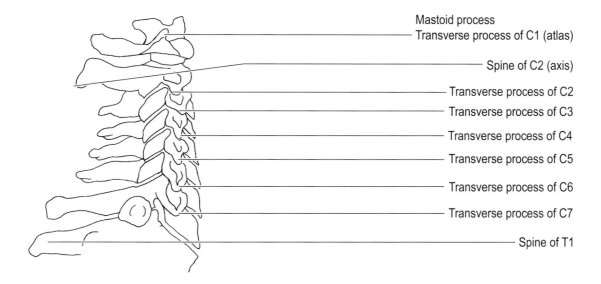

Mastoid process
Transverse process of C1 (atlas)

Spine of C2 (axis)

Transverse process of C2
Transverse process of C3
Transverse process of C4
Transverse process of C5
Transverse process of C6
Transverse process of C7

Spine of T1

Fig. 4.5 (b)
Bones of the neck (lateral aspect)

Normally the thick muscles covering the transverse processes need to be moved aside to facilitate palpation. More 'feel' of the transverse processes is available if the subject adopts a supine position with the occiput cradled in the hands of the examiner who stands at the head of the plinth facing the subject's feet. With the fingers of either hand resting on the posterolateral part of the neck, the head is moved from side to side, the axis of movement being an anteroposterior axis through the lower skull. Apply gentle pressure to the transverse process with your fingers on the opposite side to that being examined. This opens up the side of interest with the space between the transverse processes increasing, facilitating their identification.

The facet joints of this side are also being gapped, causing a greater convexity to the side being examined. It will be noticed that slight rotation to the opposite side will occur during this movement (see Fig. 4.7a, b). This technique can be used from C1 down to T1. In the lower section of the neck these transverse processes can be palpated from the front, although it is slightly uncomfortable. Occasionally, the costal element (the anterior segment of the transverse process) of C7 projects more anterolaterally than usual and can be palpated 2 cm above and 2 cm lateral to the medial end of the clavicle. This is often referred to as a 'cervical rib'.

SELF ASSESSMENT

Page 234

1. Is the skull broader anteriorly or posteriorly?

2. Name the bones which form the vault of the skull.

3. Name the suture which passes transversely across the skull behind the anterior bone.

4. In which area is Bregma sited?

5. Which suture runs anteroposteriorly along the centre of the skull superiorly?

6. Where is the Lambda site located?

7. Name the two sutures which run downwards and backwards from Lambda.

8. With what structure is the skull covered superficially?

9. What is the anterior attachment of this covering?

10. To what structure is it attached posteriorly?

Page 235

11. Which bone forms the major part of the back of the head?

12. Name the bone this joins on either side.

13. In which bone is the foramen magnum formed?

14. What bony prominence can be palpated 5 cm below the point Lambda?

15. Name the three lines which radiate laterally, on either side, from this bony prominence.

16. The mastoid process is part of which bone?

17. Where can the mastoid process be located?

18. Which muscle attaches to this bony prominence?

Page 236

19. List the bones which contribute to the formation of the eye orbit?

20. In which bone are the upper teeth located?

Please complete the labels below.

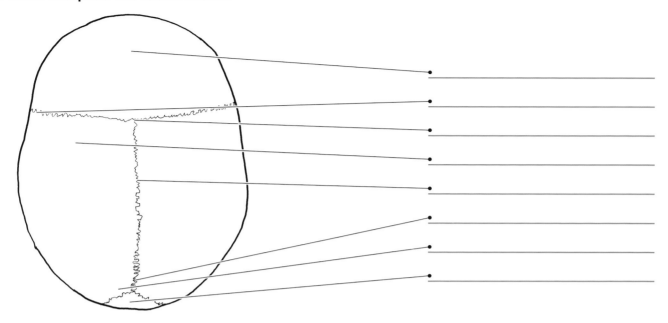

Fig. 4.1 (a) The skull (superior aspect)

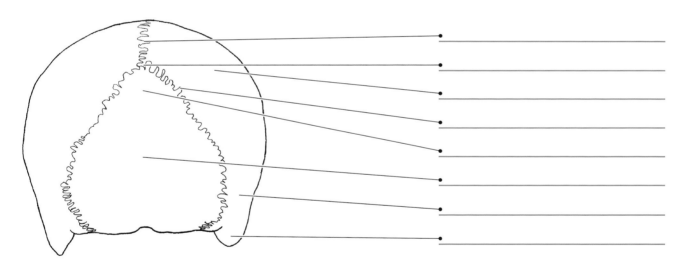

Fig. 4.1 (c) The skull (posterior aspect)

21. Which bone presents the sockets for the inferior teeth?

22. Give the name of the notch at the upper rim of the eye orbit.

23. With which bones does the temporal bone articulate?

24. Which part of the mandible articulates with the maxilla?

25. What joint is formed by these two bones?

Page 237

26. Where is the external auditory meatus located?

27. Describe what is meant by the tragus.

28. Name the bony arch anterior to the tragus.

29. Which bone does this arch meet anteriorly?

30. Is the angle of the mandible more prominent in men or in women?

31. Name the small tubercle situated on either side of the fusion of the two halves of the mandible inferiorly.

Page 238

32. List, from superior to inferior, the bony and cartilaginous structures which are situated at the anterior aspect of the neck.

33. Which muscle lies on either side of these structures?

34. What is the general name for these structures?

35. During swallowing, what happens to these structures?

36. Describe the shape of the hyoid bone.

Page 239

37. Describe the greater and lesser cornua.

38. In which area is the thyroid notch located?

39. What is the medical term for the 'Adam's Apple'?

Please complete the labels below.

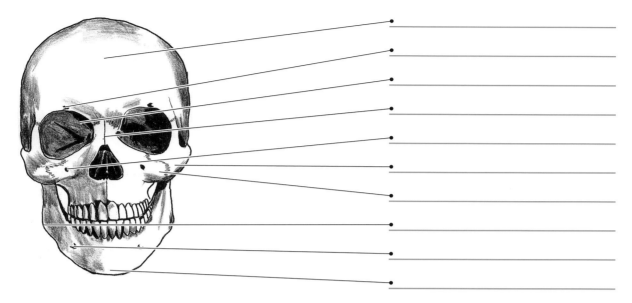

Fig. 4.2 (b) The skull (anterior aspect)

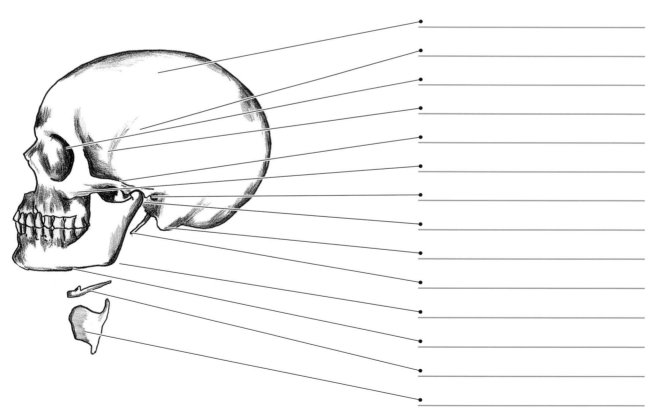

Fig. 4.2 (d) The skull (lateral aspect)

40. Where can the cartilaginous rings of the trachea be palpated?

Page 240

41. How many cervical vertebra are there?

42. Describe the features of a typical cervical vertebra.

43. List the exceptions in the cervical spines.

44. Which part of C1 transfers the weight of the head to C2?

45. What takes the place of the spine of C1?

46. Describe the transverse processes of C1.

47. By what other name is C1 known?

48. How does the body of C2 differ from those of the other cervical vertebrae?

49. Describe the spine of C2.

50. By what other name is C2 known?

51. What is the common name of C7.

52. Which structure is palpable approximately 3 cm below the external occipital protuberance?

Page 241

53. Name the two bony prominences centrally situated posteroinferiorly at the base of the neck.

Page 242

54. Where can the tip of the transverse process of C1 be palpated?

55. Name the long thin bony process situated just deep and anterior to the mastoid process.

Page 243

56. What is an alternative name for the facet joints in the spine?

57. Describe a method by which palpation of the transverse processes of the cervical spine may be facilitated.

58. Describe the meaning of the term 'cervical rib'.

Please complete the labels below.

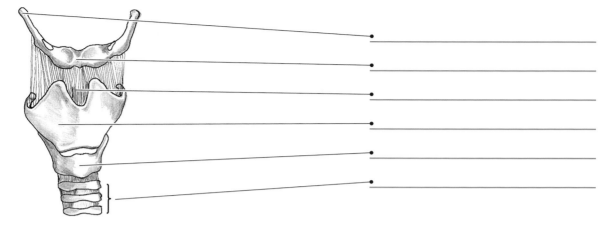

Fig. 4.3 (b) Bones of the neck (anterior aspect)

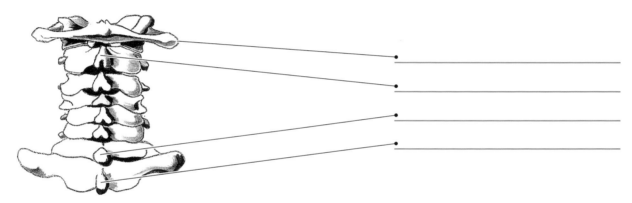

Fig. 4.4 (b) Bones of the neck (posterior aspect)

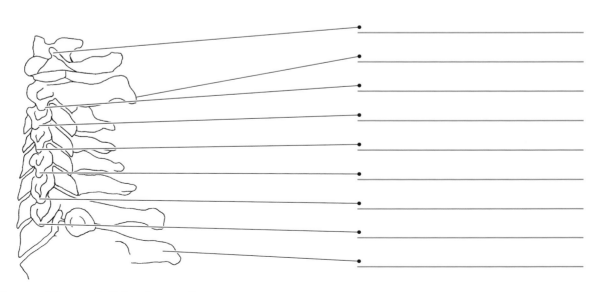

Fig. 4.5 (b) Bones of the neck (lateral aspect)

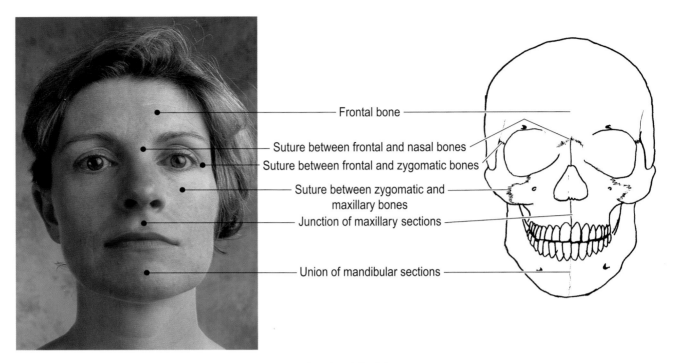

Frontal bone

Suture between frontal and nasal bones

Suture between frontal and zygomatic bones

Suture between zygomatic and maxillary bones

Junction of maxillary sections

Union of mandibular sections

Fig. 4.6 (a), (b)
The joints of the head (anterior aspect)

JOINTS

The skull [Fig. 4.6]

Most of the plates of bone which contribute to the vault of the skull are united by fibrous joints in the form of sutures. These are often visible on the surface and were described and palpated in the section on bones (see pages 234 and 235). Other suture lines which can be palpated are those between the parietal and temporal bones, between the temporal and zygomatic bones and between the two halves of the mandibles.

The first suture lies at the upper edge of the squamous portion of the temporal bone. It arches convexly upwards from the depression just lateral to the eye orbit to just anterior to the upper part of the pinna of the ear. If the subject clenches the teeth the temporalis muscle can be palpated contracting above the zygomatic arch (see page 000). At the curved upper part of this muscle, the line of the suture can be identified.

The second suture can be palpated approximately halfway along the zygomatic arch. If the finger is run anteroposteriorly, the suture can be felt as a

raised ridge crossing the arch vertically. The third can be palpated between the two halves of the mandible, running vertically downwards from the centre of the lower lip to the inferior border between the two mental tubercles. It is often marked by a sharp ridge.

Accessory movements of the joints of the skull

In the unborn child and infant these plates of bone can allow considerable movement and, on occasions, even override each other. There is slight movement throughout childhood and early adult life, but from the twenties through to middle age there is gradual fusion of the various sutures, beginning with the sagittal suture (Palastanga, Field and Soames 1998). Some authorities believe that the movement of one plate of bone on another influences the structures below and can be used as a therapeutic technique.

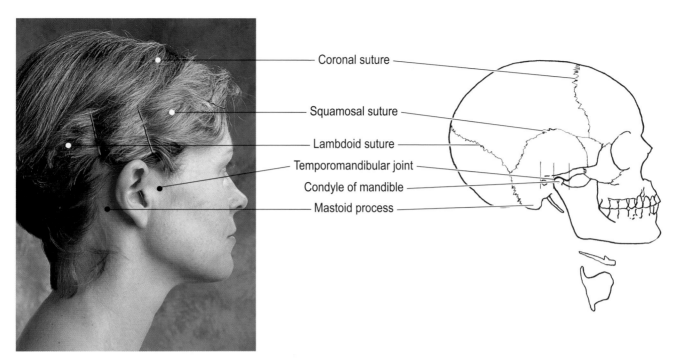

Fig. 4.6 (c), (d)
The joints of the head (lateral aspect)

The *temporomandibular joint* [Fig. 4.6c and d]

This is a bicondylar articulation taking place between the mandibular fossae of the temporal bone and the condylar processes of the mandible, the two joints being linked by the mandible.

Palpation

From the tragus of the ear, trace forwards under the posterior section of the zygomatic arch for 2 cm, where a small tubercle on the condyle of the mandible can be palpated. The line of the joint lies just above this tubercle, running forwards for approximately 2 cm concave downwards posteriorly and convex downwards anteriorly. If the subject opens the mouth, the line of the joint becomes clearer as the condyle first rotates and then moves forward on the under surface of the temporal bone.

Accessory movements

This joint is capable of many physiological movements, mainly involved in mastication. Its only true accessory movement, however, is distraction. This can be produced by placing the thumbs in the mouth on the lower molar teeth on both sides, with the fingers of each hand supporting the underside of the mandible from outside. Downward pressure is then applied to the teeth via the thumbs, using the fingers to hold the anterior part of the mandible stationary. This creates the necessary leverage to pull the condyles away from the temporal bone. Complete relaxation of the muscles of mastication is essential for any gapping to occur.

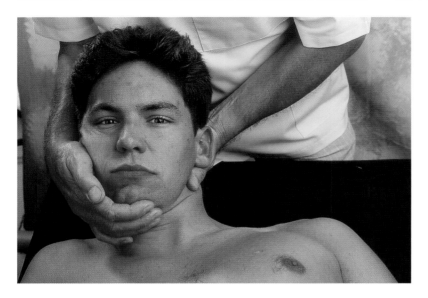

Fig. 4.7 (a)
Right lateral movement of the
cervical spine

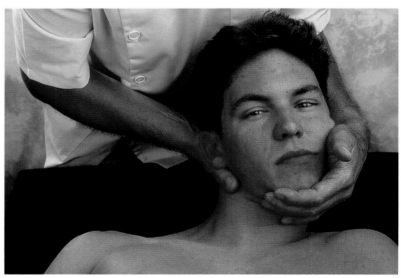

Fig. 4.7 (b)
Left lateral movement of the
cervical spine

The cervical spine [Figs 4.7 and 4.8]

With the exception of the joints between the occiput and C1, and C1 and C2, the cervical vertebrae articulate by a series of fibrous discs centrally, synovial zygapophyseal joints between the articular processes laterally, and synovial uncovertebral joints between the lateral margins of adjacent vertebral bodies.

The occipital condyles either side of the foramen magnum articulate with the facets on the superior surface of the atlas (C1) as a bicondylar joint. The atlas articulates with the axis (C2) via plane joints either side of the dens and a single central pivot joint between the dens and the anterior arch of the atlas, in front, and with the transverse ligament, behind. All of these are synovial joints.

Palpation

It is difficult to palpate any joints in the cervical region owing to their depth and location. Movements of many can be achieved by pressure on the bones that take part, but actual joint lines are normally impossible to determine and feel.

Find the articular pillars of C2–C7 lying 2 cm lateral to the spines (see pages 242 and 243). With deep but sensitive palpation, the lines of the lower zygapophyseal joints can be detected level with the tip of the spinous process of the same vertebra.

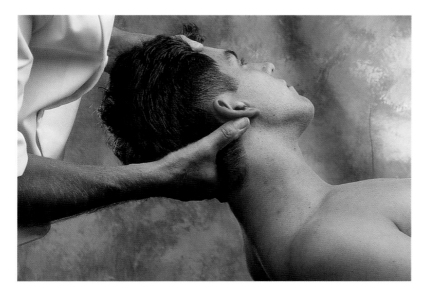

Fig. 4.7 (c)
Anterior movement of the cervical spine

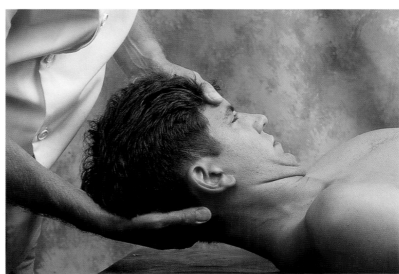

Fig. 4.7 (d)
Posterior movement of the
cervical spine

Accessory movements

Traction on the cervical spine (C2–C7), either mechanically or manually, is a true accessory movement, as it is a movement that the subject cannot perform alone. It can be carried out in extension, flexion, rotation or any combination of these, depending on the results required. It produces parting of the surfaces of the zygapophyseal and central joints with a stretching of the disc, the surrounding ligaments and muscles. There will be a decrease in the pressure within the disc, and an increase in the size, particularly in flexion, of the intervertebral foramen, through which the cervical nerves emerge.

Traction on the joints between the occiput, C1 and C2 is best obtained when the neck is slightly extended. Its use, however, is normally restricted as it can produce undesirable and dangerous effects, due to the complex nature of these joints, particularly concerning the ligaments around the dens. The ligaments remain taut in all movements, thereby maintaining the relationship of the dens with the atlas and occiput. Accessory movement,

necessary for gliding to occur, is only possible because of the precise curvatures of the articular surfaces.

With the subject lying supine, a sideways movement of the whole neck can be achieved by holding the head between the two hands and moving it from side to side while maintaining its longitudinal position (Fig. 4.7a, b).

A similar movement forwards and backwards can be achieved by placing one hand over the forehead and the other hand behind the occiput and moving the head forwards and backwards, again maintaining its longitudinal position (Fig. 4.7c, d).

Using a sagittal axis, passing through the nose, the side-to-side movement can be localized to the joints between the condyles of the occipital bone and the lateral masses of the atlas. Using a frontal axis through the centre of the skull, localized forward and backward gliding can also be achieved (Fig. 4.7c, d).

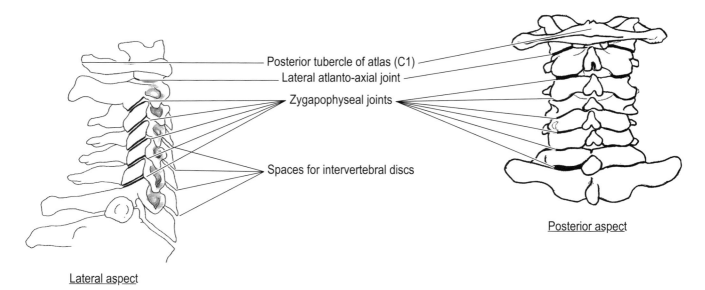

Posterior tubercle of atlas (C1)

Lateral atlanto-axial joint

Zygapophyseal joints

Spaces for intervertebral discs

<u>Posterior aspect</u>

<u>Lateral aspect</u>

Fig. 4.8 (a), (b)
Joints of the cervical spine

Other movements of the cervical vertebrae, often considered to be accessory movements, are very similar to normal physiological movements. Nevertheless, certain elements are exaggerated and therefore worthy of note.

With the subject lying prone, forward gliding of a whole vertebra on its neighbour can be achieved by pressure applied with the thumbs on the tip of the spinous process. Movement is greatest around C4 and least between C7 and T1. Pressure on the spine of C2 produces no movement between C1 and C2, as the dens is in contact with the anterior arch of C1; however, slight forward gliding will be achieved between the occiput and C1, due to the two bones moving together.

Pressure on the inferior articular pillar of C3–C7 produces a forward gliding of the inferior articular surface and a slight gapping of the superior zygapophyseal joint in a rotation-type movement. If a similar pressure is applied to the posterior aspect of the transverse process of C1, similar gliding of the lateral mass of that side against the occipital condyle and upper facet of C2 occurs.

With the subject lying supine, side-to-side movement of the vertebrae can be produced by cradling the head in the palms, as described on pages 252 and 253, with the fingers of one side applying pressure to the transverse process of the chosen vertebra. The fingers of the opposite side will then feel the transverse processes opening up, as an accompaniment to the gapping of the zygapophyseal joint.

Rotation of one vertebra on another can be taken to its limit by carefully fixing the lower vertebrae with the fingers and thumb and rotating the head with the other hand. These movements can be

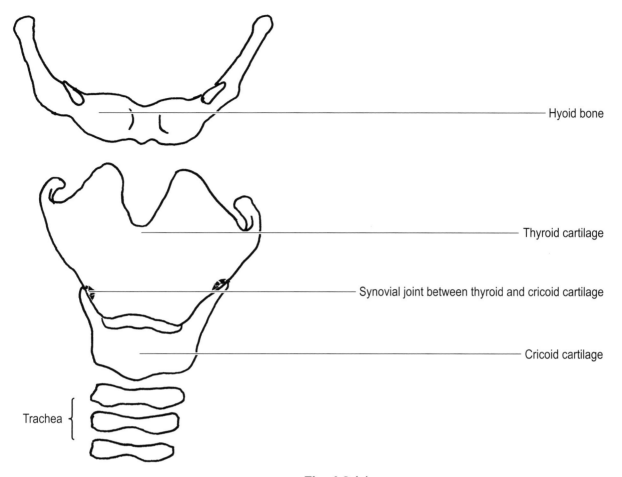

Hyoid bone

Thyroid cartilage

Synovial joint between thyroid and cricoid cartilage

Cricoid cartilage

Trachea

Fig. 4.8 (c)
Anterior structures of the neck

produced between any two cervical vertebrae, and even to some extent between the occiput and C1, producing gapping of their surfaces.

Most accessory movements of the cervical spine are difficult to perform without a great deal of knowledge and practice. It can be highly dangerous for an unskilled therapist to employ these procedures in this area, and it is recommended that the student must be carefully monitored by an experienced practitioner, who should test for contraindications prior to any movement being performed.

For further information, it is suggested that the reader consults the literature on manipulation and mobilization (Grieve 1986, Maitland 1991).

Anterior aspect of the neck

The hyoid bone and the thyroid and cricoid cartilages can all be moved from side to side approximately 1 cm using the finger and thumb alternately. They are linked by muscle and ligaments to the mandible and temporal bone above and the upper part of the trachea below.

Between the inferior cornua of the thyroid cartilage and the arch of the cricoid cartilage are small synovial joints which can be located just above the posterior projections of the cricoid cartilage. These possess a capsule and can, at times, give pain and distress when they become inflamed or degenerated.

SELF ASSESSMENT

Page 250

1. What type of joint is found between the plates of bone of the skull?

2. Where in the skull can these joints be palpated?

3. Describe the arrangement of these joints in the formation of the skull.

4. At what period in life are the plates most mobile?

5. Which ligaments are involved in the structure of these joints?

6. What is the link between the shape of the bony edge and the name of the type of joint?

Page 251

7. Give the class and type of the temporomandibular joint.

8. Describe and name the two bony processes which take part in this joint.

9. In which area is this joint located?

10. Describe the movement which can be palpated at this joint when the subject opens the mouth?

11. Which is the only accessory movement possible at this joint?

12. Describe how this accessory movement is produced.

Page 252

13. Name the class and type of joints found between two typical cervical vertebrae.

14. In what ways do they differ in their structure?

15. Explain their differing function.

16. List the joints that exist between the occiput and C1.

17. Describe the joints which exist between the Atlas C1 and the Axis C2.

18. What class and type are the joints between C1 and C2?

19. Which joints in the cervical spine is it, sometimes, possible to palpate?

20. How are these joints best located?

Please complete the labels below.

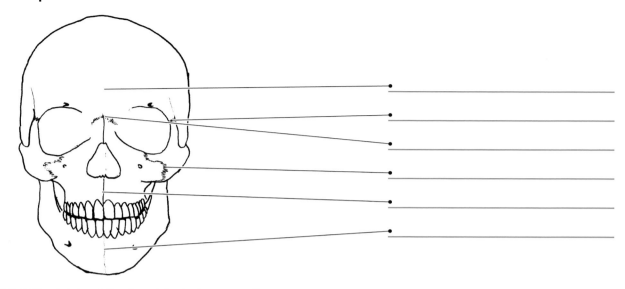

Fig. 4.6 (b) The joints of the head (anterior aspect)

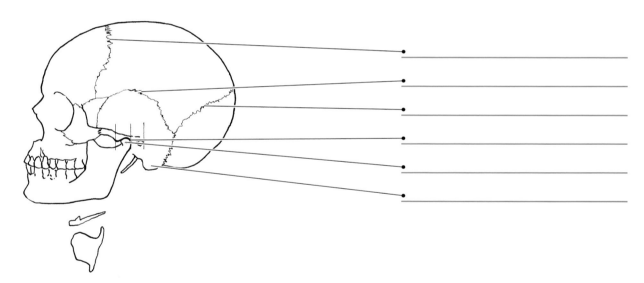

Fig. 4.6 (d) The joints of the head (lateral aspect)

Page 253

21. Name one true accessory movement of these joints.

22. How can this movement be varied?

23. What is the resultant movement produced by the application of this accessory movement?

24. How does this affect the cervical disc?

25. Performed in flexion, how does this affect the intervertebral foramen?

26. Why is it undesirable to apply too much traction to the upper cervical region?

27. Describe the procedure for obtaining lateral movement of the cervical spine.

28. Describe the technique for producing forward and backward movement of the cervical spine.

29. During forward and backward gliding of the cervical spine, state the region in which most movement occurs.

30. Where does least movement occur?

31. What type of movement occurs at a zygapophyseal joint when pressure is applied to the posterior aspect of the inferior element of the joint?

Page 254

32. Describe how forward gliding of a whole vertebra on its neighbour can be achieved?

33. Where is this movement greatest and least?

34. Why does forward pressure on the spine of C2 produce no movement between C1 and C2?

Page 255

35. From superior to inferior, name the bones and cartilages found in the anterior aspect of the neck.

36. When are these structures seen to move?

37. Can they be moved passively?

38. Describe how they are linked to the mandible and temporal bone above.

39. What is the continuation of these structures below?

Please complete the labels below.

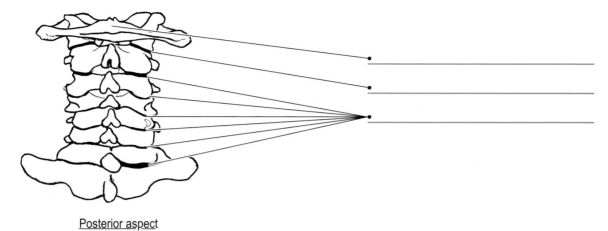

Posterior aspect

Fig. 4.8 (b) Joints of the cervical spine

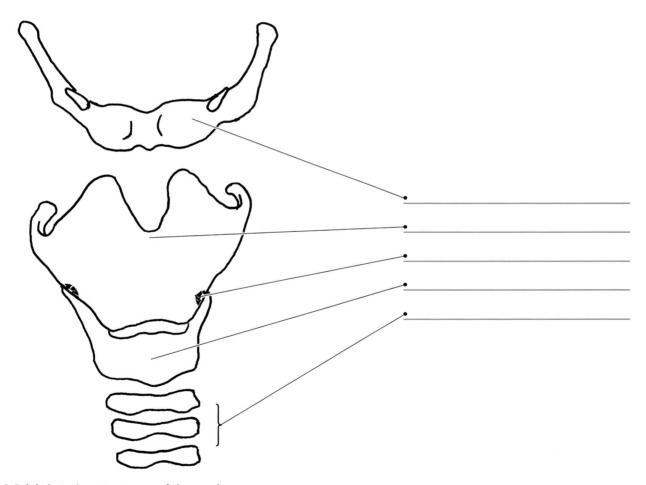

Fig. 4.8 (c) Anterior structures of the neck

40. Are there any joints between these structures?

_____

41. If so, state their location and type.

_____

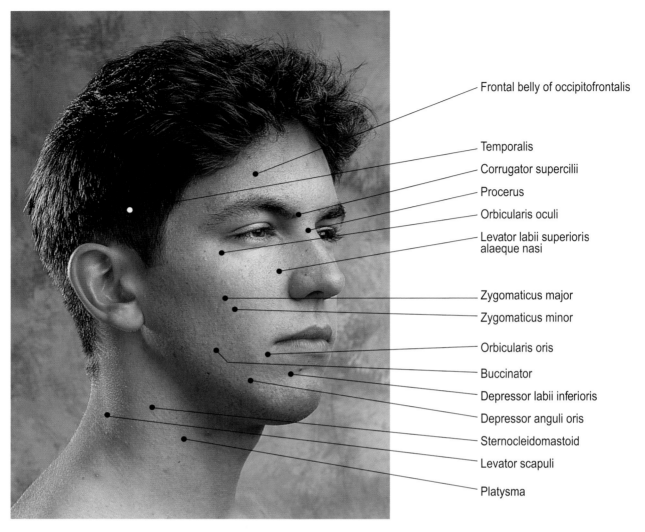

- Frontal belly of occipitofrontalis
- Temporalis
- Corrugator supercilii
- Procerus
- Orbicularis oculi
- Levator labii superioris alaeque nasi
- Zygomaticus major
- Zygomaticus minor
- Orbicularis oris
- Buccinator
- Depressor labii inferioris
- Depressor anguli oris
- Sternocleidomastoid
- Levator scapuli
- Platysma

Fig. 4.9 (a)
Muscles of the head and neck
(lateral aspect)

MUSCLES

Muscles of facial expression [Figs 4.9–4.11]

The muscles associated with the skull are mainly situated anteriorly, where they produce facial expressions, and laterally, where they produce the movements of mastication. The muscles are, however, very difficult to palpate unless they are contracting. Most muscles of the face arise from broad bony and fibrous attachments and pass to the fascia deep to the skin.

Their attachments at both ends are normally highly complex, sending fibres to blend with surrounding muscles, thus influencing the action which produces the many expressions possible in the human face. Because of this complexity only the basic attachments will be given in this text, but enough to demonstrate the action of the muscle.

Palpation

The muscle bellies of occipitofrontalis (Figs 4.9, 4.10a, b) attach superiorly via a fibrous aponeurotic sheet which passes over the scalp. Anteriorly the muscle attaches to the upper margin of the fascia over the eye orbit and posteriorly to the superior nuchal line. If the subject raises and lowers the eyebrow several times, the scalp can be felt moving forwards and backwards, with the posterior and anterior bellies contracting alternately.

Corrugator supercilii (Fig. 4.10c, d) can be palpated above the nose at the medial end of the eyebrow. If the subject frowns, short almost vertical ridges are produced as the muscle contracts.

Orbicularis oculi (Fig. 4.10e, f) closes the eye. The muscle can be palpated easily if the subject closes the eye and, with the examiner's fingers gently resting on the eyelids, the subject then

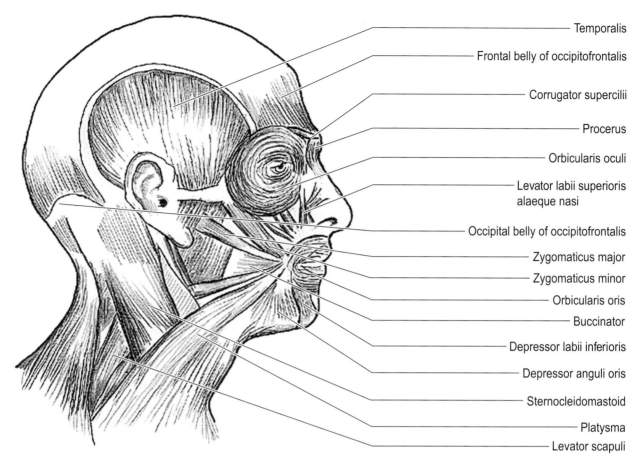

Temporalis

Frontal belly of occipitofrontalis

Corrugator supercilii

Procerus

Orbicularis oculi

Levator labii superioris
alaeque nasi

Occipital belly of occipitofrontalis

Zygomaticus major

Zygomaticus minor

Orbicularis oris

Buccinator

Depressor labii inferioris

Depressor anguli oris

Sternocleidomastoid

Platysma

Levator scapuli

Fig. 4.9 (b)
Muscles of the head and neck
(lateral aspect)

squeezes the eyes shut tightly. A hard muscular covering can be felt.

If the fingers are placed over the corner of the nose and the upper lip when the subject sneers, the contraction of levator labii superioris alaeque nasi (Fig. 4.10g, h) can be felt. The alae of the nose will also be raised and move apart while the upper lip is raised at its centre.

When the subject smiles, the corners of the mouth are drawn upwards and laterally. This movement is produced by contraction of levator anguli oris and zygomaticus major and minor (Figs 4.9 and 4.11a, b) all of which are palpable between the angle of the mouth and the zygomatic bone (the point of the cheek).

Depressor anguli oris (Fig. 4.11c, d) can be palpated just below the angle of the mouth,

particularly when it is drawn downwards, as in the expression of sadness. Contraction of depressor labii inferioris (Fig. 4.11c, d) is palpable between the lower lip and the chin. It curls the whole lower lip downwards, thereby exposing the lower teeth.

If the lips are closed tightly, the hard ring of muscle surrounding the mouth, orbicularis oris (Fig. 4.11e, f) can be palpated and when the subject tries to blow through the closed mouth, contraction of buccinator (Fig. 4.11e, f) can be felt in the cheeks.

If the teeth are now clenched together, as in a 'snarling' expression, platysma (Fig. 4.11g, h) can be palpated anywhere between the mandible and the superior part of the chest. This muscle appears to expand the neck volume and is also brought into action when resistance is given to hands being tightened around the neck.

Occipitofrontalis

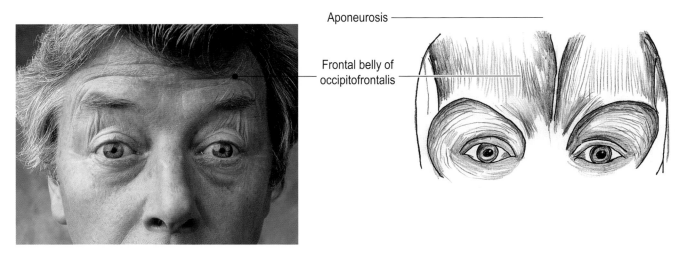

Fig. 4.10 (a), (b)
Muscles raising the eyebrows (surprise)

Frontal belly attaches to the fascia over the upper eye orbit. Posterior belly attaches to the lateral two-thirds of the superior nuchal line. Both bellies attach superiorly to the aponeurosis covering the scalp.

Corrugator supercilii

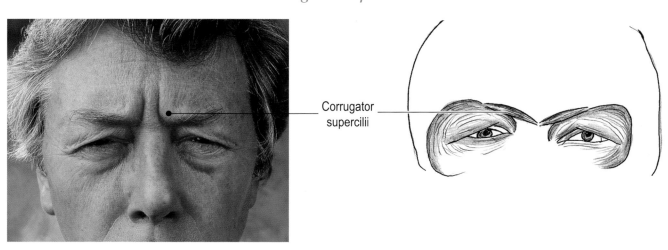

Fig. 4.10 (c), (d)
Muscles drawing the eyebrows together (frowning)

Medially attaches to bone at the medial end of the superciliary arch. Laterally attaches to the skin over mid point of the eye orbit.

Orbicularis oculi

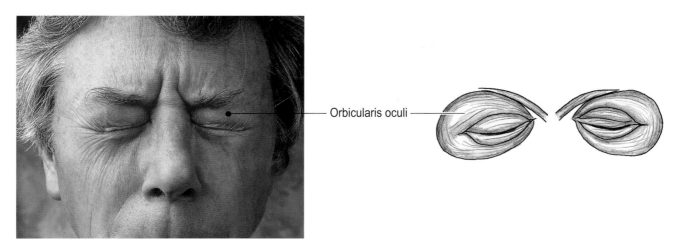

Fig. 4.10 (e), (f)
Muscles closing the eyes

Elliptical muscle attaching to the bone surrounding the eye orbit.

Levator labii superioris alaeque nasi and levator labii superioris

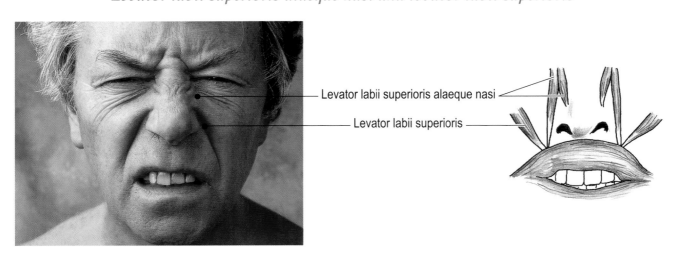

Fig. 4.10 (g), (h)
Muscles raising the upper lip and opening the nasal cavity (sneering)

Levator labii superioris alaeque nasi attaches above to the maxillary bone and below to the greater alar cartilage and skin covering it.

Levator labii superioris attaches above to the maxilla and zygomatic bone and below to the upper lip halfway between the angle of the mouth and the mid point.

Levator anguli oris

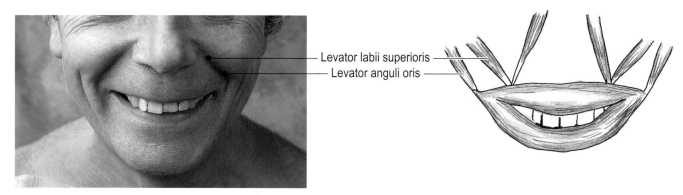

Fig. 4.11 (a), (b)
Muscles raising the corners of the mouth (smiling)

The levator anguli oris attaches above to canine fossa just below the infraorbital foramen of maxilla and attaches below to the corner of the mouth.

Depressor anguli oris and depressor labii inferioris

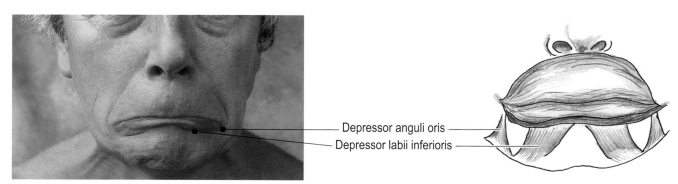

Fig. 4.11 (c), (d)
Muscles pulling the corners of the mouth and lower lip downwards (indicating sadness)

Depressor anguli oris attaches to the mental tubercle of the mandible below and to the angle of the mouth above.

Depressor labii inferioris attaches below to the oblique line close to the mental foramen and above to the centre of the lower lip.

Orbicularis oris and buccinator

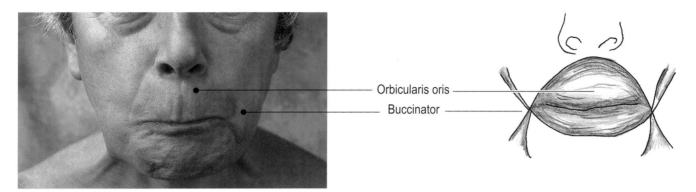

Fig. 4.11 (e), (f)
Muscles closing or pursing the lips

Orbicularis oris is a highly complex raphe of fibres surrounding the mouth composed of eight blending sections and functionally acting in four quadrants. In addition it receives fibres from all the surrounding muscles.

Buccinator basically attaches to the molar area of the maxilla and mandible. Its fibres pass forwards blending with the orbicularis oris, its upper fibres into the upper lip, its lower fibres into the lower lip, but its middle fibres crossing at the corners of the mouth.

Platysma

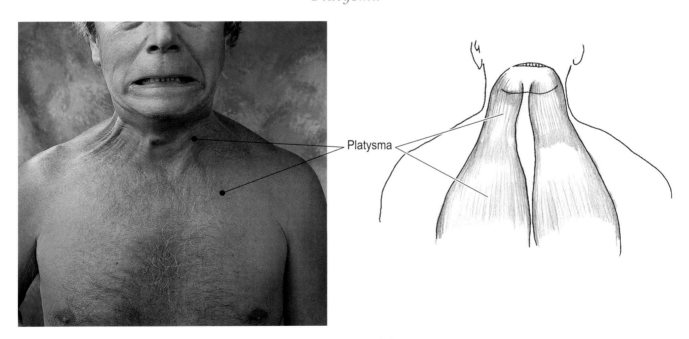

Fig. 4.11 (g), (h)
Muscles drawing fascia around the mouth downwards (protecting the structures in the neck and producing a snarling expression).

Attaches below to the fascia covering the upper part of pectoralis major and deltoid. Above it attaches to the inferior border of the mandible with some of its lateral fibres passing over to the lower lip and its medial fibres crossing over to the opposite side.

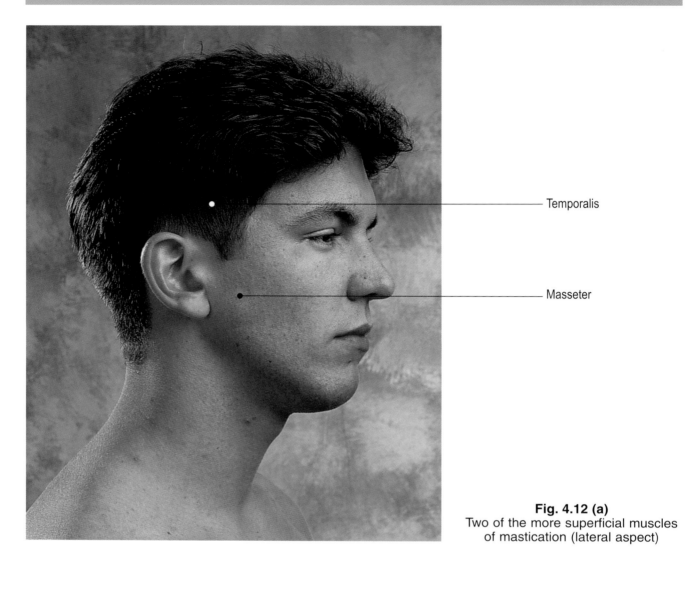

Temporalis

Masseter

Fig. 4.12 (a)
Two of the more superficial muscles
of mastication (lateral aspect)

Muscles of mastication [Fig. 4.12]

These are powerful muscles situated more deeply on the lateral side of the face. Temporalis is a fan-shaped muscle attaching above to the lateral side of the temporal bone, reaching as high as the suture between it and the parietal bone. The muscle passes down under the zygomatic arch to the coronoid process of the mandible. Masseter attaches above to the zygomatic arch, its fibres passing downwards and backwards to attach to the lateral surface of the mandible close to its angle.

The medial and lateral pterygoid lie deep to the upper part of the ramus and coronoid of the mandible. The medial pterygoid attaches above to the medial side of the lateral pterygoid plate and palatine bone to pass downwards and backwards to the medial side of the ramus and angle of the mandible. The lateral pterygoid attaches above to the lateral side of the lateral pterygoid plate and the temporal bone and passes backwards to attach to the neck of the mandible and the capsule and disc of the temporomandibular joint.

Palpation

With the fingers placed just above the zygomatic arch, alternately clench and relax the teeth. Although hidden to a certain extent by the thick fascia which covers it, the contraction of the fan-shaped belly of temporalis can be palpated. Passing almost vertically deep to the zygomatic arch to the mandible, its fibres become too deep to palpate.

The same action with the fingers over the side of the mandible just above and in front of the angle enables the powerful masseter muscle to be felt contracting and relaxing. A series of ridges can be palpated, indicating the direction and power of its fibres. In some subjects, particularly lean males, the coarse muscle fibres can be seen crossing the side of the jaw obliquely. The lower fibres can be traced as far as the lower border of the mandible, inferiorly, and the anterior end of the zygomatic arch superiorly.

Palpation of the medial and lateral pterygoid muscles is impossible, as they are too deeply situated.

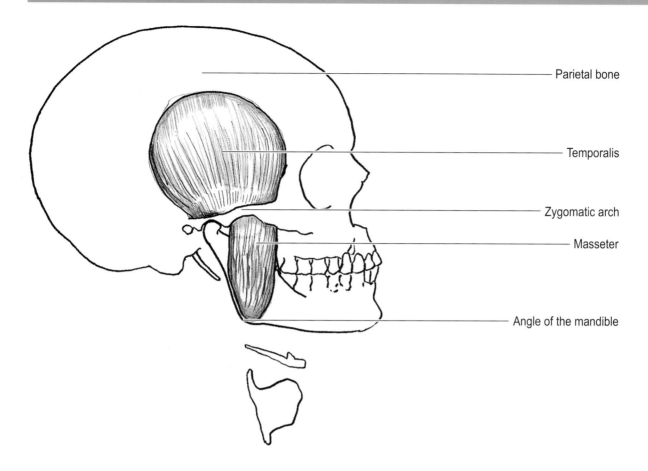

Fig. 4.12 (b)
Two of the more superficial muscles
of mastication (lateral aspect)

It will be noted that the temporalis and the masseter muscles are concerned with closing the mouth and with powerful biting. Although the mandible acts as a third-order lever in the initial bite, as the food moves backwards between the molars it changes so that the food is first in line with the muscle pull and then nearer to the temporomandibular joint than the muscles. The mandible then becomes a second-order lever, with its decrease in range but increase in power. It is at this point that the act of chewing takes place.

Give the subject a piece of steak to eat, for example, and while he or she is doing so place your fingers over the posterior part of the cheeks. As the steak makes its way backwards, the muscles contract harder and the jaw moves from side to side in a grinding action utilizing the pterygoid muscles. If the steak is tough, these muscles will ache.

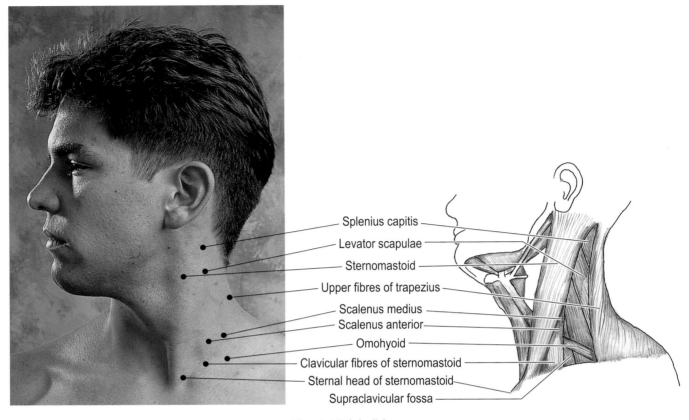

Splenius capitis
Levator scapulae
Sternomastoid
Upper fibres of trapezius
Scalenus medius
Scalenus anterior
Omohyoid
Clavicular fibres of sternomastoid
Sternal head of sternomastoid
Supraclavicular fossa

Fig. 4.13 (a), (b)
Muscles of the neck (lateral aspect, posterior group)

Muscles of the neck [Fig. 4.13]

The neck is surrounded by layers of muscle. These vary in their function which may include moving the neck itself, moving the head, mastication, swallowing and moving the shoulder girdle. Some are involved in a combination of several of these functions.

The more superficial muscles tend to be the more powerful and are therefore easier to find and palpate. However, because of their size they do tend to cover the smaller, deeper muscles.

Some of the muscles are only attached to different parts of the vertebral column, some attach the column to the head and thoracic cage. Others, usually the longer, attach to the head and the thoracic cage. All the attachments are complex, but have a direct bearing on the resultant movement and function. All attachments are essential knowledge in anatomy, and further study must be made beyond this palpation and surface marking text (see *Anatomy and Human Movement*, Palastanga, Field and Soames 1998, *Gray's Anatomy*, Williams, Warwick, Dyson and Bannister 1995).

Palpation

With the subject sitting, place your hands over the posterosuperior area of the neck, halfway between the occiput and the acromion process. When the subject raises the pectoral girdle, as in a shrugging movement, the powerful upper fibres of trapezius (Fig. 4.13a, b) can be felt contracting. The muscle can be traced superiorly to its aponeurotic attachment to the medial third of the superior nuchal line, external occipital protuberance and the sides of the ligamentum nuchae. Inferiorly it can be traced to its attachments to the posterior border of the lateral third clavicle, medial border of the acromion and lateral part upper lip of the spine of the scapula. The central muscular fibres sometimes appear to be stringy and are often quite tender, particularly after a period of sustained activity.

Sternomastoid (sternocleidomastoid) (Fig. 4.13a, b) attaches to the mastoid process above, and the upper surface of the medial end of the clavicle and upper border of the sternum below. To palpate the muscles, place your fingers over the lower attachment. When the subject turns the head to

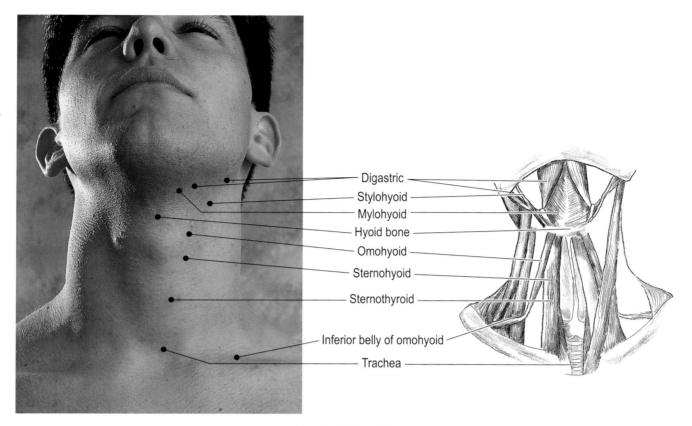

Digastric
Stylohyoid
Mylohyoid
Hyoid bone
Omohyoid
Sternohyoid
Sternothyroid
Inferior belly of omohyoid
Trachea

Fig. 4.13 (c), (d)
Muscles of the neck (anterior aspect, anterior group)

the opposite side, two distinct attachments can be felt, one more cord-like from the sternum and the other more aponeurotic from the clavicle. These appear to twist on each other as they are traced upwards. The thick strap-like sternomastoid stands away from the neck when contracted. It becomes cord-like again as it approaches and attaches to the mastoid process, spreading as a sheet to the lateral part of the superior nuchal line. Both sternomastoid muscles contract strongly and are easily palpable if the subject raises the head when lying supine. (Contraction of both sterno-mastoid and trapezius can be produced by resisting movement of the head and neck to the same side – lateral flexion – or rotating the head to the opposite side.)

The scalene muscles (Fig. 4.13a, b) lie just behind and deep to sternomastoid, and with the subject seated can be palpated deep in the hollow between it and the upper fibres of trapezius in the posterior triangle of the neck. These cord-like muscles, running down to attach to the first and

second ribs, appear to be continuously contracted while the head is in the upright position. During coughing, it is often possible to palpate the infe-rior belly of the omohyoid muscle (Fig. 4.13a, b) as it crosses the lower anterior part of the poste-rior triangle of the neck. Posterosuperior to this is scalenus anterior, and a little higher, scalenus medius. On elevation of the pectoral girdle, the fibres of levator scapulae can be palpated nearer the top of the posterior triangle (Fig. 4.13a, b).

During swallowing, the muscles between the mandible, hyoid, thyroid cartilage and sternum contract and relax. Consequently, if the fingers are placed on either side of the throat between the mandible and the hyoid during swallowing, mylohyoid can be observed contracting and lifting the hyoid bone (Fig. 4.13c, d).

Sternohyoid is difficult to palpate during swal-lowing, but in yawning its fibres can be observed on either side of the thyroid cartilage passing downwards towards the sternum.

SELF ASSESSMENT

Page 260

1. Which two main groups of muscles exist on the face?

2. Describe the ways in which these muscles differ in their function.

3. Describe the location where the frontal belly of occipitofrontalis is found.

4. Where does this muscle attach anteriorly?

5. Describe its posterior attachment.

6. How are the two muscle bellies linked?

7. What facial expression is produced when occipitofrontalis contracts?

8. Where is corrugator supercillii located?

9. What expression is produced by its contraction?

10. What is the main action of obicularis occuli?

11. Describe the deformity if orbicularis occuli ceased to function. (fr)

12. Explain how this muscle is best palpated.

13. Name its bony attachment.

Page 261

14. What muscle is put into action on the side of the nose when the subject adopts a sneering expression?

15. Describe what happens to the ala of the nose when this muscle contracts.

16. Name two muscles which are active in the facial expression of smiling.

17. State their bony attachment.

18. In which area are these muscles palpable?

19. Which muscle draws down the corners of the mouth, as in sadness?

20. Name the muscle which draws the whole lower lip downwards.

21. What is the action of obicularis oris?

22. Describe the disability which occurs if this muscle ceases to function. (fr)

Please complete the labels below.

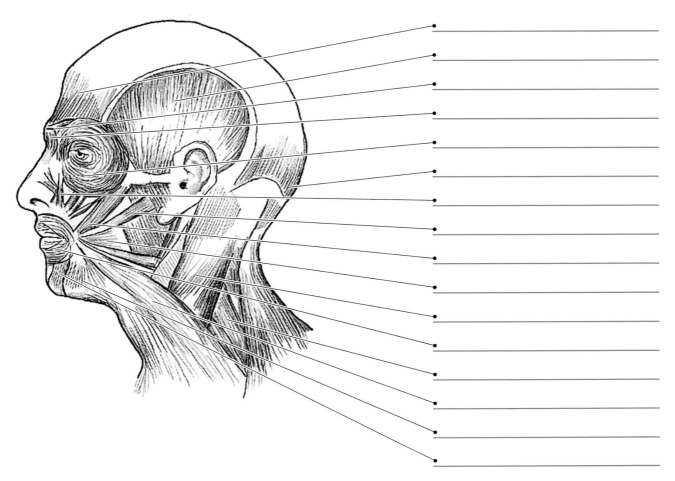

Fig. 4.9 (b) Muscles of the head and neck (lateral aspect)

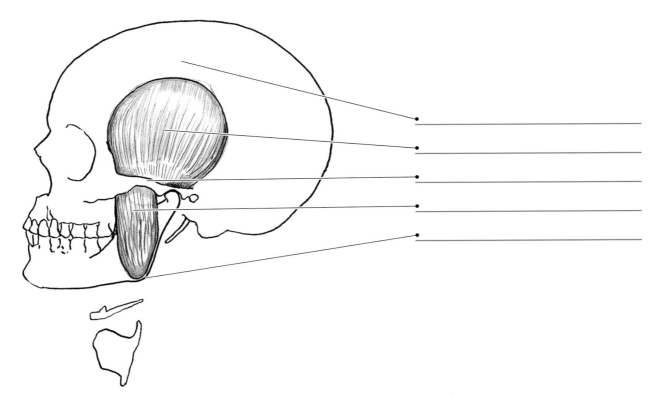

Fig. 4.12 (b) Two of the more superficial muscles of mastication (lateral aspect)

23. Which muscle is involved in expelling air through closed lips, as in playing a trumpet?

24. In the expression of snarling, which muscle is brought into action?

25. In which area can this muscle be palpated?

Page 266

26. List the muscles involved in the act of mastication.

27. Where are these muscles situated?

28. Describe their function.

29. What are the attachments of the muscle which passes under the zygomatic arch?

30. List the attachments of any one other of the group.

31. Describe how the mandible changes its order of lever in chewing. (fr)

Page 268

32. Give a reasoned account of the differing functions produced by the muscles of the neck.

33. List the most powerful muscles.

34. Which muscle can be palpated between the occiput and the acromion process of the scapula?

35. Describe its attachment to the occiput.

36. Where does this muscle attach to the scapula and clavicle?

Page 269

37. Describe the upper and lower attachments of the sternocleidomastoid muscle.

38. In which movements of the neck do both the above muscles participate?

39. What movements are produced by the left sternomastoid contracting alone?

40. List the muscles which can be palpated, above the hyoid bone, during the act of swallowing.

41. Describe their location.

Please complete the labels below.

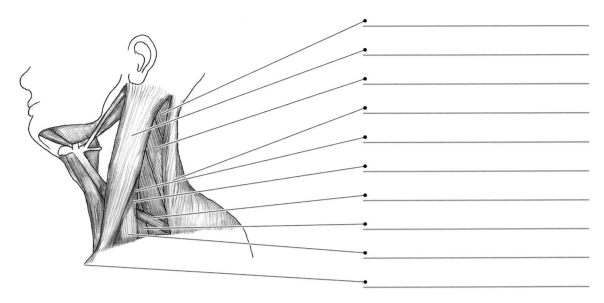

Fig. 4.13 (b) Muscles of the neck (lateral aspect, posterior group)

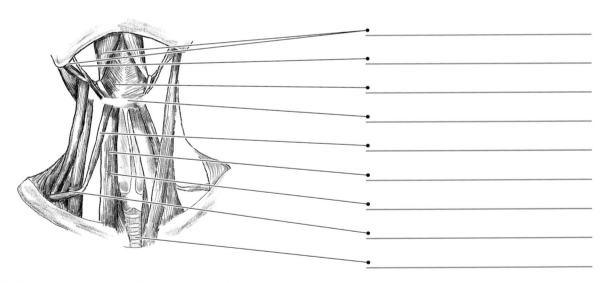

Fig. 4.13 (d) Muscles of the neck (anterior aspect, anterior group)

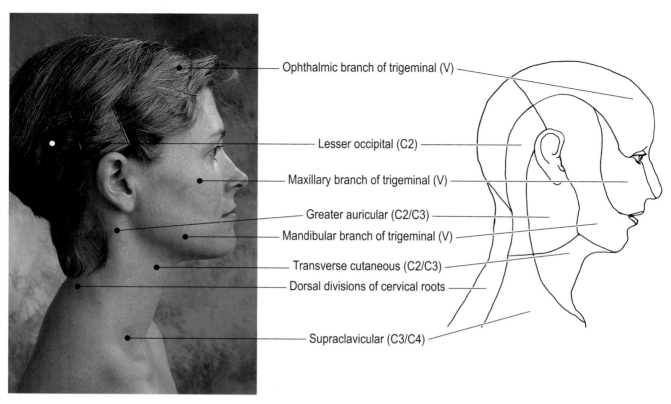

Fig. 4.14 (a), (b)
Cutaneous supply of the head and neck (lateral aspect)

NERVES [Fig. 4.14]

The cutaneous innervation of the face, including forehead, is by the cranial nerves, mainly by the ophthalmic, maxillary and mandibular branches of the trigeminal. The occipital, temporal and posterior part of the parietal regions are supplied by the greater auricular, and greater and lesser occipital, branches of the cervical plexus. The neck is supplied almost entirely through the anterior and posterior rami of the cervical nerve roots, via the transverse cutaneous and supraclavicular branches of cervical plexus (Fig. 4.14a, b). The muscles of facial expression are supplied by the facial nerve (cranial VII), the muscles of mastication via the mandibular branch of the trigeminal (cranial V). All the muscles of the neck are supplied by the cervical nerve roots via the cervical or brachial plexuses. Some of these roots receive communication from other cranial nerves, for example the glossopharyngeal (cranial IV), accessory (cranial XI) and hypoglossal (cranial XII).

Palpation

Very few nerves are palpable in the head and neck region. Usually only the terminal branches reach the surface and even these are difficult to find. Posteriorly it is possible to palpate the greater occipital nerve (root value C2) as it passes vertically to supply the skin over the back of the skull as far forwards as the vertex (Fig. 4.14a, b). This cord-like structure can be palpated over the lower part of the occipital bone approximately 3 cm from the midline. Pressure on the nerve either by the examiner's fingers or muscle tension due to poor posture, or long periods of continuous contraction, can lead to unpleasant sensations and headaches. Care should, therefore, be taken with this examination procedure. Massage to relieve the tension of the muscles surrounding the nerve can produce almost immediate relief from the resulting headache.

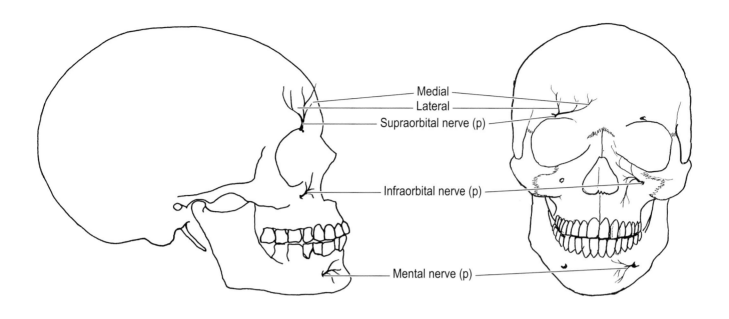

Fig. 4.14 (c), (d)
Cutaneous branches emerging onto the face (lateral and anterior aspect) (p, palpable)

Pressure on the supraorbital nerve as it crosses the superomedial rim of the orbit and on the infraorbital nerve as it emerges from the maxilla just below the centre of the eye orbit (Fig. 4.14c, d) causes discomfort over these areas and the area supplied by the nerves. They are, however, quite difficult to palpate.

On the anterior surface of the mandible, approximately 1 cm lateral to the midline and approximately 1 cm above the inferior border, the mental nerve, a continuation of the inferior dental nerve, emerges on to the surface (Fig. 4.14c, d). The nerve is often palpable in this region, and if pressure is applied to the area an unpleasant feeling is experienced by the subject. It is worth noting that this is the area which appears to become numb first when the dentist gives an anaesthetic injection for drilling the bottom teeth. Just above the central part of the clavicle in the supraclavicular fossa, a series of 'cord-like' structures can be palpated running downwards and laterally. These are the trunks of the brachial plexus emerging from between scalenus anterior and scalenus medius before passing deep to the clavicle to enter the axilla. Pressure in this area will cause discomfort locally and possibly also result in a 'tingling', pain or numbness over the distribution of these nerves in the upper limb.

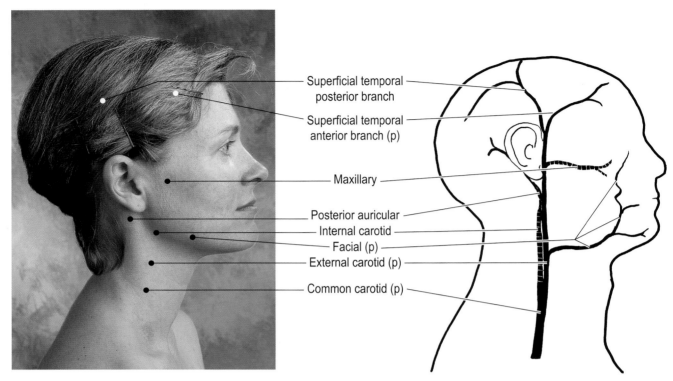

Fig. 4.15 (a), (b)
Main arteries of the head and neck, lateral aspect (p, palpable)

ARTERIES [Fig. 4.15]

The left **common carotid** artery arises from the arch of the aorta, while the right is a division of the brachiocephalic artery. They pass up on either side of the neck deep to sternomastoid to the level of the upper border of the thyroid cartilage, where each divides into the **internal** and **external carotid** arteries.

The former passes superiorly, anterior to the upper three transverse processes, to enter the skull through the carotid canal. Each supplies the cerebral hemisphere, orbit and nose of its own side.

The external carotid artery passes vertically from the upper border of the thyroid cartilage, deep to the parotid gland behind the ramus of the mandible, where it divides into the **superficial temporal** and **maxillary** arteries (Fig. 4.15a, b).

Palpation

The common carotid artery can be palpated on either side of the thyroid cartilage deep to sterno-mastoid. The muscle has to be moved laterally so that the fingers can be slipped from the anterior aspect into the cleft between the cartilage and the muscle. On the lateral side of the upper part of the thyroid cartilage, close to the greater cornua of the hyoid bone, the pulsations of the artery, as it divides, can easily be palpated. This point is important for checking the pulsations of the carotid arteries and is worth spending some time practising.

Between the tragus of the ear and the neck of the mandible the pulsations of the superficial temporal artery can be felt. It can also be palpated above the upper limit of temporalis. The maxillary artery, just below the zygomatic bone, is not quite so obvious as it is covered by muscle and fascia, although to the practised professional it is palpable running anteriorly.

The **facial artery** (Fig. 4.15a, b) can be palpated as it crosses the lower border of the body of the mandible, halfway between the angle of the mandible and the mental tubercle. With care, it can be traced upwards to the corner of the mouth and cheek. Finally, above the eye the pulsations of the supraorbital artery can be palpated as it

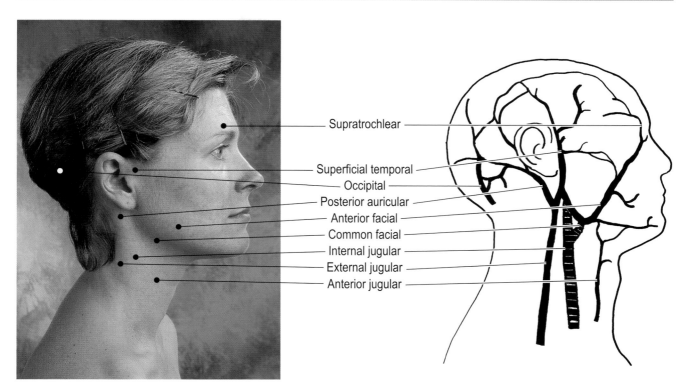

Fig. 4.16 (a), (b)
Veins of the head and neck (lateral aspect)

crosses the medial superior margin of the orbit. It is at this point that injuries, particularly in the sport of boxing, occur. The artery is often ruptured and large quantities of blood pulse out on to the eye and face. It is worth remembering that if pressure were applied to this point for just a few minutes, this loss of blood would cease and the area could be cleaned up, exposing the injury which is usually just a minor trauma.

VEINS [Fig. 4.16]

The veins of the head, neck, and face are divided into two main groups: (a) those that drain the exterior of the cranium and deep tissues of the face, and (b) those that drain the brain, the neck and the superficial areas of the face. The former mainly drain into the **external jugular vein**, while the latter mainly drain into the **internal jugular**.

Palpation

None of these veins is easy to palpate. The lower part of the external jugular contains two sets of valves 4 cm apart, the lower as it joins the subclavian vein. The valves do not prevent regurgitation of blood, and the area between the two sets often bulges and is termed 'the sinus'.

The surface marking of the external jugular is from the angle of the mandible to the middle of the clavicle.

The surface marking of the internal jugular vein can be marked by a broad line drawn from the lobe of the ear to the medial end of the clavicle. It also contains a valve at its junction with the subclavian vein and is often distended just above; however, this lies deep to sternocleidomastoid and cannot be palpated.

SELF ASSESSMENT

Page 274

1. Which group of nerves innervate the skin of the head and face?
   _____

2. Give the names of nerves involved?
   _____

3. Describe the innervation of the skin of the anterior, lateral and posterior aspects of the neck.
   _____

4. Name the branches involved.
   _____

5. From which plexus are these nerves derived?
   _____

6. Which nerve supplies the muscles of facial expression?
   _____

7. The muscles of mastication are supplied by which nerve?
   _____

8. Which plexuses supply all the muscles of the neck?
   _____

9. From which cranial nerves do some of the cervical roots receive communication?
   _____

10. Why are nerves of the head and neck difficult to find?
    _____

11. Which nerve is palpable on the lower posterior part of the occiput?
    _____

12. From which root does it derive its fibres?
    _____

13. Which area of skin over the skull does it supply?
    _____

14. Why must too much pressure on this area be avoided?
    _____

15. What procedure may produce immediate relief from any symptoms?
    _____

Page 275

16. Name the nerve which can be palpated crossing the medial aspect of the superior rim of the eye orbit.
    _____

17. Where does the infraorbital nerve emerge?
    _____

18. When the dentist anaesthetizes the inferior dental nerve, where is numbness usually first observed?
    _____

19. Name this nerve.
    _____

Please complete the labels below.

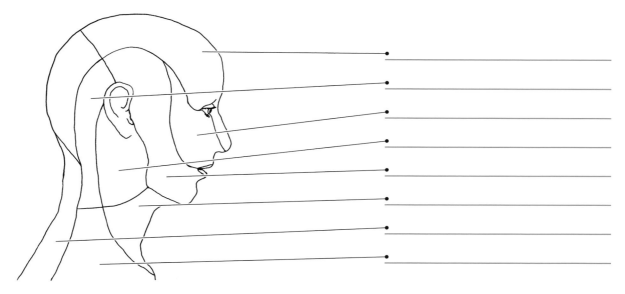

Fig. 4.14 (b) Cutaneous supply of the head and neck (lateral aspect)

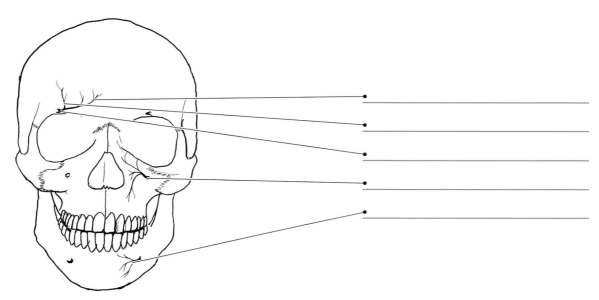

Fig. 4.14 (d) Cutaneous branches emerging onto the face (lateral and anterior aspect) (p, palpable)

20. By what name are the cord-like structures just posterior to the central part of the clavicle in the supraclavicular fossa known?

_____

21. Between which two muscles do these cord-like structures pass?

_____

22. What bony structure lies below these nerves?

_____

Page 276

23. Describe the differences in the origin of the left and right carotid arteries.

24. These arteries pass up the neck deep to which muscle?

25. In which area do they divide into internal and external carotid arteries?

26. Describe the course of the internal carotid artery as it enters the skull.

27. Through which foramen does it enter? (fr)

28. To what structure does it supply blood in the skull?

29. Name the two branches that are given off from the external carotid artery just posterior to the ramus of the mandible.

30. Where on the body can the common carotid artery be palpated?

31. In which area of the body can the superior temporal artery be palpated?

32. Where may the facial artery be palpated?

33. Which artery can be palpated crossing the superomedial part of the orbit?

Page 277

34. List the two main groups of veins that are found in the head and neck.

35. Describe the area of drainage of each group.

36. Which two main veins receive the blood from the head and neck?

37. What structures are found in the lower part of the external jugular vein?

38. What is the term used for this area?

39. Describe the surface marking of the external jugular vein.

40. What is the surface marking of the internal jugular vein.

41. The junction between the internal jugular and subclavian veins is deep to which muscle?

Please complete the labels below.

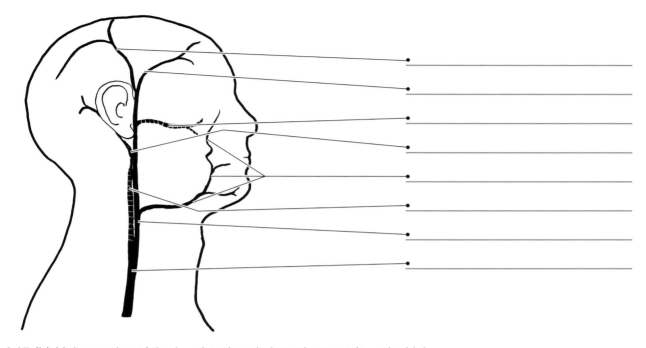

Fig. 4.15 (b) Main arteries of the head and neck, lateral aspect (p, palpable)

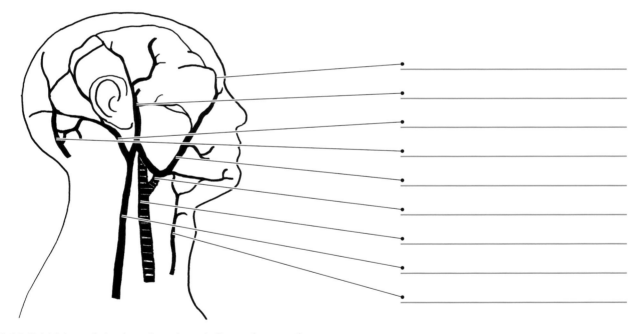

Fig. 4.16 (b) Veins of the head and neck (lateral aspect)

5

The thorax

Contents

At the end of this chapter you should be able to:

A. Find, recognize and name the constituent bony components of the thorax including the clavicle, scapula, ribs and vertebrae noting their size and position.

B. Palpate many of the bony features, being able to relate one to another.

C. Locate, name or number the spines and transverse processes of all the thoracic vertebrae.

D. Recognize and palpate all 12 of the ribs noting their extent.

E. Name all the joints in which the clavicle, scapula, ribs, sternum and vertebrae are involved and palpate the joint lines where possible.

F. Give the class and type of all the joints named.

G. Demonstrate any accessory movements which may be possible in the joints of the thorax.

H. Locate and name the muscles which cover the thorax.

I. Be able to draw the shape of the muscle on the surface and give its attachments.

J. Demonstrate the actions of all of the muscles covering the thorax.

K. Describe the position and attachments of the diaphragm.

L. Give an account of its actions and functional significance.

M. Demonstrate the cutaneous distribution of the thoracic nerves giving an outline of the course each takes.

N. Describe the arrangement of chambers in the heart.

O. Be able to give the surface markings of the main boundaries of the heart.

P. Describe the arrangement of the main arteries in the thorax giving their surface markings.

Q. Describe the arrangement of the main veins in the thorax giving their surface markings.

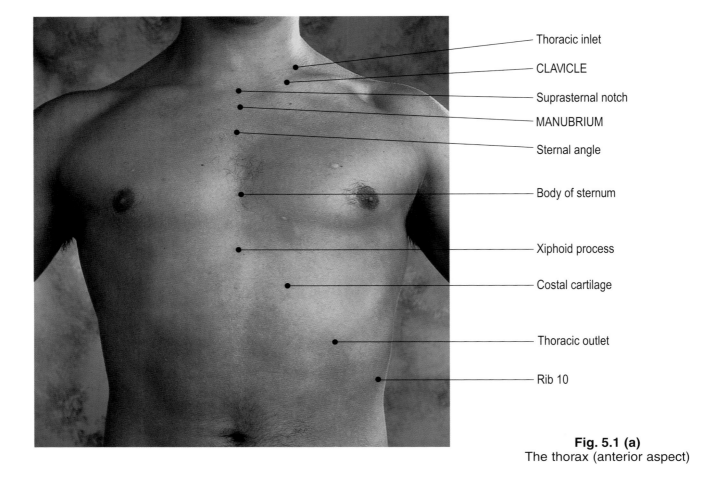

Thoracic inlet

CLAVICLE

Suprasternal notch

MANUBRIUM

Sternal angle

Body of sternum

Xiphoid process

Costal cartilage

Thoracic outlet

Rib 10

Fig. 5.1 (a)
The thorax (anterior aspect)

BONES

The thoracic cage

The bony structure of the thoracic cage consists of the sternum [*stereos* (Gk) = solid, hard], anteriorly, the twelve thoracic vertebrae [vertebra (L) = joint; from verto-I turn] posteriorly, the first being the smallest and the twelfth the largest (Figs 5.2–5.4), and the twelve ribs on either side linking the vertebrae with the sternum. The sternum is angled forward at the manubriosternal joint and angled backwards at the xiphisternal joint, forming a concavity backwards. The ribs are concave inwards and the vertebral column is concave forwards in this region. This forms a large cavity for the protection of vital organs such as the heart and lungs.

The rib spaces are filled with a musculofibrous sheet made up of the intercostal muscles and membrane forming a sealed unit in front, to the sides and behind. There are, however, openings at the top and bottom. The former is smaller and consists of the first thoracic vertebra posteriorly, the first rib on either side and the manubrium anteriorly. This is termed the 'thoracic inlet'. Below there is a much larger opening, termed the 'thoracic outlet', which consists of the twelfth

thoracic vertebra posteriorly, the xiphoid anteriorly and the costal cartilages of ribs 7, 8, 9 and 10, the tip of rib 11 and the full length of rib 12.

The sternum

The sternum lies centrally at the front of the chest and comprises three flat plates of bone, the manubrium [*manubrium* (L) = a handle; the sternum, as a whole, resembles a sword] superiorly, the body centrally and the pointed xiphoid [*xiphos* (Gk) = a sword] process inferiorly. The xiphoid usually remains cartilaginous until approximately the age of 40 years.

The clavicle and scapula

The clavicle lies almost horizontal, articulating with the superolateral part of the manubrium. Posterolaterally the scapula rests on the second to eighth ribs, with the acromion at the lateral end of the spine articulating with the lateral end of the clavicle at the acromioclavicular joint (Fig. 2.7).

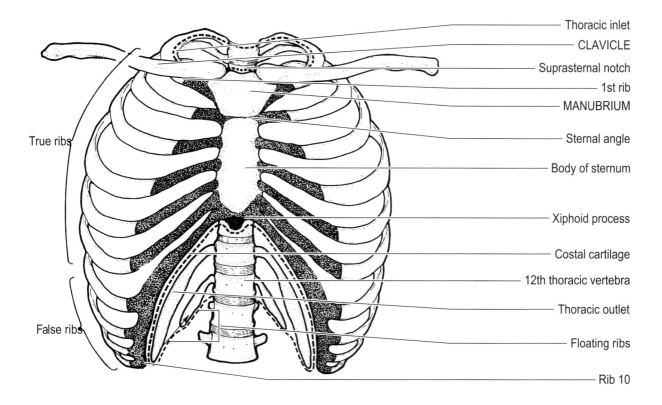

Fig. 5.1 (b)
Bones of the thorax (anterior aspect)

Palpation

Find the suprasternal notch at the upper border of the manubrium (Fig. 5.1a, b). On either side, the medial ends of the clavicle project above the line of the manubrium. Just below the medial end of the clavicle, the manubrium appears to be enlarged laterally. This is actually the anterior end of the first rib and, with careful palpation, the joint between it and the manubrium can be located running vertically, concave laterally 1 cm below and 1 cm lateral to the medial end of the clavicle. Trace down the anterior surface of the manubrium until you find a raised horizontal line; this is where it joins the body of the sternum at the manubriosternal (sternal angle) joint (Fig. 5.1a, b). The reflex angle between the manubrium and body of the sternum is of the order of 200°, changing some 5–7° between full inspiration and full expiration. On either side of the manubriosternal junction the costal cartilages of the second ribs can be palpated, with the lateral border of the manubrium just above.

Continue to trace down either side of the sternum and identify the third to sixth ribs and their costal cartilages, with the lateral border of the sternum lying between their medial ends. The sternum narrows inferiorly and usually dips inwards to join the cartilaginous xiphoid process. The costal cartilage of the seventh rib usually articulates with the sternum at the xiphisternal junction. The whole of the sternum is subcutaneous and is commonly used to take samples of bone marrow. The xiphoid process varies in its formation; it may appear to be pointed, double pointed or even rounded. Normally it projects forwards and therefore can easily be palpated. Occasionally it projects downwards and backwards and is then difficult to palpate.

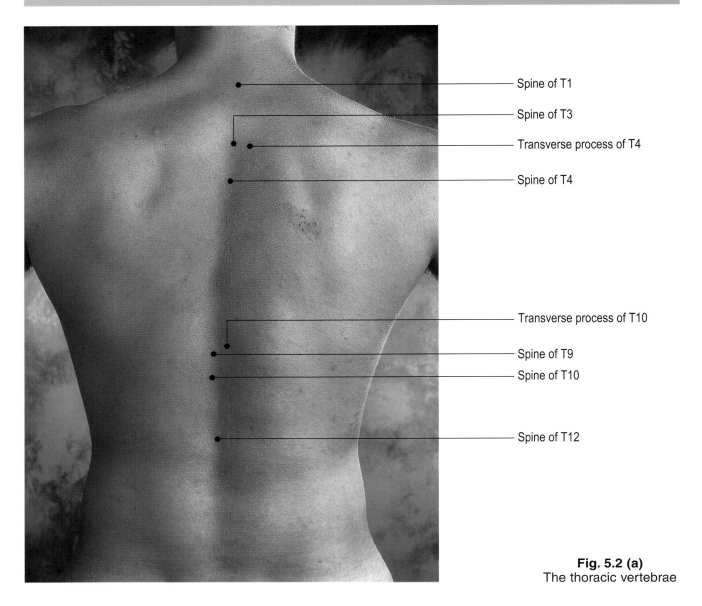

Spine of T1

Spine of T3

Transverse process of T4

Spine of T4

Transverse process of T10

Spine of T9

Spine of T10

Spine of T12

Fig. 5.2 (a)
The thoracic vertebrae

The vertebrae

The thoracic part of the vertebral column can only be palpated posteriorly, where it presents spines and transverse processes. However, these either overlap each other or are covered with strong, thick muscles and fascia, proving difficult even for the experienced palpator to identify with ease.

The spines form a line of tubercles down the midline of the thorax. They are not uniform in length, but pass downwards and backwards with a tendency to overlap the spine below. Those near the upper part of the thorax have their tips level with the upper surface of the vertebral body below, while the lower half have longer spines which reach to the lower border of the vertebra

below. The tip of the spine of T3 is roughly level with the root of the spine of the scapula, and that of T7 level with the inferior angle of the scapula. The spine of T12 is not typical, as it is squared posteriorly and resembles that of a lumbar vertebra; it is level with the disc between T12 and L1. Accurate location of these spines must therefore be carried out by palpation, normally, counting down from an identifiable point above or below.

The transverse processes are much more difficult to palpate as they are covered by strong, thick muscles even in the thinner subject. The tips of the transverse processes are level with the upper border of their own vertebral body (Fig. 5.2).

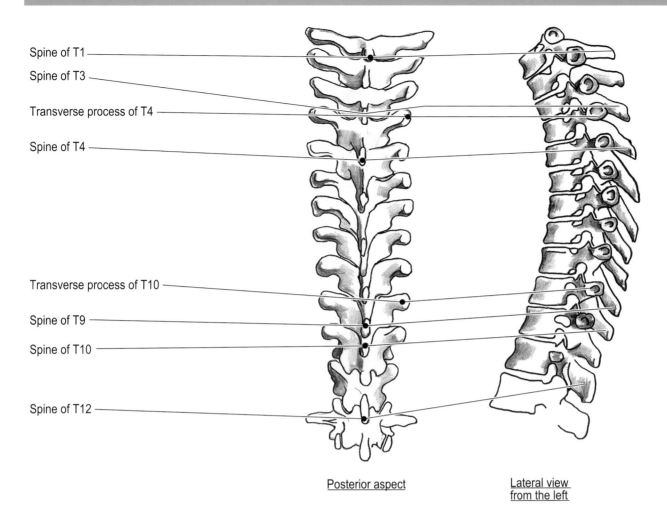

Spine of T1

Spine of T3

Transverse process of T4

Spine of T4

Transverse process of T10

Spine of T9

Spine of T10

Spine of T12

Posterior aspect

Lateral view
from the left

Fig. 5.2 (b)
The thoracic vertebrae

Palpation

With the subject in slump sitting, and rounding the back by placing the chin on the chest, the tips of the spines become more identifiable. Find the spines of C7 and T1, these being the two most prominent spines at the base of the neck.

With great care, count down the tips of the spines, being sure to mark the upper spine with the fingers of one hand while seeking the spine below with the other. Each spine will appear quite pointed until the level of T12, where a flattened appearance is noted, being similar to that of a lumbar spine. If palpation is difficult, use the technique suggested on page 0, where the fingertips are moved rapidly up and down the spine, in a scanning manner. This type of palpation is a useful method of locating and mapping structures which lie below the surface. It is rarely used, as it gives the impression of merely moving the skin on the underlying structures. It amounts to the building up of a total picture by adding together many disparate bits of information.

Use the pads of all fingers of one hand, the most sensitive if possible, to sweep across an area, allowing the fingers to move the skin and superficial fascia on the deeper structures. The palpator will be building up a picture in a similar manner to the scanning beam of a video camera. The other hand will be used to mark certain points and mark from where the previous information was obtained. Finer palpatory techniques can then be used on selected areas.

The lateral tips of the transverse processes lie 3 cm lateral and parallel to the spines. The tip of the spine, however, lies 1 cm below the level of the transverse process of the vertebra below. This measurement remains constant because the shorter spines in the upper thorax are compensated for by the transverse processes being slightly raised. Lateral to the tips of the transverse processes is a groove marking the line of the costotransverse joints.

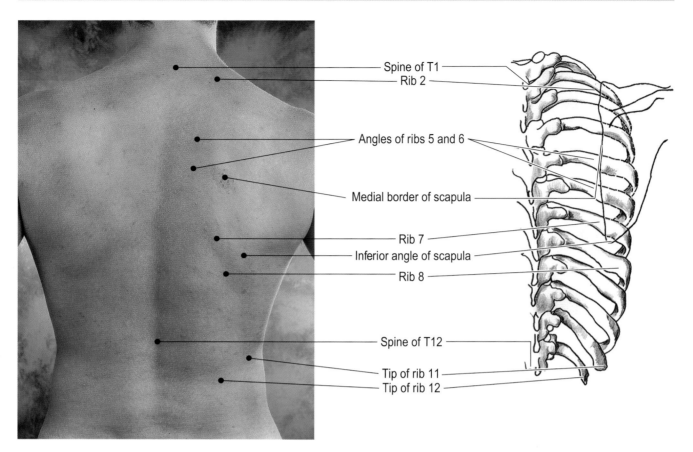

Fig. 5.3 (a), (b)
The ribs of the right side (posterior aspect)

The ribs

There are 12 ribs on either side, convex outwards, the eighth being the longest and the twelfth the shortest. The upper seven ribs articulate with the vertebral bodies and transverse processes posteriorly by the facets on their heads and tubercles. The first, tenth, eleventh and twelfth ribs have only one facet, the rest two. The eleventh and twelfth ribs have no tubercles. The ribs articulate with the sternum anteriorly via a varying length of costal cartilage. These are termed 'true' ribs. The three ribs immediately below that are the eighth to tenth, which articulate anteriorly via their costal cartilage with the costal cartilage above, and are termed 'false' ribs. The two lowest ribs do not articulate with their transverse process posteriorly and are free anteriorly and are therefore termed 'floating' ribs (Fig. 5.1).

Palpation

To enable the back muscles to relax, the subject is best examined in a prone-lying position. Just lateral to the tip of each transverse process the posterior section of each rib can be palpated, being separated from the transverse process by a depression. With the subject's arm hanging over the side of the couch (i.e. the pectoral girdle in protraction), find and trace the first to tenth ribs laterally. The rib angle lies approximately 3–4 cm lateral to the tips of the transverse processes and can readily be palpated in the mid-thoracic region, becoming less clear above and below. The first rib does not possess an angle and those of the eleventh and twelfth ribs are slight if present.

Each rib, together with the intercostal spaces above and below, can be traced anteriorly to where it joins the sternum. The second to seventh or

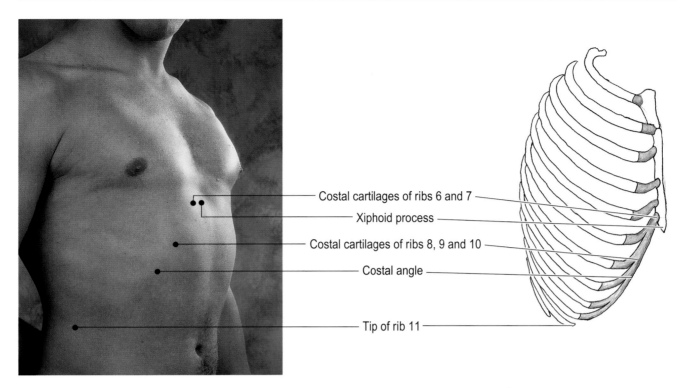

Costal cartilages of ribs 6 and 7

Xiphoid process

Costal cartilages of ribs 8, 9 and 10

Costal angle

Tip of rib 11

Fig. 5.3 (c), (d)
The ribs of the right side (lateral aspect)

eighth ribs are usually hidden posterolaterally by the scapula, while the eleventh and twelfth ribs only exist posterolaterally.

The first rib is the most difficult to palpate. It lies deep to the clavicle anteriorly, and deep to trapezius and levator scapulae posteriorly. If deep pressure is applied immediately below the clavicle, 1 cm lateral to its medial end, the junction of the rib with the manubrium can be palpated.

Above the middle of the clavicle in the supra-clavicular fossa, it is possible, using deep pressure, to feel the lateral border of the first rib, but this area is particularly tender and may produce unpleasant reactions in the upper limb due to pressure on the trunks of the brachial plexus and subclavian artery.

Posteriorly, the neck and tubercle of the first rib can be palpated running downwards and laterally approximately 2 cm lateral to the tip of the spine of the seventh cervical vertebra. This, however, is dependent on the thickness of the upper fibres of trapezius.

The costal cartilages at the anterior end of the eighth to tenth ribs form the anterior part of the costal margin, running superomedially to join the xiphoid process. At the level of the ninth costal cartilage an angle and projection are formed, the 'costal angle'. This lies on a level with the trans-pyloric plane, in common with the spine of L1 and the tip of the twelfth rib. Just above the twelfth, the eleventh rib can easily be identified, ending in a point just anterior to the mid-axillary line.

SELF ASSESSMENT

Page 284

1. Describe the formation of the bony structure of the thorax.

2. List the three sections of the sternum.

3. How many ribs take part in the formation of the thorax?

4. Describe the function of the thoracic cage.

5. Explain how the sternum is adapted for its function.

6. List the vital organs that are protected by the thoracic cage.

7. Which tissue changes the rib cage into a sealed container?

8. Describe the thoracic inlet.

9. Name three differing structures which pass through this opening.

10. Describe the formation of the thoracic outlet.

11. Name two differing structures which pass through this opening.

12. For how long does the xyphoid normally remain cartilaginous?

13. With which bones does the clavicle articulate?

14. How many ribs are in contact with the scapula when the upper limb is at rest?

15. Name the two joints in which the clavicle participates.

Page 285

16. Describe the technique for locating the joint of the first rib with the manubrium.

17. Give the surface marking of the joint between the first rib and the manubrium.

18. In degrees, what is the angle between the manubrium and the sternum?

Please complete the labels below.

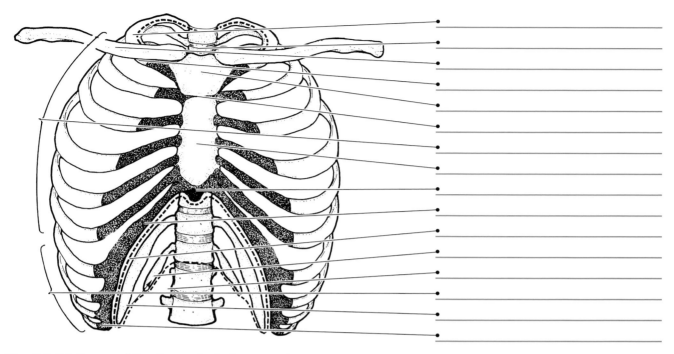

Fig. 5.1 (b) Bones of the thorax (anterior aspect)

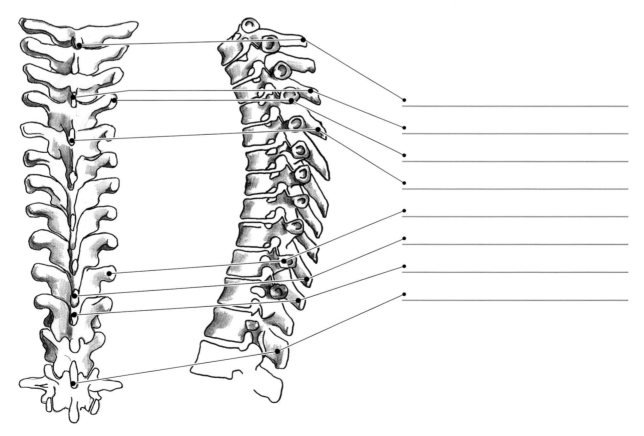

Fig. 5.2 (b) The thoracic vertebrae

19. How many degrees does this vary from full inspiration to full expiration?

20. Explain the reasons why this movement is necessary.

21. Which structure may be palpated on either side of the manubriosternal joint?

22. When tracing down the lateral border of the sternum, which structures can be palpated?

23. To which structure does the sternum join inferiorly?

24. Which cartilage normally joins the sides of the xyphysternal joint?

Page 286

25. Of the thoracic vertebral column, which structures can usually be palpated posteriorly?

26. Explain the reasons why these structures may be difficult to palpate.

27. In the upper thorax, describe the relationship of the tip of the spine of one vertebra with the body of the vertebra below.

28. Explain how this relationship differs in the lower thoracic vertebrae.

29. Which of the thoracic vertebrae has a spine shaped differently from the other vertebrae?

30. The tip of which thoracic vertebra lies at a level of the root of the spine of the scapula?

31. The inferior angle of the scapula lies on a level with the tip of the spine of which vertebra?

32. Describe the relationship between the tips of the transverse processes and the body of the vertebra.

Page 287

33. Describe a technique whereby the tips of the spines of the thoracic vertebrae can be made more prominent.

34. Which two spines are more prominent in a normal spinal column?

35. Describe a procedure for facilitating the palpation of these spines.

Please complete the labels below.

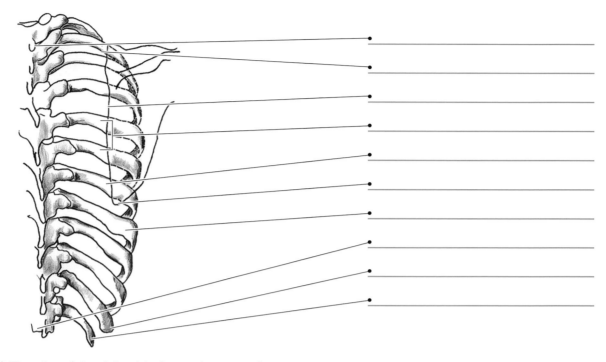

Fig. 5.3 (b) The ribs of the right side (posterior aspect)

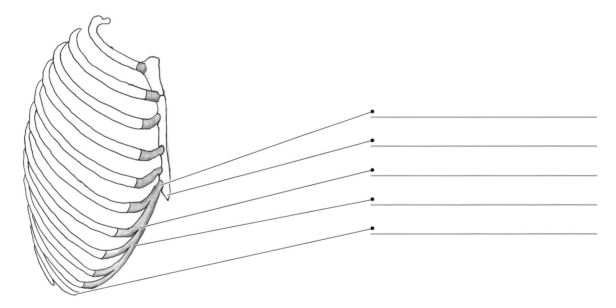

Fig. 5.3 (d) The ribs of the right side (lateral aspect)

36. What is the distance between the tip of the spine and the tip of the transverse process of the same vertebra in the thoracic area?

_____

37. Explain the reason why this distance remains constant.

_____

38. Which joints lie in the groove lateral to the transverse processes?

_____

Page 288

39. State the numbers of the longest and shortest ribs.

_____

40. Which ribs have only one articular facet on their heads and why?

_____

41. On which ribs are there no tubercles?

_____

42. Describe what is meant by a 'true' rib.

_____

43. Which ribs are termed 'false' ribs and why?

_____

44. Explain what is meant by a 'floating rib'?

_____

45. Which ribs belong to this category?

_____

46. How far do the rib angles lie laterally to the tips of the transverse processes and where are they best palpated?

_____

47. Which ribs do not possess an angle?

_____

Page 289

48. In palpating the lateral side of the first rib just above the middle third of the clavicle, explain the reason why great care must be taken and what may result.

_____

49. Which muscle overlies the posterior part of the first rib?

_____

50. What structure is interposed between the 'true' ribs and the sternum?

_____

51. Describe how the costal angle is formed.

_____

52. List three structures which lie on the same level as the costal angle.

_____

53. Where can the tip of the eleventh rib be palpated?

_____

Please complete the labels below.

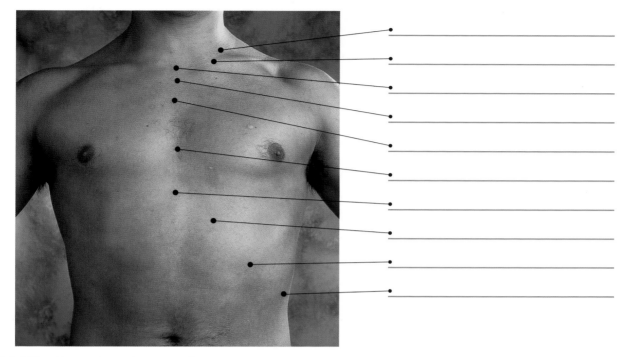

Fig. 5.1 (a) The thorax (anterior aspect)

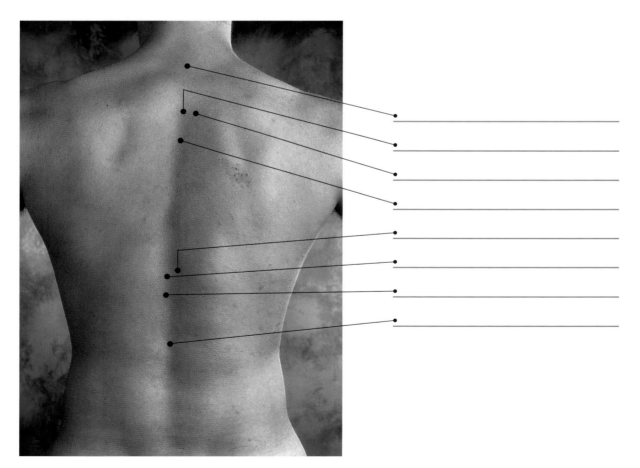

Fig. 5.2 (a) The thoracic vertebrae

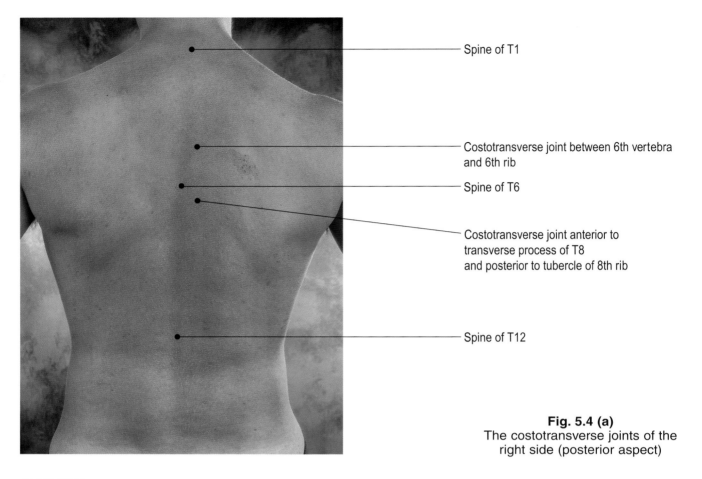

Spine of T1

Costotransverse joint between 6th vertebra and 6th rib

Spine of T6

Costotransverse joint anterior to transverse process of T8 and posterior to tubercle of 8th rib

Spine of T12

Fig. 5.4 (a)
The costotransverse joints of the right side (posterior aspect)

JOINTS

The thoracic vertebral column [Fig. 5.4]

The joints of the thoracic vertebral column are similar to those in the cervical region except that there are no uncovertebral joints and there are facets on the side of all of the bodies and the upper ten transverse processes, for the articulation of the ribs. The vertebral bodies articulate centrally, by a series of intervertebral discs, which are complex cartilaginous symphyses made up of an outer ring of fibrous bands passing obliquely from one body to the other (the annulus fibrosus) and a central nucleus (the nucleus pulposus) composed of a soft highly hydrophilic substance. These discs are supported by many ligaments including the very strong anterior and posterior longitudinal ligaments.

On either side there are the zygapophyseal joints (Fig. 5.4d, e) between the articular facets, two above and two below. In addition there are the costovertebral joints (Fig. 5.4c), between the heads of the ribs and the side(s) of the body of the vertebrae and the costotransverse joints, between the tubercle of the rib and the transverse process (Fig. 5.4a–c). The zygapophyseal, costovertebral and costotransverse joints are all synovial, surrounded by a capsule which is lined with synovial membrane and supported by ligaments. (For detailed study refer to Palastanga, Field and Soames 1998.)

Palpation

All but the costotransverse and possibly the zygapophyseal joints are impossible to palpate. The costotransverse joints lie in the furrow between the transverse processes and the ribs and can be located either by following backwards along the line of a known rib to the point where it is obscured by the transverse process or by finding the tip of the spinous process of a known vertebra and tracing out laterally to the furrow mentioned above. Due to the length of the spines in the thoracic area the transverse process you can feel is that of the vertebra below.

The joints between the articular facets lie at the upper edge of the lamina as it meets the lamina above. The joint is virtually impossible to palpate, but the lamina can be traced a little laterally from the spines if the model is completely relaxed in prone lying and the fingers are slipped down the side of the spinous process. It must be remembered, however, that the lamina you feel is that of the vertebra below. The use of quick, gliding movements of the fingers (see page 8) and positioning the model with the spine in flexion will aid palpation.

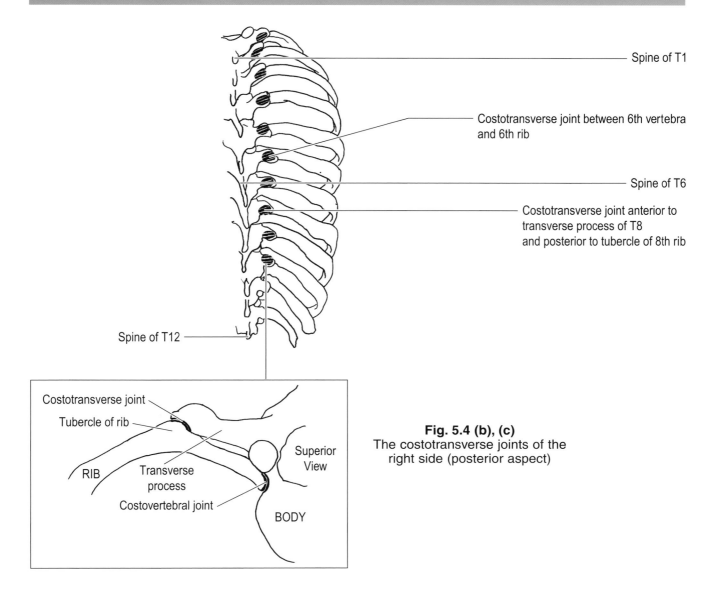

Fig. 5.4 (b), (c)
The costotransverse joints of the
right side (posterior aspect)

Labels in figure: Spine of T1; Costotransverse joint between 6th vertebra and 6th rib; Spine of T6; Costotransverse joint anterior to transverse process of T8 and posterior to tubercle of 8th rib; Spine of T12; Costotransverse joint; Tubercle of rib; RIB; Transverse process; Costovertebral joint; Superior View; BODY

Accessory movements

As stated above, pressure on the lamina of one vertebra can part the zygapophyseal joint surfaces above and compress those below on the ipsilateral side (Fig. 5.4c).

Posterior-to-anterior pressure applied to the tip of the spine causes it to act as a lever, parting the upper zygapophyseal joint and compressing the lower (Fig. 5.4f, g). Pressure applied to the lateral side of the spinous process causes rotation of the body of the vertebra to the opposite side, resulting in gapping of the upper zygapophyseal joint on the side to which the spine is moved, but compressing the lower joint. It has the opposite effect on the joints of the ipsilateral side.

Traction on the thoracic intervertebral joints is difficult to produce, resulting in virtually no movement. However, movement certainly occurs, to a limited extent, during lumbar or cervical traction.

Laterally, the heads of the ribs articulate with the bodies of the vertebrae and the tubercles of the ribs articulate with the transverse processes of the vertebrae (Fig. 5.4).

With the subject lying prone, pressure on the angle of the rib will part the costotransverse joint. If the thumbs are moved a little medially to an area just lateral to the joint, the gapping is increased. However, if the pressure is applied even more medially, it will encroach upon the back of the transverse process, producing exactly the opposite effect and resulting in compression of the costotransverse joint (Fig. 5.4c).

Posterior aspect

Shaded area shows joint surface deep to
inferior articular processes

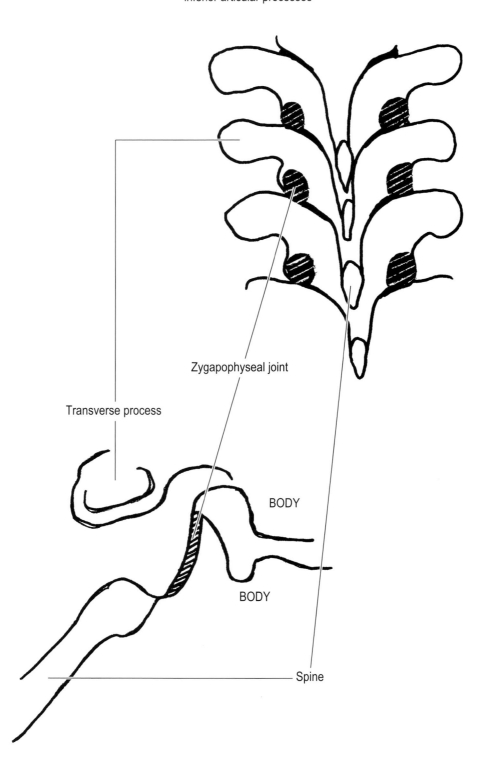

Zygapophyseal joint

Transverse process

BODY

BODY

Spine

Lateral aspect

Fig. 5.4 (d), (e)
Zygapophyseal joints of thoracic spine. Shaded areas show joint surface deep to inferior articular processes

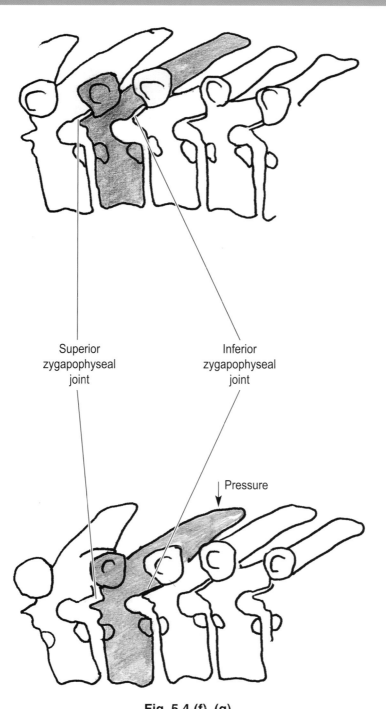

Superior
zygapophyseal
joint

Inferior
zygapophyseal
joint

↓ Pressure

Fig. 5.4 (f), (g)
Vertebrae in horizontal position showing effect of pressure on spine in direction of arrow

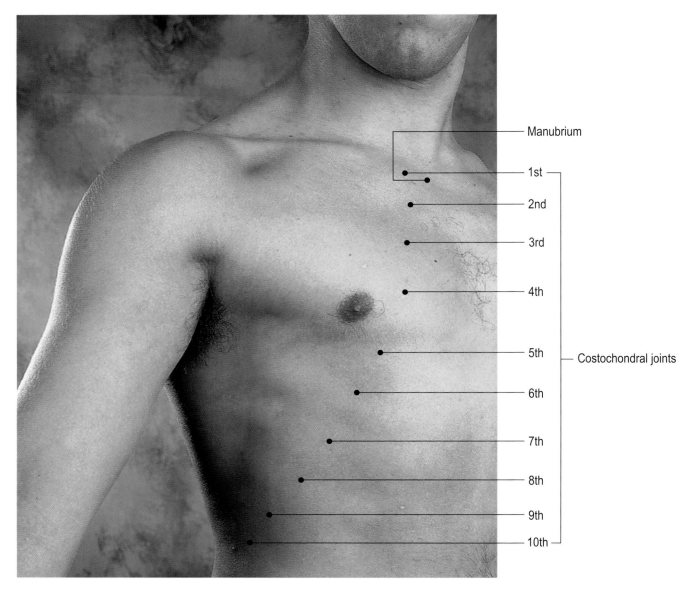

Fig. 5.5 (a)
Costochondral joints of the right side (anterior aspect)

The joints of the anterior end of the ribs

Anteriorly, the upper seven ribs articulate with the sternum via their costal cartilages. These are termed true ribs. The costal cartilages of ribs eight to ten articulate with the costal cartilage above, and are termed false ribs, and the two lower ribs are only capped with costal cartilage and do not link up with the sternum, and are termed floating ribs. There are three sets of joints in this area, namely, the costochondral, the interchondral and the sternocostal joints.

The costochondral joints

These joints are really the junction between the rib and its anterior end which has not yet ossified.

The rounded end of the cartilage fits into the depressed roughened end of the rib. Its periosteum is continuous with its perichondrium.

Palpation

The costochondral joints (Fig. 5.5a, b) can be identified, in some subjects, lying approximately 3 cm lateral to the sternum at the second rib, progressing to some 12 cm from the xiphoid at the seventh rib and approximately 18 cm from the xiphoid process at the tenth rib. Pressure on the anterior surface of these joints can often be unpleasant and too much palpation may lead to a very tender area which may last for some time.

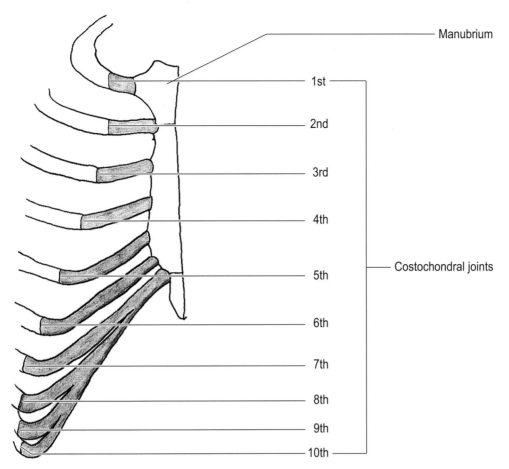

Fig. 5.5 (b)
Costochondral joints of the right side (anterior aspect)

Accessory movements

With the subject lying supine and applying pressure to the sternal area of the chest, quite marked compression can be achieved. This is due in part to the flexibility of the ribs and costal cartilage and in part to the slight gliding and bending movements occurring between the costochondral, interchondral, sternocostal and intersternal joints.

Movement of each individual joint can be achieved by applying pressure, normally with two thumbs, to the rib or to the costal cartilage close to either side of the joint. The movement is minimal in some joints, such as that of the first and second ribs with the sternum, but quite considerable lower down the thorax, particularly at the interchondral joints.

Some of these joints can be traumatized and become inflamed, usually following a blow on the chest or stress on the rib cage due to resting heavily against a beam or bar. This causes an acute pain over that area of the chest. If the pain is over the area of the heart, it may erroneously be associated with a heart attack.

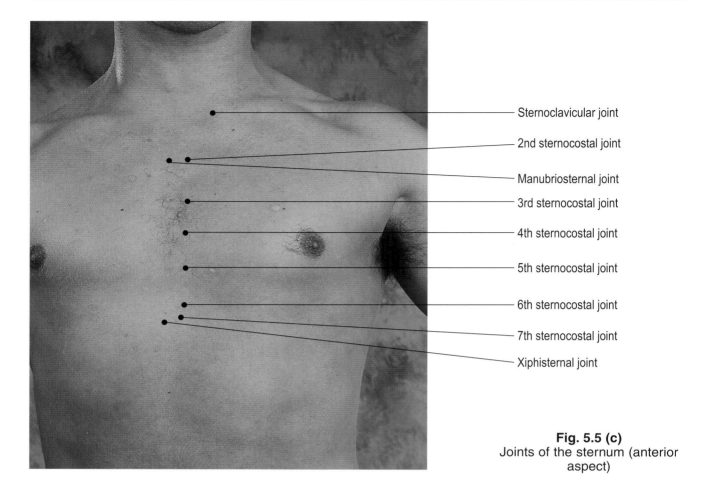

Sternoclavicular joint

2nd sternocostal joint

Manubriosternal joint

3rd sternocostal joint

4th sternocostal joint

5th sternocostal joint

6th sternocostal joint

7th sternocostal joint

Xiphisternal joint

Fig. 5.5 (c)
Joints of the sternum (anterior aspect)

The sternocostal (chondrosternal) joints [Fig 5.5c and d]

These are the joints between the anterior rounded end of the costal cartilages of the upper seven ribs and the small hollow cavities on the side of the sternum.

The first articulates with the side of the manubrium just below the clavicular notch. It is a synarthrosis, having a similar structure to a symphysis and therefore forms a fairly rigid union. It is close to the midline of the body, a location where most symphyses are found.

The second to the seventh are all synovial joints, being surrounded by a capsule which is lined with synovial membrane and supported by ligaments that radiate from the front of the cartilage on to the anterior aspect of the sternum (the sternocostal radiate ligaments). The second costal cartilage joins the sternum at the side of the manubriosternal joint and has the extra support of an interosseous ligament which attaches to the disc of the manubriosternal joint. The seventh costal cartilage joins a small shallow facet formed by the lower part of the sternum and the xiphoid process. It is supported front and back by costoxiphoid ligaments. This synovial joint is often replaced by a symphysis.

Palpation

At the side of the manubriosternal joint, approximately 7 cm below the sternal notch, the articulation of the second costal cartilage, the manubrium (Fig. 5.5b) and body, can be palpated as a small V-shaped notch, with the concavity facing laterally. Below this, on either side, the third to seventh ribs and their costal cartilages can be palpated as they articulate with the lateral border of the sternum at the costosternal or chondrosternal joints. The section of the sternum between each costal cartilage is concave laterally, being the anterior limit of the intercostal spaces. The joint between the first rib and the manubrium lies 1 cm below, and 1 cm lateral to, the medial end of the clavicle and is more difficult to identify; nevertheless, the anterior limit of the rib can be palpated.

The costal cartilage of the eighth to tenth ribs can be identified articulating medially, with the costal cartilage above, at the interchondral joints and forms the costal margin.

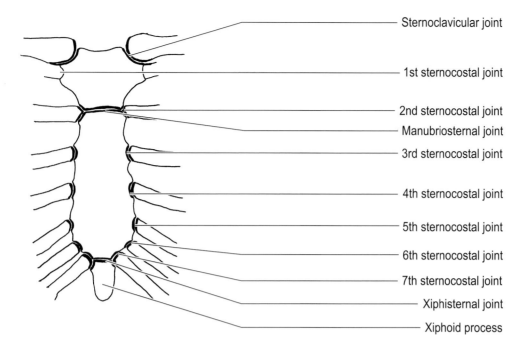

Sternoclavicular joint

1st sternocostal joint

2nd sternocostal joint

Manubriosternal joint

3rd sternocostal joint

4th sternocostal joint

5th sternocostal joint

6th sternocostal joint

7th sternocostal joint

Xiphisternal joint

Xiphoid process

Fig. 5.5 (d)
Joints of the sternum (anterior aspect)

Joints of the sternum

The sternum is composed of three segments: the manubrium superiorly, the body centrally, and the small, pointed xiphoid process inferiorly. The joints between these sections are secondary cartilaginous symphyses.

Palpation

The manubriosternal joint is easy to identify (Fig. 5.5c, d) as it is some 7 cm below the upper border of the sternum at the sternal angle. It is level with the articulation of the second costal cartilage with the sternum.

The joint between the body and the xiphoid process (Fig. 5.5c, d) is more difficult to palpate, although the body and the xiphoid are both easily identifiable.

Accessory movements

There is very little accessory movement of the manubriosternal joint, although pressure on either the body or the manubrium, close to the joint, will produce slight angling of the two sections. At the xiphisternal joint, however, the xiphoid process can normally be moved backwards some considerable distance by pressure applied to its anterior surface. This produces an angling at the joint.

SELF ASSESSMENT

Page 296

1. Which joints exist between the bodies of cervical but not thoracic vertebrae?

2. Which ribs do not articulate with their transverse processes?

3. Describe the joints which exist between two thoracic vertebral bodies.

4. Name the regions of the discs and describe their structure.

5. List the ligaments which support these discs.

6. What is the length and direction of the fibres of these ligaments?

7. Describe the zygapophyseal joints and state the direction of their facets.

8. Where do the costovertebral joints exist and how do some of these differ from the standard?

9. Between which bony surfaces are the costotransverse joints found?

10. Which joints of the thoracic spine may it be possible to palpate?

Page 297

11. If pressure is applied to the lamina of one vertebra, describe how this will affect the zygapophyseal joint above.

12. How will this procedure affect the zygapophyseal joint below?

13. If posterior to anterior pressure is applied to the tip of a thoracic spine, describe how this will affect the zygapophyseal joints above.

14. If pressure is applied to the lateral side of the spine of a thoracic vertebra, what movement occurs in the vertebral body?

15. What movement occurs at the zygapophyseal joints on the ipsilateral side of the spine?

16. Pressure on the angle of the rib will affect which joint?

17. Describe how this procedure will affect the joint.

18. Explain the reasons why pressure must be applied accurately in this area.

Please complete the labels below.

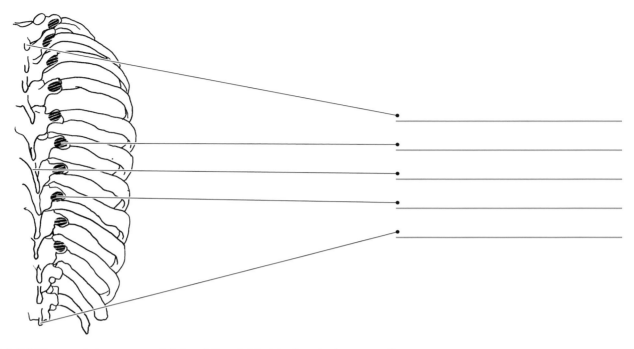

Fig. 5.4 (b) The costotransverse joints of the right side (posterior aspect)

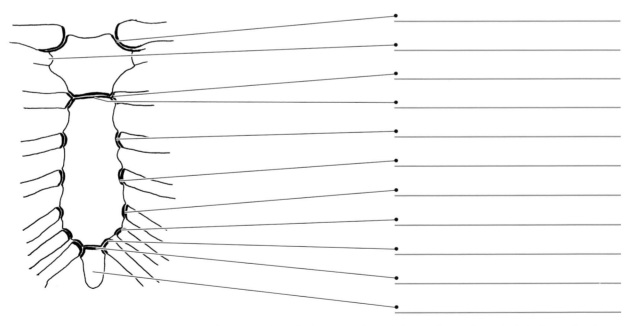

Fig. 5.5 (d) Zygapophyseal joints of thoracic spine. Shaded areas show joint surface deep to inferior articular processes

Page 300

19. How many ribs articulate almost directly with the sternum?

20. Name the class and type of these joints.

21. In how many joints does a 'false' rib participate?

22. List the ribs which fit into this category?

23. In how many joints does a 'floating rib' participate?

24. Describe the structure of a costochondral joint.

25. Approximately, how far are these joints situated lateral to the sternum and zyphoid process?

26. Explain the consequences of over palpation of these joints.

Page 302

27. What type of joint exists between the first rib and the sternum?

28. Explain how this joint differs from the other costosternal joints.

29. How does the second sternocostal joint differ from the other joints?

30. What distance, in centimetres, is the sternal angle below the sternal notch?

31. Which structures can be palpated just lateral to the sternum?

32. Describe the surface markings of the first sternocostal joint.

33. With what structure do the costal cartilages of ribs 8,9 and 10 articulate?

34. What do these costal cartilages form?

Page 303

35. List the three parts of the sternum.

36. What type of joints exist between these segments?

Please complete the labels below.

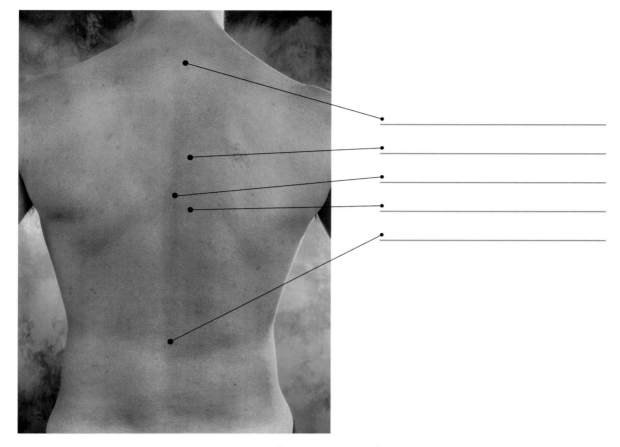

Fig. 5.4 (a) The costotransverse joints of the right side (posterior aspect)

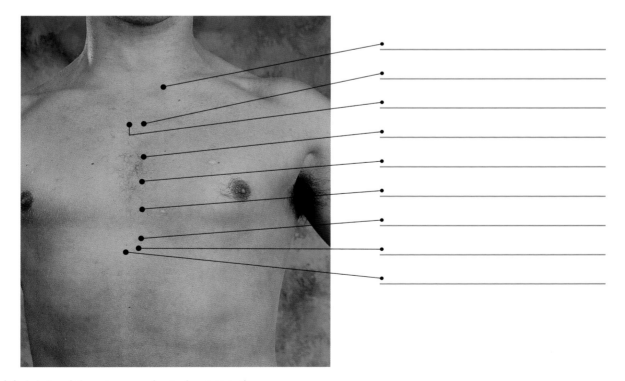

Fig. 5.5 (c) Joints of the sternum (anterior aspect)

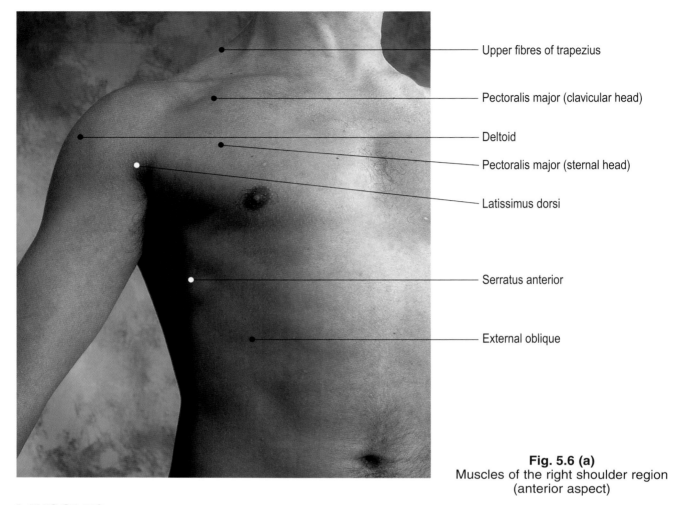

Upper fibres of trapezius

Pectoralis major (clavicular head)

Deltoid

Pectoralis major (sternal head)

Latissimus dorsi

Serratus anterior

External oblique

Fig. 5.6 (a)
Muscles of the right shoulder region
(anterior aspect)

MUSCLES

The anterior aspect of the chest

The muscle that dominates the upper part of the chest is pectoralis major. Lying deep to it are pectoralis minor and the upper intercostal muscles. In the lower part of the chest, rectus abdominis and the external oblique muscle of the abdomen have their upper attachment (see Fig. 6.5).

The pectoralis minor is a triangular muscle with its base attaching to the third, fourth and fifth ribs at approximately the mid-clavicular line and its apex attaching to the coracoid process of the scapula. It is very difficult to palpate. The intercostal muscles attach to the lower border of the rib above and to the upper border of the rib below. They are easier to palpate in the lower region of the chest (see page 311). The external oblique muscle attaches above to the external surface of the lower border of the lower eight ribs. You will be able to feel the contraction of the muscle if you place your fingers under the lower border of the rib cage, on the right, just lateral to the costal angle and ask the sitting model to turn to the left. The rectus abdominis attaches above to the fifth, sixth and seventh costal cartilages just lateral to the sternum. Place your fingers just below the rib cage just lateral to the xiphoid process and ask

the sitting model to lean backwards. Immediately the powerful contraction of the muscle will be palpated. (See also pages 358 and 359.)

Pectoralis major

Pectoralis major (Figs 5.6 and 5.7) is a large, thick triangular muscle situated on the upper anterior area of the chest wall. It is composed of two main groups of fibres, clavicular and sternal. The clavicular fibres attach medially to the anterior surface of the medial half of the clavicle. Its sternal fibres attach to *its* side of the sternum, the anterior surface of the upper seven costal cartilages and the upper part of the aponeurosis covering the abdominal muscles. Both sets of fibres pass laterally, leaving a small space between them, and join together laterally to form a bilaminar tendon which attaches to the lateral lip of the intertubercular groove. The lower sternal fibres tend to fold up behind the upper fibres to form the double bilaminated tendon. The muscle forms a pleasantly shaped lower border, which becomes the anterior border of the axilla laterally.

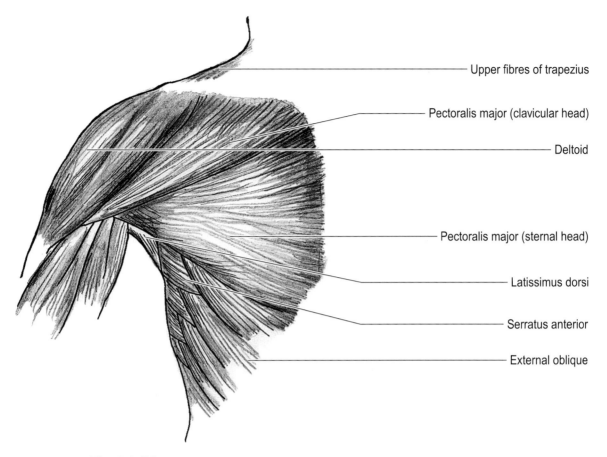

- Upper fibres of trapezius
- Pectoralis major (clavicular head)
- Deltoid
- Pectoralis major (sternal head)
- Latissimus dorsi
- Serratus anterior
- External oblique

Fig. 5.6 (b)
Muscles of the right shoulder region
(anterior aspect)

Palpation

Pectoralis major is easily recognizable and palpable in even the less muscular subject. If the subject presses the hands against the iliac crest, the whole of the muscle contracts. The lower border of the anterior wall of the axilla is rounded, due to the lower sternal fibres of pectoralis major twisting upwards posterior to its upper fibres. The muscle can be traced medially and inferiorly on to the anterior aspect of the chest as far down as the costal cartilage of the seventh rib and xiphoid process.

The bulk of the muscle forms a rounded shape on the upper anterior chest wall and is the muscle that men try to develop to give a pleasant shape to the upper part of the chest. It is almost entirely covered by the breast in the female, particularly in its lower section. If the arms are flexed against resistance, the clavicular fibres can easily be identified, just below the medial half of the clavicle, as a column of muscle standing clear of the chest wall (Fig. 5.7a, b) passing downwards and laterally.

During extension against resistance from the flexed position, the lower sternal fibres become apparent as a thick triangular shape forming the lower boundary of the muscle (Fig. 5.7c, d). To observe the two sets of fibres clearly, the subject's arm should be held at about 45° of flexion and he or she should then be asked to first raise and then pull down the arm against resistance. The tendon can be traced laterally to its attachment to the humerus.

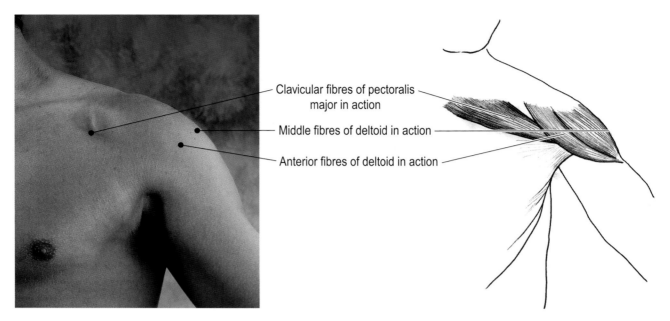

Fig. 5.7 (a), (b)
Sternal fibres of pectoralis major and deltoid of left shoulder (anterior aspect)

Functional anatomy

It is interesting to note that pectoralis major has two functionally distinct sets of fibres, a bilaminal tendon, and is supplied through two nerves (lateral and medial pectoral). In addition, it is involved in two actions which appear to oppose each other. The clavicular fibres will flex and the sternal fibres will extend the shoulder joint. In prone kneeling, both sets of fibres act to stabilize the upper trunk posture, preventing sway either forwards, backwards or from side to side; and in crawling, the limb is taken forwards by the clavicular fibres and

backwards by the sternal fibres. This important muscle must have had a greater importance in our evolution, and recognition of its residual function may help in its re-education.

In patients suffering from respiratory embarrassment, pectoralis major may be used as an accessory muscle of inspiration. In this case the arms have to be fixed, as in gripping a post or beam, thus fixing the lateral attachment of the muscle to the humerus. The medial attachment of the muscle may then be used to expand the chest a little more.

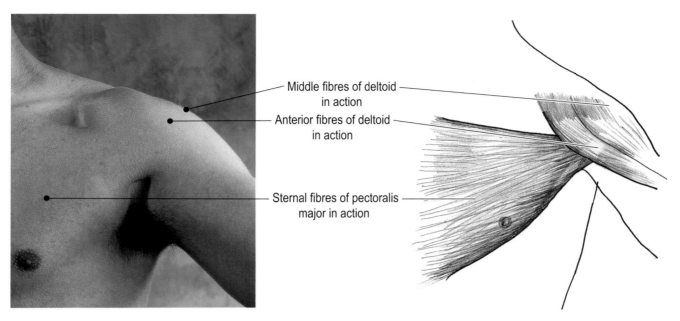

Middle fibres of deltoid
in action

Anterior fibres of deltoid
in action

Sternal fibres of pectoralis
major in action

Fig. 5.7 (c), (d)
Sternal fibres of pectoralis major and deltoid of left shoulder (anterior aspect)

Comparative anatomy

The pectoralis muscle(s) also play an important role in the animal, bird, fish, reptile and insect worlds. In the quadruped it acts as a stabilizing muscle for the forelimb in the standing position, similar to that in the human prone kneeling position, and because of its shape takes part in both the propulsive and recovery phase of the forelimb in locomotion. It also acts as a sling for the thorax holding it up between the two limbs. In the bird and insect it creates the enormous thrust for take-off and flight, while at the same time controlling the intricate movements of the wings. In the fish it controls the fine movements of the pectoral fin in a comparatively simple up-and-down motion, but occasionally may have fibres which are extended into the neck region. The pectorals in the forelimb of a reptile normally have the adaptability of being functional in water and on the land.

Biceps brachii and coracobrachialis

Running vertically from the coracoid process (see pages 15 and 17), the combined tendon of the biceps brachii and coracobrachialis can be palpated just below the coracoid process but is soon hidden by the broad tendon of the pectoralis major. It emerges below and can be identified passing down into the antero-medial aspect of the arm and splitting into its anterior (bicipital) and posterior (coracobrachialis) section.

The intercostals

If the fingers are placed between the ribs, a tight membranous sheet can be palpated. This consists of the external and internal intercostal muscles and their covering fascia. These are best palpated just below the pectoralis major and slightly lateral to the line of the nipple. On muscular subjects they are more hidden by larger, more superficial muscles.

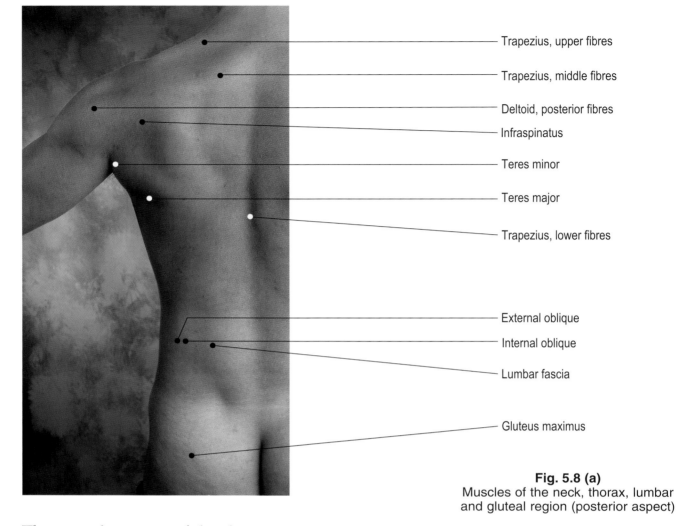

Trapezius, upper fibres

Trapezius, middle fibres

Deltoid, posterior fibres

Infraspinatus

Teres minor

Teres major

Trapezius, lower fibres

External oblique

Internal oblique

Lumbar fascia

Gluteus maximus

Fig. 5.8 (a)
Muscles of the neck, thorax, lumbar
and gluteal region (posterior aspect)

The posterior aspect of the chest

Trapezius [Fig. 5.8a and b]

The two trapezius muscles cover most of the posterior aspect of the neck and upper thorax connecting the skull, ligamentum nuchae, seventh cervical and all the thoracic spines to the lateral end of the clavicle, acromion and superior border of the spine of the scapula. Their upper fibres can be palpated halfway between the external occipital protuberance and the acromion process, forming the pleasant contour of the upper lateral aspect of the shoulder. Its middle fibres can be palpated between the upper border of the spine and the lower cervical and upper thoracic regions. The lower fibres are more difficult to identify as they pass from the lower thoracic spines to the medial end of the spine of the scapula. The upper fibres are easier to identify if the shoulder girdle is raised, the middle fibres if the shoulder girdle is retracted and the lower fibres if the shoulder girdle is depressed.

Levator scapulae and the rhomboids

These muscles lie deep to the trapezius. Levator scapulae attaches above to the transverse processes

of the upper four cervical vertebrae and below to the upper part of the medial border of the scapula. The rhomboid muscles attach above to the lower part of the ligamentum nuchae, the spine of the seventh cervical vertebra and the spines of the upper five thoracic vertebrae. They pass downwards and laterally to attach to the lower two-thirds of the medial border of the scapula. These muscles add bulk to the area between the scapula and lower neck and can be palpated in this region when the shoulders are raised and braced back.

Supraspinatus and infraspinatus

Supraspinatus arises from the supraspinous fossa of the scapula, passing laterally to the top of the greater tuberosity of the humerus. Infraspinatus arises from the infraspinous fossa, passing laterally to the posterior aspect of the same tuberosity.

When the subject begins to raise the arm from the side, supraspinatus can be identified just above the spine of the scapula in the supraspinous fossa. Below the spine, infraspinatus can be felt contracting when the arm is laterally rotated.

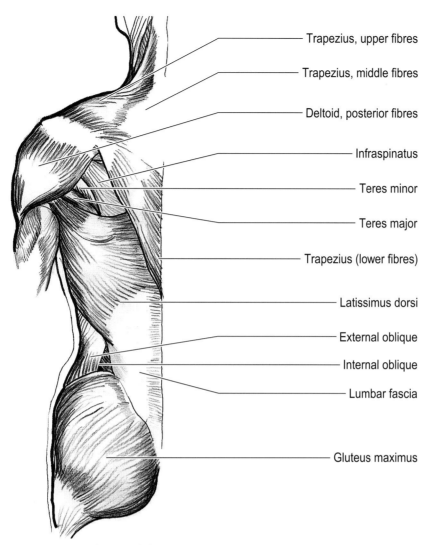

Trapezius, upper fibres

Trapezius, middle fibres

Deltoid, posterior fibres

Infraspinatus

Teres minor

Teres major

Trapezius (lower fibres)

Latissimus dorsi

External oblique

Internal oblique

Lumbar fascia

Gluteus maximus

Fig. 5.8 (b)
Muscles of the neck, thorax, lumbar
and gluteal region (posterior aspect)

Teres major and latissimus dorsi

These two muscles are triangular in shape and cover the lateral border of the scapula, teres major actually arising from the border. Latissimus dorsi comes from an extensive attachment to the spines of the lower six thoracic vertebrae, the thoracolumbar fascia and the posterior section of the iliac crest. It passes over the inferior angle of the scapula, taking a few fibres of origin, and then twists under the axilla, with teres major, to attach to the floor of the intertubercular groove with teres major attaching to its medial lip.

If the arm is extended against resistance from a flexed position, teres major and latissimus dorsi can be felt contracting. The triangular bulk of teres major lies over the lateral border of the scapula, while the tendon of latissimus dorsi can be traced, laterally and forwards, forming the posterior wall of the axilla. This tendon can be traced to its muscle fibres medially over the dorsum of the chest and lumbar area and can readily be identified if the subject coughs.

Serratus anterior [Fig. 5.6a and b]

Serratus anterior is a flat but powerful muscle attaching to the whole of the medial border of the scapula. Passing deep to the scapula, it attaches anteriorly to the lateral aspect of the first to eighth ribs at the mid-axillary line. Most of the muscle is concealed beneath the scapula, but palpation of its anterior attachment to the ribs is possible. If, during protraction, the fingers are placed behind the mid-axillary line but in front of the scapula, its anterior attachment to the ribs can be identified. Care must be taken to observe the contraction when the pectoral girdle is retracted and begins to move forwards. Once the lateral border of the scapula has passed beyond the mid-axillary line, the muscle is hidden.

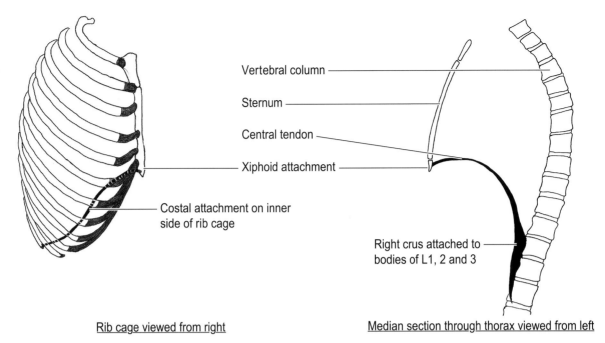

Rib cage viewed from right

Vertebral column

Sternum

Central tendon

Xiphoid attachment

Costal attachment on inner
side of rib cage

Right crus attached to
bodies of L1, 2 and 3

Median section through thorax viewed from left

Fig. 5.9 (a), (b)
Attachments of the diaphragm

The diaphragm [Figs 5.9 and 5.10]

The diaphragm is a musculotendinous sheet separating the thoracic and abdominal cavities. It forms a double cupola within the thorax, with the heart resting upon its central tendinous part. Anteriorly it attaches to the xiphisternum, laterally to the inner aspect of the lower six ribs on a line with the inner surface of the costochondral joints, and posteriorly to the vertebral column. It is the main muscle of inspiration and moves according to the state of respiration. It is therefore more useful to indicate its surface markings after full expiration and then after a deep inspiration. The attachments to the xiphisternum, ribs and vertebral column remain constant, but the two cupolae and central tendon vary in height. It must also be remembered that the position of the diaphragm is influenced by other factors: it lies at a higher level with respect to the rib cage when lying supine than when standing; its downward movement is restricted by food and gas in the stomach, and by increased pressure in the abdominal cavity, for example during pregnancy; in side lying it is pushed up into the thoracic cavity on the lower side by the contents of the abdomen; and in prone lying the liver tends to restrict its downward movement on the right side.

On full expiration, the right cupola rises to the level of the fourth rib, the left to the fourth intercostal space and the central tendon to the level of

the fifth costal cartilage. On full inspiration, which may produce a 6 cm descent of the cupolae, the diaphragm may reach the level of the sixth or seventh ribs. In quiet respiration, the diaphragm normally only moves up and down 1–2 cm.

The attachment of the diaphragm to the inside of the chest wall can be marked by an oblique line drawn from the xiphoid process, anteriorly, downwards and laterally slightly concave downwards. It follows the line of the sixth costal cartilage attaching to the inner surface anterior end of the sixth to tenth ribs (Fig. 5.9a). It then attaches to the inner surface of the eleventh and twelfth ribs with its vertebral attachment being marked by a line running down the lateral side of the bodies of the first and second lumbar vertebrae on the left and the first to third lumbar vertebrae on the right (Fig. 5.10b). These can be marked by two vertical lines, 2 cm lateral to the first and second lumbar spines on the left and the first to third lumbar spines on the right.

Palpation

It is impossible to palpate the diaphragm. On full inspiration there is a bulging of the abdomen between the two costal margins. Although this is produced by the diaphragm, it is actually the upper section of the abdominals.

(a)

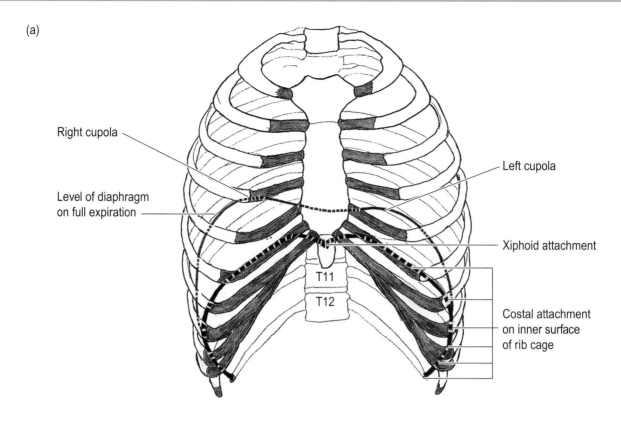

Right cupola

Level of diaphragm on full expiration

Left cupola

Xiphoid attachment

T11

T12

Costal attachment on inner surface of rib cage

(b)

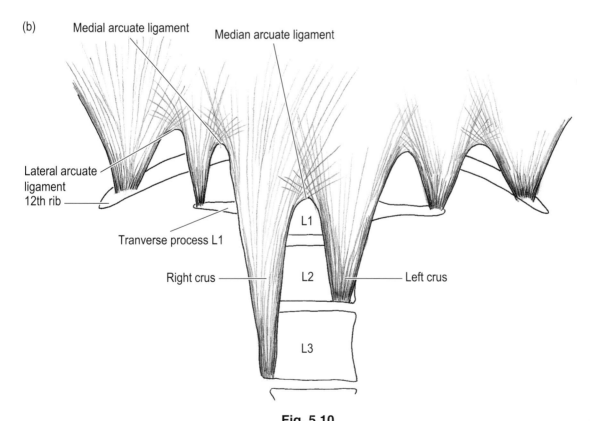

Medial arcuate ligament

Median arcuate ligament

Lateral arcuate ligament 12th rib

Tranverse process L1

L1

Right crus

L2

Left crus

L3

Fig. 5.10
The diaphragm. (a) The rib cage (anterior aspect). (b) Attachments of diaphragm to the vertebrae and 12th rib (anterior aspect viewed from inside rib cage)

SELF ASSESSMENT

Page 308

1. Describe the shape of the pectoralis minor muscle.

2. State its proximal and distal attachments.

3. Explain the reasons why this muscle is difficult to palpate.

4. Describe the general arrangement of the intercostal muscles.

5. How does the external oblique muscle attach to the rib cage?

6. What is the action of the external oblique muscle?

7. Where is it easiest to palpate the external oblique muscle?

8. To which ribs is the rectus abdominis muscle attached?

9. Explain how this muscle is most easily palpated.

10. Describe the shape of pectoralis major and state its location.

11. Name the two main groups of fibres.

12. Where do these groups of fibres attach?

13. Describe the arrangement of the tendon's attachment.

14. To which space does the pectoralis major form the anterior border?

Page 309

15. Describe how a contraction of the whole of the pectoralis major can be produced.

16. Explain the reasons why this muscle is difficult to palpate in the female.

17. In what ways do the two sets of fibres vary in their action?

18. How can this variation be demonstrated?

Page 310

19. Discuss the possible evolutionary development of the pectoralis major muscle. (fr)

20. Describe a way in which this muscle can be used as an accessory muscle of inspiration. (fr)

Please complete the labels below.

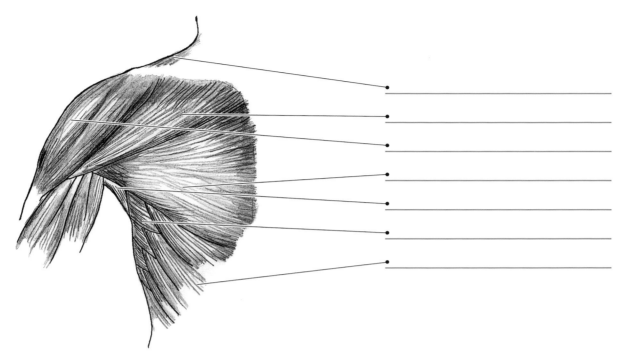

Fig. 5.6 (b) Muscles of the right shoulder region (anterior aspect)

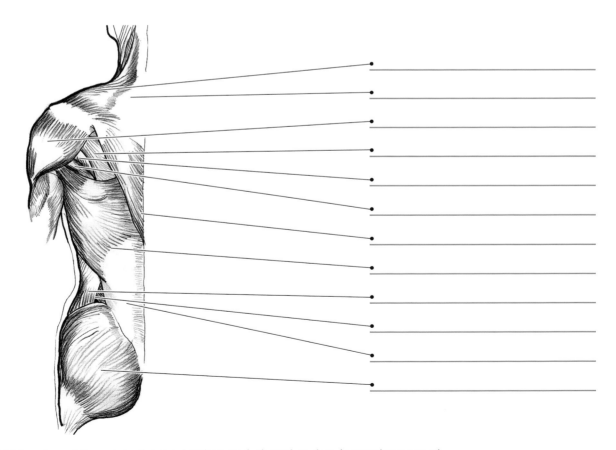

Fig. 5.8 (b) Muscles of the neck, thorax, lumbar and gluteal region (posterior aspect)

Page 311

21. Discuss the actions of pectoralis major in the quadruped. (fr)

22. Discuss the actions of pectoralis major in the bird. (fr)

23. Discuss the actions of pectoralis major in the insect. (fr)

24. Discuss the actions of pectoralis major in the reptile. (fr)

25. Compare the similarities between the attachments of the coracobrachialis and biceps brachii muscles.

26. In which area can these two tendons be palpated?

27. Where can the intercostal muscles be palpated and where is this best carried out?

Page 312

28. Describe the extensive attachments of the trapezius centrally.

29. Give its attachment to the shoulder girdle.

30. In which region can the upper fibres be palpated?

31. The middle fibres are palpable, where?

32. Outline the actions of the trapezius muscle.

33. Describe the location of the levator scapulae.

34. State the attachments of the levator scapulae.

35. What are the attachments of the rhomboid major muscle?

36. Where does the rhomboid minor attach?

37. In which area of the body can the supraspinatus muscle be palpated?

38. Describe how this muscle may be put into action.

39. Where can infraspinatus be palpated?

40. What is the action of infraspinatus?

Please complete the labels below.

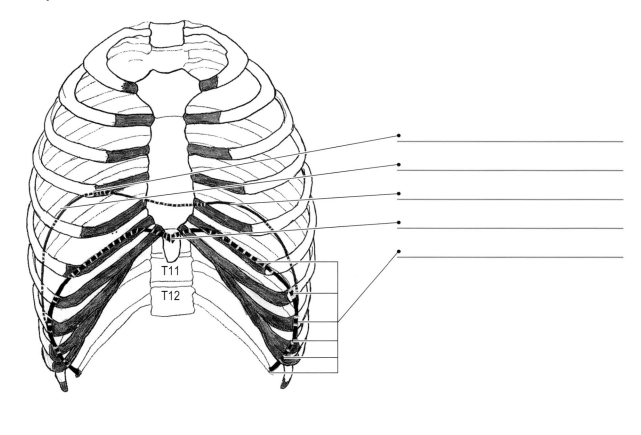

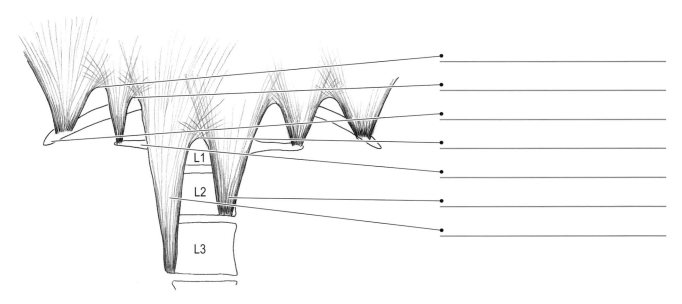

Fig. 5.10 The diaphragm. (a) The rib cage (anterior aspect). (b) Attachments of diaphragm to the vertebrae and 12th rib (anterior aspect viewed from inside rib cage)

Page 313

41. List the attachments, to the trunk, of the latissimus dorsi muscle.

_____

42. Describe its peculiar form of attachment to the humerus.

_____

43. Of what does it form the posterior wall?

_____

44. In which area can the teres major muscle be palpated?

_____

45. Describe the functional activity of the latissimus dorsi.

_____

46. What is the shape and position of the serratus anterior?

_____

47. Where is the serratus anterior attached anteriorly?

_____

48. Explain the reasons why it is difficult to palpate the serratus anterior.

_____

Page 314

49. Between which two cavities is the diaphragm situated?

_____

50. Of what is the diaphragm composed?

_____

51. Describe its general shape and form.

_____

52. To what structure is it attached anteriorly?

_____

53. List its lateral and posterior attachments.

_____

54. What is its main function?

_____

55. List the factors which may influence its position in the body.

_____

56. On full expiration, to what level do the two cupolae rise on either side?

_____

57. On full expiration, to what level does the central tendon rise?

_____

58. What distance can each of the cupolae descend on full inspiration?

_____

59. How far may the diaphragm descend on quiet respiration?

_____

60. State the surface marking of the attachments of the diaphragm.

_____

61. To which vertebrae does the diaphragm attach?

_____

Please complete the labels below.

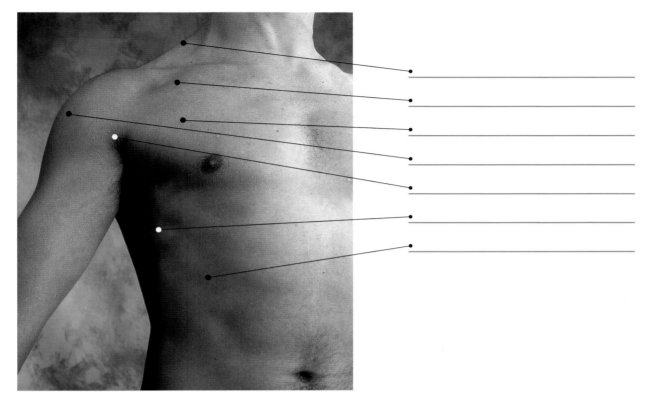

Fig. 5.6 (a) Muscles of the right shoulder region (anterior aspect)

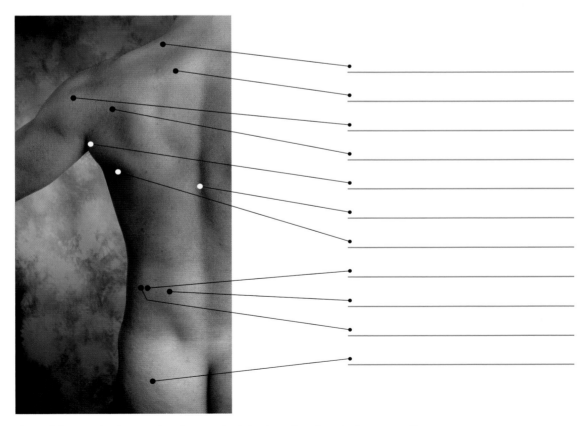

Fig. 5.8 (a) Muscles of the neck, thorax, lumbar and gluteal region (posterior aspect)

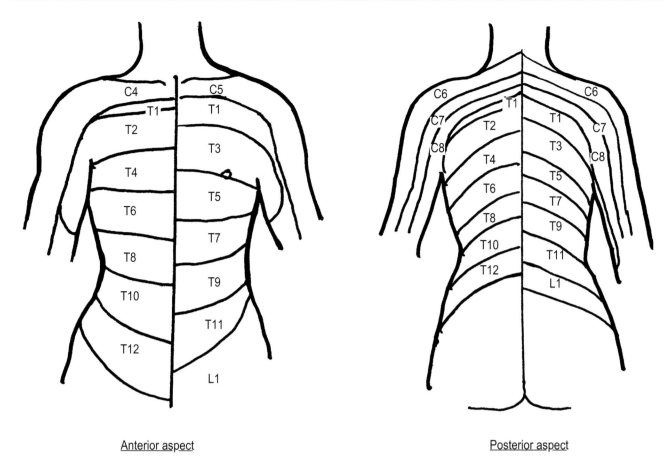

Anterior aspect   Posterior aspect

Fig. 5.11 (a), (b)
Cutaneous nerve supply to the thorax

NERVES [Figs 5.11 and 5.12]

The only nerves that become superficial in the thoracic region are those that supply the skin covering the ribs and intercostal spaces. By the time they reach the surface they are fine filaments and impossible to palpate.

Each intercostal nerve passes around the inside of the rib cage deep to the internal intercostal muscle, normally giving off a lateral branch at approximately the mid-axillary line. The area of skin supplied by each nerve usually includes that covering the rib above and below, including the external intercostal muscle passing between. Therefore there is an area of overlap of the cutaneous nerves, so that the loss of sensation from one nerve only leaves an area of paraesthesia not anaesthesia.

Below the sixth rib the nerves continue obliquely around the abdominal wall in the same direction as the ribs between which they commenced.

In the condition herpes zoster (shingles), the sensory component of an individual thoracic nerve is often affected by the virus and this leads to small pustules appearing over the area supplied by this particular nerve. The patient presents with a strip around the chest or abdomen following the line of its distribution (Fig. 5.11). Although this condition commonly appears to affect a single thoracic nerve it may affect any nerve in the body.

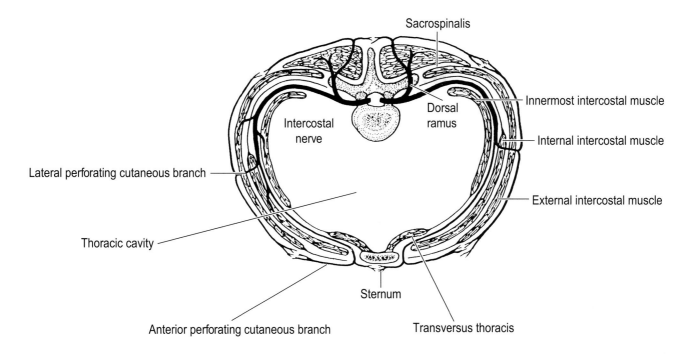

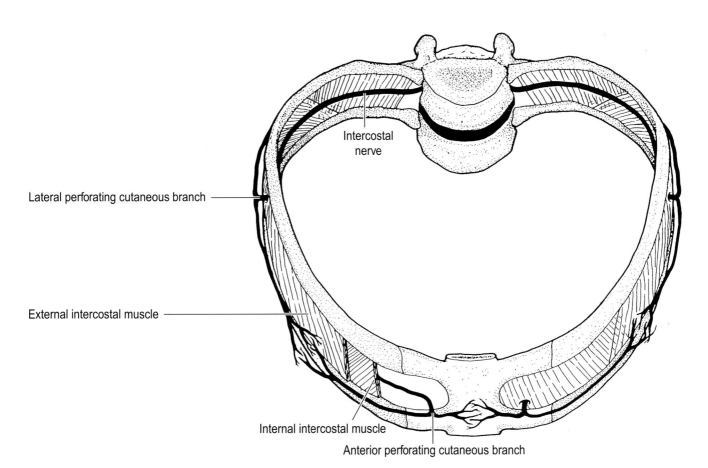

Fig. 5.12 (a), (b)
The course and distribution of a typical intercostal nerve

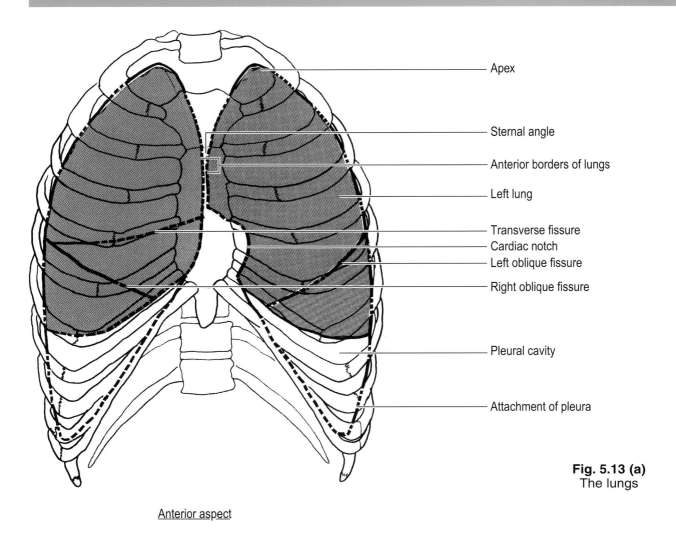

— Apex

— Sternal angle

— Anterior borders of lungs

— Left lung

— Transverse fissure
— Cardiac notch
— Left oblique fissure

— Right oblique fissure

— Pleural cavity

— Attachment of pleura

Fig. 5.13 (a)
The lungs

Anterior aspect

STRUCTURES WITHIN THE THORACIC CAGE

Although the structures contained within the thoracic cage are almost totally hidden by the ribs, sternum and vertebral column, it is of some importance to be able to indicate the surface markings of the major organs and vessels. Owing to considerable movement during life, no surface marking can be constant; nevertheless, each organ stays within certain boundaries. These will be indicated by the markings given.

The lungs [Fig. 5.13]

The lungs almost totally fill the thorax either side of the heart. The apex of each lung can be palpated, on deep inspiration, as it rises behind the middle third of the clavicle. These are the only areas of the lungs which are palpable and may prove to be elusive in some individuals. Each lung takes on the shape of the deep surface of the rib cage and intercostal muscles, being convex laterally and concave medially and inferiorly. Each lung presents anterior posterior and inferior borders

medially. The borders divide the lung into lateral, medial and inferior surfaces.

Surface markings

The surface markings of the anterior borders of the two lungs differ slightly. Both descend from the apex of the lung, behind the sternoclavicular joint of the appropriate side, to come together behind the sternal angle. They then pass downwards close to the midline until the level of the fourth costal cartilage, where the left anterior border passes laterally in a C-shaped curve concave medially (the cardiac notch) to reach the inferior border behind the sixth costal cartilage in the mid-clavicular line. The right medial border passes straight downwards, reaching the inferior border at the sixth chondrosternal joint (Fig. 5.13a).

The posterior borders of both lungs pass vertically downwards in front of the necks of the ribs, approximately 2 cm either side of the spines of the vertebrae, from the apex of the lung to the level of the tenth rib (Fig. 5.13c).

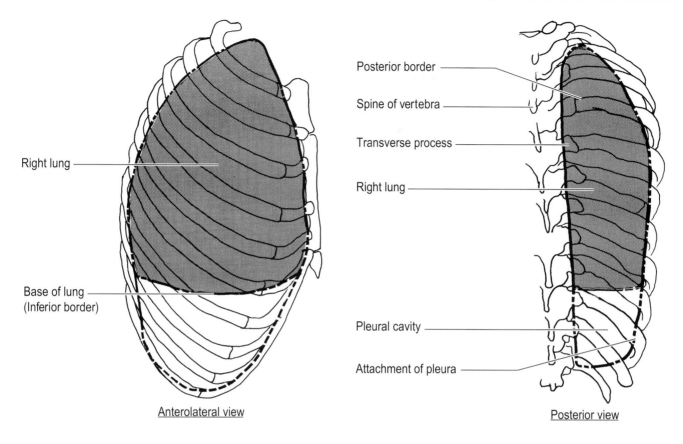

Anterolateral view

Fig. 5.13 (c)
The lungs

Posterior view

Fig. 5.13 (b)
The lungs

The inferior border of each lung passes almost horizontally around the chest wall, being level with the sixth costal cartilage anteriorly, crossing the eighth rib in the mid-axillary line and the tenth rib posteriorly. The base of the right lung is usually slightly higher than the left owing to the presence of the liver below it (Fig. 5.13a–c).

Parietal pleura lines the thoracic cage of each side and covers each lung in parts. The lower part of this pleura, however, is prolonged downwards for some 5 cm below the lower border of the lung to the twelfth rib posteriorly, the tenth rib at the mid-axillary line and the sixth costal cartilage anteriorly (Fig. 5.13a, c). This is termed the pleural cavity.

The fissures of the lungs

Each lung is marked by an oblique fissure; the right lung, in addition, has a transverse fissure.

These mark the junctions between the various lobes of each lung; the left therefore possesses two lobes, upper and lower, while the right possesses three, upper, middle and lower. Each oblique fissure can be marked on the chest wall by a line drawn obliquely downwards and forwards from a point 2 cm lateral to the spine of T3, crossing the mid-axillary line at the fifth rib, to reach the inferior border of the lung at the costal cartilage of the sixth rib, 7 cm from the midline (Fig. 5.13a). A good guide for the direction of this line is given by the medial border of the scapula when the arm is raised above the head.

Only the right lung has a transverse fissure, which marks the division of the upper and middle lobes. It is indicated by a line from the fifth rib in the mid-axillary line to the fourth costal cartilage 3 cm from the median plane, essentially running along the lower border of the fourth rib.

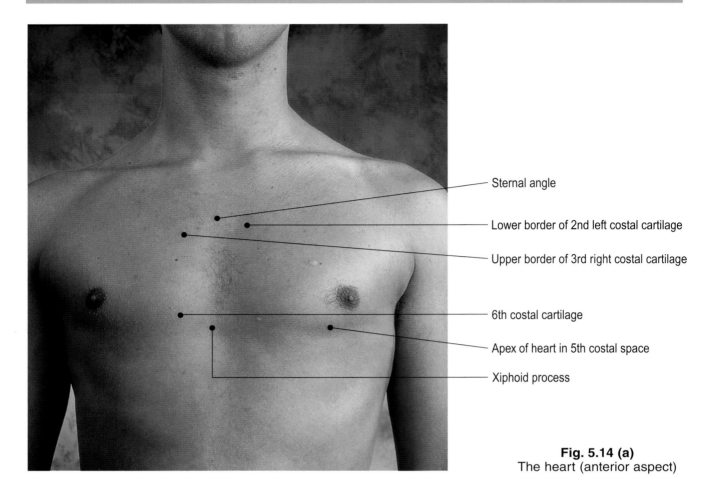

Sternal angle

Lower border of 2nd left costal cartilage

Upper border of 3rd right costal cartilage

6th costal cartilage

Apex of heart in 5th costal space

Xiphoid process

Fig. 5.14 (a)
The heart (anterior aspect)

The heart

The heart is a roughly cone-shaped double muscular pump situated behind the sternum with its apex downward and to the left and its base upward and to the right. It is composed of specialized contractile muscular tissue (myocardium) contained within a double layer of serous pericardium, which is joined around the area where the great vessels enter the heart. The outer layer of the pericardium is attached to the central part of the upper surface of the diaphragm and the inner layer is connected to the heart musculature. The two pumps, although pumping together, are completely separate and are often referred to as the 'left heart' and the 'right heart'. Each pump is composed of an upper receiving chamber called the atrium and a lower more powerful muscular chamber called the ventricle.

The heart is a rhythmically contractile tissue, which is controlled by nerve impulses. The upper chambers or atria are completely separated from the lower ventricles by a fibrous non-conductive layer. The only communication between the two is by a bundle of specialized tissue.

Location

The position of the heart within the thorax is variable, to some extent, depending on the posture adopted, so that its surface markings are slightly higher when lying compared with standing and sitting.

The projection of the heart on to the anterior surface of the chest is as follows (Figs 5.14 and 5.15). The apex of the heart points downwards and to the left and can be palpated 9 cm from the midline in the fifth left intercostal space. The pulsations are enhanced if the subject is sitting and leans slightly forward, as the apex of the heart is pressed

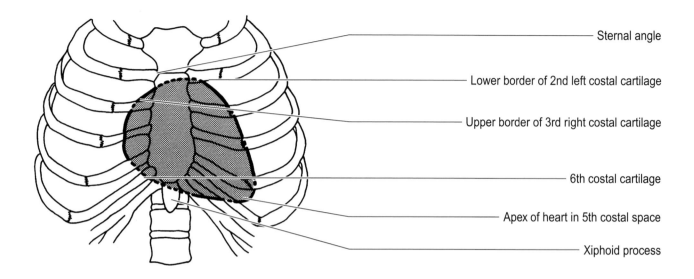

Sternal angle

Lower border of 2nd left costal cartilage

Upper border of 3rd right costal cartilage

6th costal cartilage

Apex of heart in 5th costal space

Xiphoid process

Fig. 5.14 (b)
The heart (anterior aspect)

against the chest wall. The upper limit of the heart is marked by two points, one at the lower border of the second left costal cartilage 3 cm to the left of the midline, and the other at the upper border of the third right costal cartilage 3 cm to the right of the midline. The lower right border of the heart can be indicated on the lower border of the costal cartilage of the right sixth rib 3 cm from the midline. The boundaries are curved, joining the above points and making an area approximately the size of the individual's clenched fist.

Function

The heart is responsible for pumping the blood around the body. The deoxygenated blood enters the right atrium from the systemic circulation through the large veins, e.g. the inferior and superior vena cava. It is then pumped down into the right ventricle through the right atrioventricular, tricuspid, valve which then contracts, sending the blood into the lungs, passing via the pulmonary valve.

Oxygenated blood is received into the left atrium from the lungs and is propelled down into the left ventricle through the left atrioventricular (mitral) valve. When full, the left ventricle contracts, pumping the blood through the aortic valve into the aorta and back into the systemic circulation.

Equal volumes of blood must be expelled from the two ventricles at each stroke, the right into the lungs and the left into the systemic circulation. This will maintain an equal rate of flow in both systems.

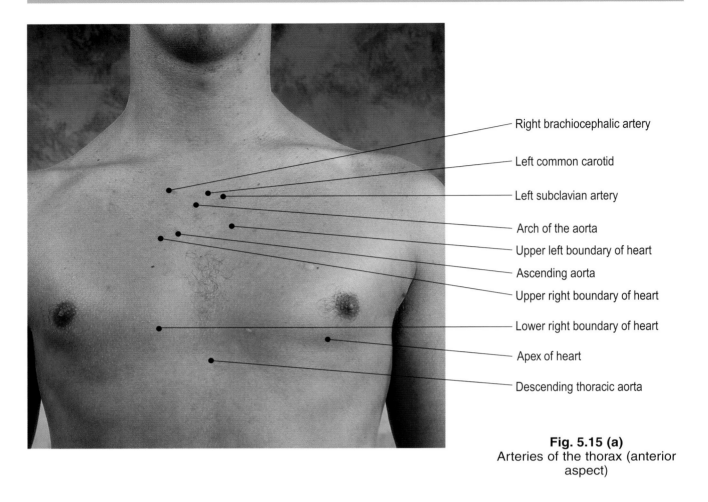

Right brachiocephalic artery

Left common carotid

Left subclavian artery

Arch of the aorta

Upper left boundary of heart

Ascending aorta

Upper right boundary of heart

Lower right boundary of heart

Apex of heart

Descending thoracic aorta

Fig. 5.15 (a)
Arteries of the thorax (anterior
aspect)

Major arteries [Fig. 5.15]

The aorta

The aorta is the main artery carrying oxygenated
blood to the body. It leaves the heart at the base of
the left ventricle, immediately giving off the two
coronary arteries which supply the heart itself
with blood. It passes upwards, slightly forwards
and to the right before arching backwards and to
the left over the right pulmonary vessels. It then
passes inferiorly through the thorax on the left
side of the vertebral bodies, behind the heart. As
it does so it gradually comes to lie more in the
midline, finally leaving the thorax in front, but
slightly to the left of the body of T12, passing
between the two crura and behind the median
arcuate ligament of the diaphragm.

Surface markings

The aortic valve lies deep to the sternum adjacent
to the third intercostal space. From here the
ascending aorta, a band 2.5 cm wide, passes
upwards and to the right as far as the second right
chondrosternal joint. The arch of the aorta then
passes behind the sternal angle (and the lower part
of the manubrium) over the heart, to end behind
the second left costal cartilage. The descending
aorta can be represented by a line extending from
this point to its exit from the thorax just left of
the midline and above the transpyloric plane,
which is on a level with the tips of the ninth costal
cartilages.

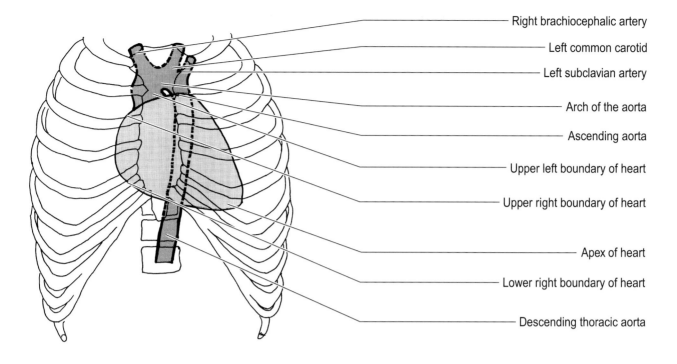

Right brachiocephalic artery

Left common carotid

Left subclavian artery

Arch of the aorta

Ascending aorta

Upper left boundary of heart

Upper right boundary of heart

Apex of heart

Lower right boundary of heart

Descending thoracic aorta

Fig. 5.15 (b)
Arteries of the thorax (anterior
aspect)

The brachiocephalic, left common carotid and left subclavian arteries

From the upper convexity of the arch of the aorta, three major vessels arise. The brachiocephalic (innominate) artery is anterior and to the right. Immediately behind and to the left is the left common carotid. Behind and to the left of the left common carotid is the left subclavian.

The brachiocephalic artery supplies oxygenated blood to the right side of the head and neck via the right common carotid artery through its internal and external branches. It also supplies blood to the right arm via the right subclavian artery. The left common carotid artery supplies blood to the left side of the head and neck via its internal and external branches. The left subclavian supplies blood to the left arm.

Surface markings

The brachiocephalic artery arises from the arch of the aorta behind the manubrium slightly right of centre and passes upwards, backwards and to the right for approximately 5 cm. It divides behind the right sternoclavicular joint into the right subclavian and right common carotid.

The left common carotid arises from the aorta just to the left of the mid point of the manubrium and passes upwards, backwards and to the left for approximately 4 cm to enter the neck behind the left sternoclavicular joint.

The left subclavian artery arises from the posterior part of the arch of the aorta behind the first intercostal space on the left, just lateral to the manubrium. It passes upwards and to the left for approximately 7 cm behind the first chondrosternal joint on the left to the inner borders of the left first rib. It passes over the rib *en route* to the left upper limb.

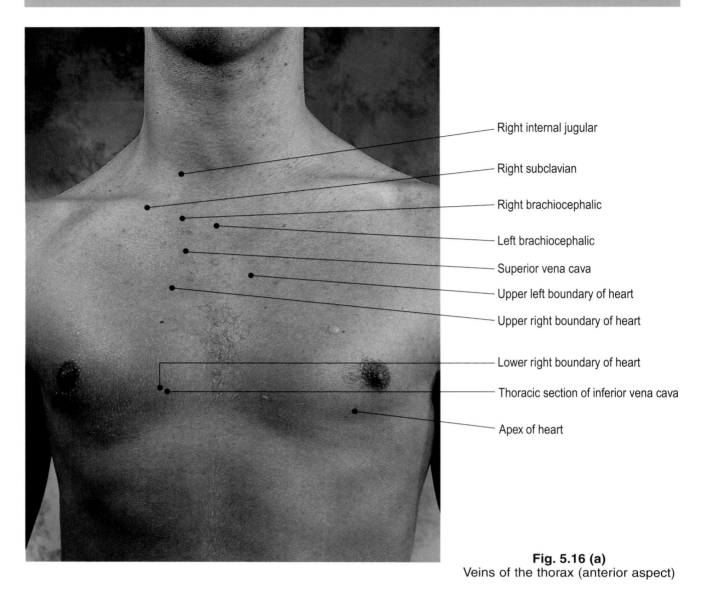

Right internal jugular

Right subclavian

Right brachiocephalic

Left brachiocephalic

Superior vena cava

Upper left boundary of heart

Upper right boundary of heart

Lower right boundary of heart

Thoracic section of inferior vena cava

Apex of heart

Fig. 5.16 (a)
Veins of the thorax (anterior aspect)

VEINS [Fig. 5.16]

The large veins of the thorax are also situated deep within the thoracic cage and are impossible to palpate. Nevertheless, it is of some value to know where they lie in relation to palpable surface markings. It must, however, be remembered that the chest wall, the heart, diaphragm and lungs are all moveable structures and this will lead to small differences in their relationship to one another. Surface markings, therefore, will be as accurate as possible but a little leeway must be expected in this area.

Outline of network

Venous blood from the head, neck, both upper limbs and upper trunk enters the left and right brachiocephalic (innominate) veins. It then passes into the superior vena cava and thus into the upper part of the right atrium of the heart.

Venous blood from the two lower limbs and lower trunk passes, via the internal and external iliac veins, into the abdominal inferior vena cava, entering the thoracic cavity, for just a short distance forming its thoracic section. This empties into the lower part of the right atrium of the heart.

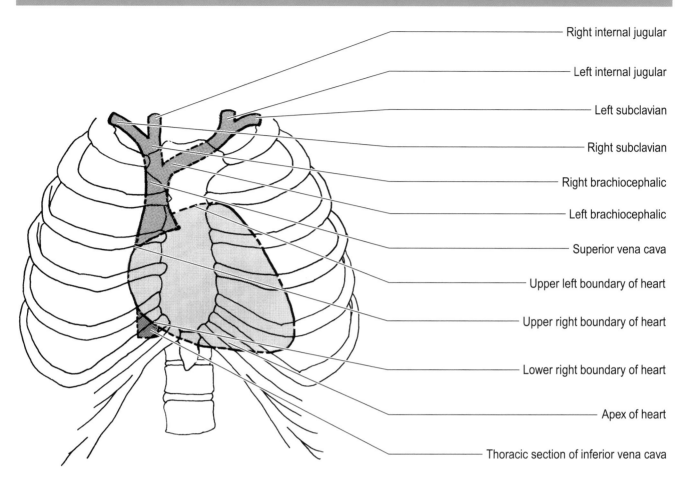

Right internal jugular

Left internal jugular

Left subclavian

Right subclavian

Right brachiocephalic

Left brachiocephalic

Superior vena cava

Upper left boundary of heart

Upper right boundary of heart

Lower right boundary of heart

Apex of heart

Thoracic section of inferior vena cava

Fig. 5.16 (b)
Veins of the thorax (anterior aspect)

Surface markings

In the upper thorax, the left and right brachio-cephalic (innominate) veins are formed by the internal jugular and the subclavian veins of their respective sides, just lateral to each sternoclavicular joint.

The left brachiocephalic vein passes downwards and to the right for approximately 6 cm to join the right brachiocephalic behind the sternal end of the first, right costal cartilage. At this point they form the superior vena cava.

The superior vena cava passes vertically down-wards for approximately 7 cm from behind the costal cartilage of the first rib on the right to enter the right atrium behind the sternal end of the third costal cartilage.

In the lower thorax, the inferior vena cava enters the thoracic cavity through the upper fibrous part of the diaphragm, entering the lower part of the right atrium of the heart almost immediately, lying behind the sternal end of the sixth right costal cartilage.

SELF ASSESSMENT

Page 322

1. Describe the general arrangement of the intercostal nerves.

2. Which area of skin is usually supplied by one intercostal nerve?

3. Explain the reasons why the loss of sensation through one nerve only causes parasthesia.

4. What signs normally appear on the chest wall in the condition of herpes zoster?

Page 324

5. Which part of the lungs may be palpated, and where?

6. Describe the general shape of the lungs.

7. What are the surface markings of the left lung?

8. Describe the differences between the surface markings of the right and left lungs.

Page 325

9. Why is the base of the right lung slightly higher than that of the left?

10. Describe what is meant by the pleural cavity.

11. What are the surface markings of the pleural cavity?

12. What are the fissures of the lungs?

13. How many fissures are there on each lung?

14. What are the surface markings of each of the fissures?

Page 326

15. Explain the reasons why the heart is often referred to as a double pump.

16. Of what tissue is the heart composed?

17. Name the main chambers of the heart.

18. What is the only conductive connection between the upper and lower chambers?

19. State the surface marking of the apex of the heart.

20. What are the surface markings of the upper part of the heart?

Please complete the labels below.

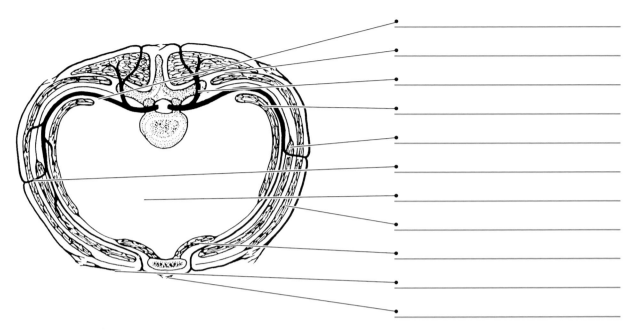

Fig. 5.12 (a) The course and distribution of a typical intercostal nerve

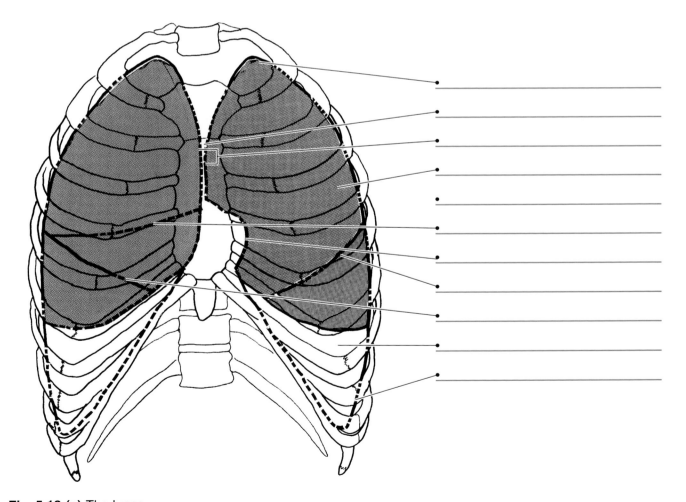

Fig. 5.13 (a) The lungs

Page 327

21. List the surface marking of the lower right side of the heart.

22. Into which chamber of the heart do the superior and inferior vena cava empty their blood?

23. Name the valve which lies between the right atrium and right ventricle.

24. To which area in the body is the blood from the right ventricle distributed?

25. Through which valve does this blood flow?

26. From where does the left atrium receive its blood?

27. Name the valve through which the blood passes from the left atrium to the left ventricle.

28. Into which large vessel is the blood pumped from the left ventricle?

29. Through which valve does this blood pass?

Page 328

30. Which arteries supply the heart tissue with blood?

31. Describe the root of the ascending, arch and descending aorta.

32. Name and state the position of the structures which surround the aorta as it leaves the thoracic cavity.

33. What is the surface marking of the aortic valve?

34. What are the surface markings of the ascending, arch and descending aorta?

Page 329

35. Name the three major vessels which arise from the arch of the aorta.

36. Describe their general relation to each other.

37. To which part of the body is the blood from the right common carotid artery distributed?

38. Supply of blood to the right arm is via which artery?

Please complete the labels below.

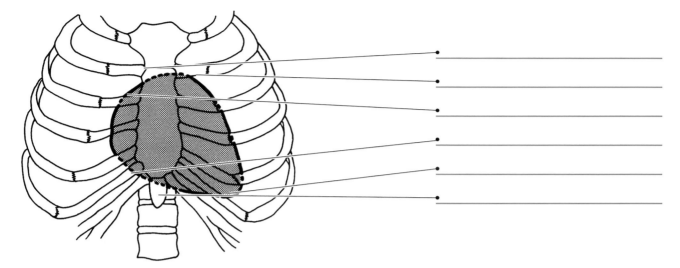

Fig. 5.14 (b) The heart (anterior aspect)

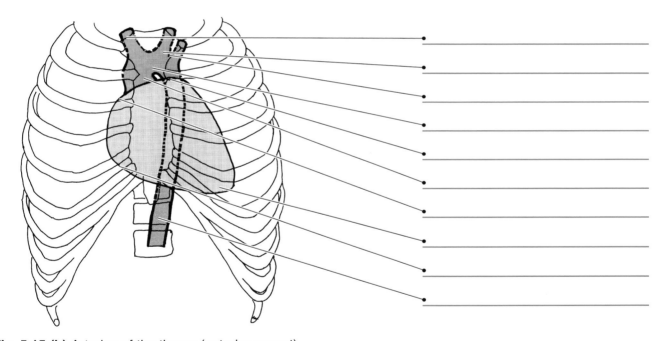

Fig. 5.15 (b) Arteries of the thorax (anterior aspect)

39. Which main artery supplies blood to the left arm?

40. In which area does the brachiocephalic artery divide into the right subclavian and right common carotid?

41. Behind what structure does the left common carotid artery enter the neck?

42. What are the surface markings of the left subclavian artery on its root to the left upper limb?

Page 330

43. Give the areas from which the right brachiocephalic vein receives its blood.

44. Through which vein is this blood passed into the heart?

45. Into which chamber does this blood enter the heart?

46. Which areas of the body are drained by the internal iliac veins?

47. Which areas are drained by the external iliac veins?

48. Through which vessels is this blood relayed to the heart?

49. Into which chamber does this blood enter the heart?

Page 331

50. Behind which joint are the brachiocephalic veins formed?

51. State the surface marking of the junction between the left and right brachiocephalic veins.

52. Which vein is formed by this union?

53. State the surface marking behind which the superior vena cava enters the right atrium.

54. Through which part of the diaphragm does the inferior vena cava pass?

55. What is the surface marking of the point at which the inferior vena cava enters the right atrium?

Please complete the labels below.

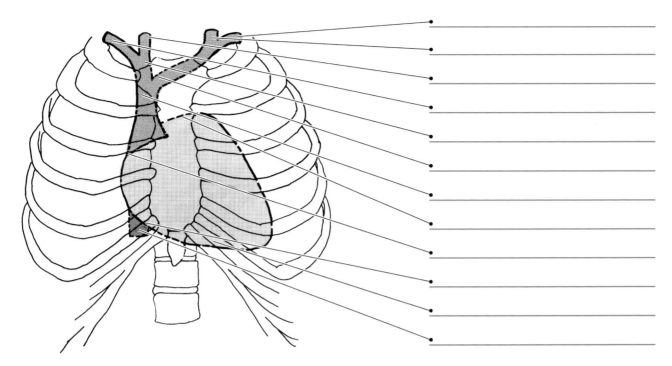

Fig. 5.16 (b) Veins of the thorax (anterior aspect)

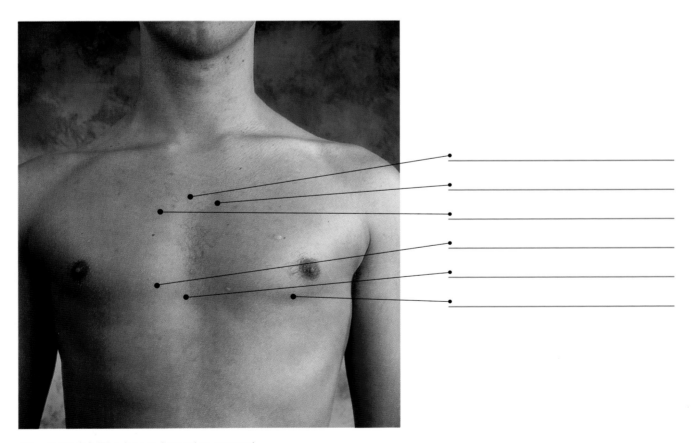

Fig. 5.14 (a) The heart (anterior aspect)

The abdomen

Contents

At the end of this chapter you should be able to:

A. Find, recognize and name the constituent bony components of the boundaries of the abdomen including the lower ribs, cartilages, xyphoid process, lumbar vertebrae and pelvic girdle.

B. Palpate many of the bony features, being able to relate one to another.

C. Locate, name or number the spines and transverse processes of all the lumbar vertebrae.

D. Recognize and palpate the main bony landmarks of the pelvis, sacrum and coccyx.

E. Name all the joints of the lumbar spine and pelvis noting their active and passive range of movement.

F. Give the class and type of all the joints named.

G. Palpate the joint lines, where possible, and give their surface markings.

H. Demonstrate any accessory movements which may be possible in the joints of the lumbar spine and pelvis.

I. Locate and name the muscles which surround the abdomen.

J. Be able to draw the shape of the muscle on the surface and give its attachments.

K. Demonstrate the actions of all of the muscles covering the abdomen.

L. Give an account of their actions and functional significance.

M. Describe the main anatomical regions of the abdomen.

N. Give the surface markings of the liver, spleen, pancreas, gall bladder, small intestine, large bowel, kidneys and bladder.

O. Demonstrate the cutaneous distribution of the nerves covering the abdomen giving an outline of the course each takes.

P. Describe the arrangement of the main arteries in the abdomen giving their surface markings.

Q. Describe the arrangement of the main veins in the abdomen giving their surface markings.

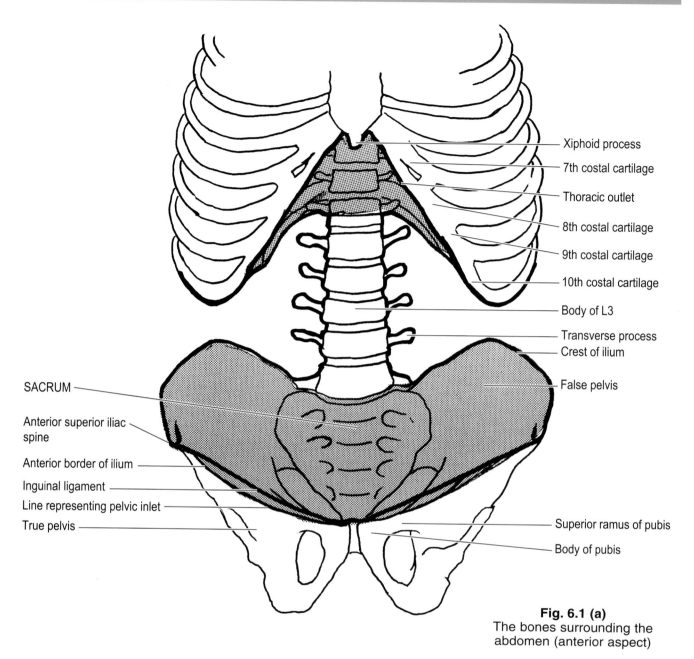

Fig. 6.1 (a)
The bones surrounding the
abdomen (anterior aspect)

BONES

The abdomen consists mainly of soft tissue contained within predominantly muscular walls. Its only bony features are the boundaries of the thoracic outlet above consisting of the xiphoid process at its centre in the front, the lower border of the seventh, eighth, ninth and tenth costal cartilages, the tip of the eleventh rib and the inferior border of the twelfth rib. Posteriorly, the body of the twelfth thoracic vertebra completes the ring. Below, the pelvic inlet comprises the pubis anteriorly, its superior rami on either side, the anterior border and the crest of the ilium and posteriorly the base of the sacrum. The vertebral column forms its posterior boundary. It is, however, important to mark out these boundaries, as they provide useful landmarks for some of the organs it contains.

The thoracic outlet [Fig. 6.1a]

Palpation

Find the xiphoid process, which is the most inferior portion of the sternum. Trace along the costal margin beyond the costal angle (the ninth costal cartilage) to its lowest extremity, which is normally the tenth rib. Continuing posteriorly, the eleventh rib becomes evident, with its tip just anterior to the mid-axillary line, with the tip of the twelfth rib slightly lower and just posterior. The tip of the twelfth rib normally lies on the same level as the spine of the first lumbar vertebra.

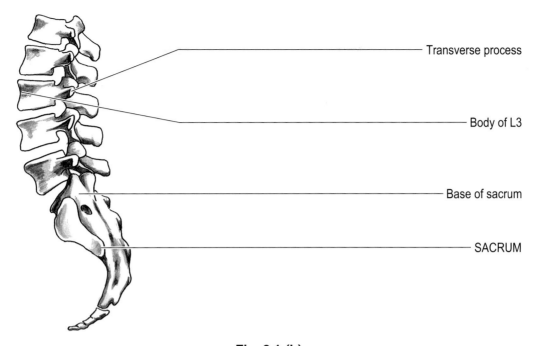

Transverse process

Body of L3

Base of sacrum

SACRUM

Fig. 6.1 (b)
The bones surrounding the abdomen (lateral aspect, viewed from left)

The pelvic girdle

Palpation

Identify the anterior superior iliac spine at the anterior extremity of the iliac crest. Trace the lateral lip of the iliac crest posteriorly, beyond the iliac tubercle to the posterior superior iliac spine and sacrum. Now, run the pads of your fingers down the central part of the abdominal wall to about 5 cm above the genitalia. The pubic tubercles become evident on either side, with each pubic crest running medially to a central space which marks the pubic symphysis. The bony ring is completed by the superior ramus of the pubis, which is difficult to palpate, and anterior border of the ilium, easily identifiable in its upper section. The inguinal ligament stretches above this region from the pubic tubercle to the anterior superior iliac spine.

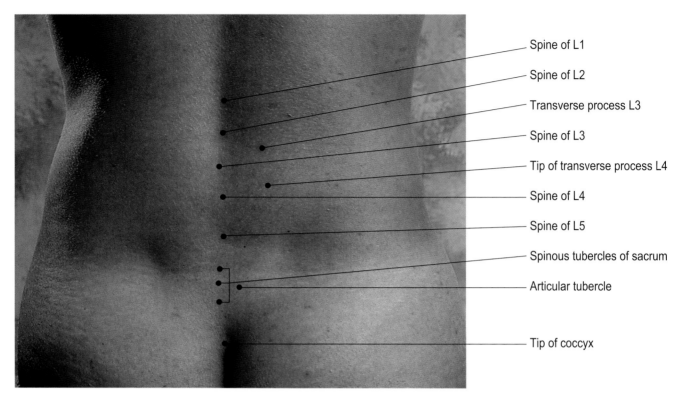

Spine of L1
Spine of L2
Transverse process L3
Spine of L3
Tip of transverse process L4
Spine of L4
Spine of L5
Spinous tubercles of sacrum
Articular tubercle
Tip of coccyx

Fig. 6.1 (c)
Lumbar vertebrae and sacrum (posterior aspect)

The lumbar vertebrae

There are five lumbar vertebrae, with L1 being the smallest and L5 the largest. As in all other vertebrae, their bodies are anterior and their spines are posterior. Laterally, they present transverse processes, the fifth being much larger than the rest. Their upper articular processes face inwards and their lower facets face outwards, those of the fifth facing more anteriorly. There is a large neural canal in the lumbar region which is more triangular in shape.

Palpation

Lumbar vertebrae. Posteriorly the spines of the lumbar vertebrae project backwards and are individually identifiable. With the subject lying prone, place a firm pillow under the abdomen which flattens the lumbar lordosis. This makes the spines of the lumbar vertebrae become more pronounced, appearing as a line of flattened edges forming a crest down the centre of the lumbar region (Fig. 6.1c, d). The spines are continuous with those of the sacrum below and the thoracic vertebrae above.

Immediately above the central part of the sacrum is a hollow, due to the spine of the fifth vertebra being shorter and the body being situated slightly more anterior than the rest. The small gaps between the spines tend to disappear when the vertebral column is flexed, owing to the tension of the supraspinous ligament.

If deep pressure is applied approximately 5 cm lateral to the vertebral spines, beyond the bulk of the erector spinae muscles, the tips of the transverse processes, particularly of the first lumbar vertebra, can be palpated. These are quite thin compared with those of the thorax and may be tender to palpate.

The sacrum

The sacrum is composed of five fused vertebrae, with S1 being the largest and S5 being the smallest. The sacrum is triangular in shape, with its base uppermost. Evidence of the separate vertebral bodies is still clear on the anterior surface. A line of spinous tubercles can be seen running vertically down the centre of its posterior surface and it is marked on either side by articular tubercles. Laterally the sacrum presents large lateral masses beyond its neural foramina. The sacrum is tilted forwards above, with its lower section projecting backwards.

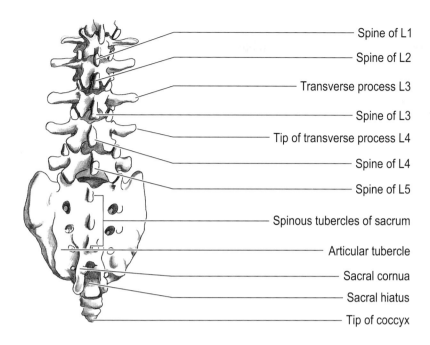

Spine of L1
Spine of L2
Transverse process L3
Spine of L3
Tip of transverse process L4
Spine of L4
Spine of L5
Spinous tubercles of sacrum
Articular tubercle
Sacral cornua
Sacral hiatus
Tip of coccyx

Fig. 6.1 (d)
Lumbar vertebrae and sacrum (posterior aspect)

Palpation

The sacrum. The posterior surface of the sacrum can be identified between the posterior borders of the two ilia. Its lower section projects backwards and is easy to palpate, while its upper section (the base) lies more anterior and is more difficult to examine. It has a central, vertical series of spinous tubercles, in line with the lumbar spines and the coccyx, accompanied on either side by a row of articular tubercles which are all palpable (Fig. 6.1c, d).

The coccyx

The coccyx comprises three or four rudimentary vertebrae normally fused into one bone, with the upper being the largest and the lowest being a very small tubercle of bone. Normally it is tilted, with its inferior tip pointing downwards and forwards.

Palpation

The coccyx. As this bone varies considerably in size and shape it may prove a little difficult to palpate. Several alternative methods can be employed:

1. Trace the spinous processes which run down the centre of the posterior surface of the sacrum to approximately 2.5 cm below the level of the posterior inferior iliac spines (see pages 126 and 127). Here, the pointed lower end of the coccyx can be palpated.
2. Gently run your fingers up the cleft between the two gluteus maximus muscles until the hard bony tip of the coccyx is found.
3. Draw an equilateral triangle with its base on the two posterior inferior iliac spines of the ilium with its apex downwards. This point should be on the tip of the coccyx.

In many subjects the coccyx is angled forwards and the finger must be pressed deep into the cleft to identify the shape. Care must be taken as pressure on the bone can cause pain, particularly if the joints between it and the sacrum have been damaged at any time.

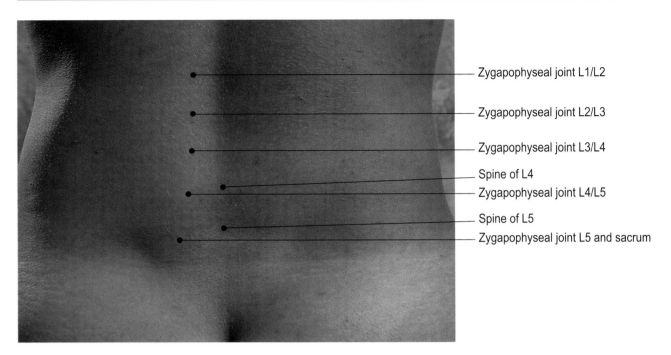

Fig. 6.2 (a)
Zygapophyseal joints of lumbar spine (posterior view)

JOINTS

The lumbar spine [Fig. 6.2]

The zygapophyseal joints are the most superficial in the lumbar region. They are nevertheless covered by thick, strong muscle, making the task of palpation extremely difficult. With the fingers pressed between the sides of the vertebral spines and the parallel-running column of muscle (sacro-spinalis), the sides of the spines and in some subjects the laminae of each vertebra may be palpated. Each is a little higher than its corresponding spine, being almost totally hidden by the thick muscle layer.

Deep pressure through the muscle, using the tips of the thumbs, applies pressure to the posterior aspect of the zygapophyseal joints, which lie 1 cm lateral and slightly lower than the vertebral spine. With great care and precision this pressure can be targeted on to the upper articular pillar of the vertebra below by moving lateral to the joint, or on to the lower articular pillar of the vertebra above by moving just medial to the joint. The lower facets of the vertebrae are convex anteriorly and fit snugly into the concave anterior edge of the upper facets of the vertebra below. Thus, anterior pressure on the lower vertebra causes its articular facet to glide forwards, slightly parting its anterior segments, whereas pressure on the upper vertebra pushes the lower facet into the socket, preventing any further movement (Fig. 6.2d, e).

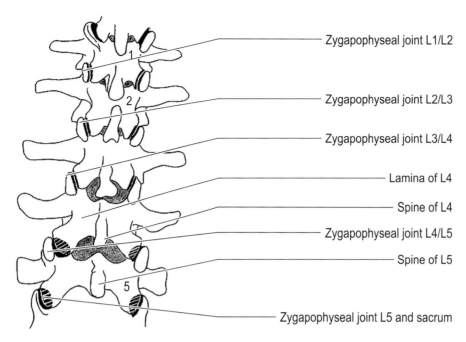

Fig. 6.2 (b)
Zygapophyseal joints of lumbar spine (posterior view)

Accessory movements

Distraction (traction) of the joints of the lumbar spine is the only true accessory movement possible. All other movements of gliding, gapping and compression of the zygapophyseal joints, together with twisting and compression of the intervertebral discs, occur in the area during normal lumbar activities.

Traction can be applied to this area in many ways, either manually or mechanically. The lumbar column, however, can be placed in many different positions to achieve the therapeutic result required.

Extension of the lumbar spine tends to create a 'close-packed' position for the individual joints, as the articular surfaces come into full contact and ligaments become taut. This, therefore, is not a desirable position in which to achieve traction. All other positions towards flexion allow space for the joint surfaces to part or glide; however, in full flexion the ligaments again become taut, preventing the required movements. Traction in full flexion is almost impossible to apply. The optimum position in which to apply traction is midway between extension and flexion.

Simple traction can be applied to the lumbar spine by applying a distraction force to either the pelvis or the lower limbs, with the subject lying either supine or prone. It is preferable to place a pillow under the abdomen in the latter position to prevent extension. Manual traction can also be applied with the subject sitting or standing, by raising the upper trunk and allowing the pelvis and lower limbs to act as the traction force.

Mechanical traction can be applied in many positions of the lumbar spine, avoiding full extension and full flexion for the same reasons as outlined above. It may be applied continuously or intermittently over a set period of time. These therapeutic traction techniques are complex and need skill and knowledge of techniques and precautions. For further study, reference should be made to literature dedicated to this subject.

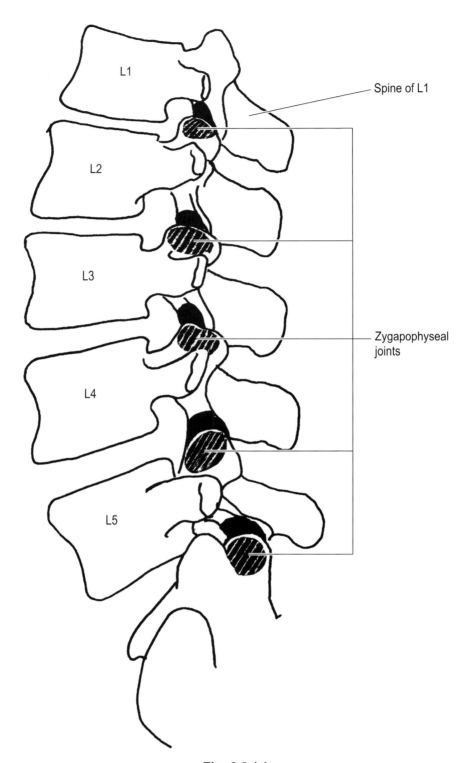

Fig. 6.2 (c)
Zygapophyseal joints of the lumbar spine (lateral aspect from left)

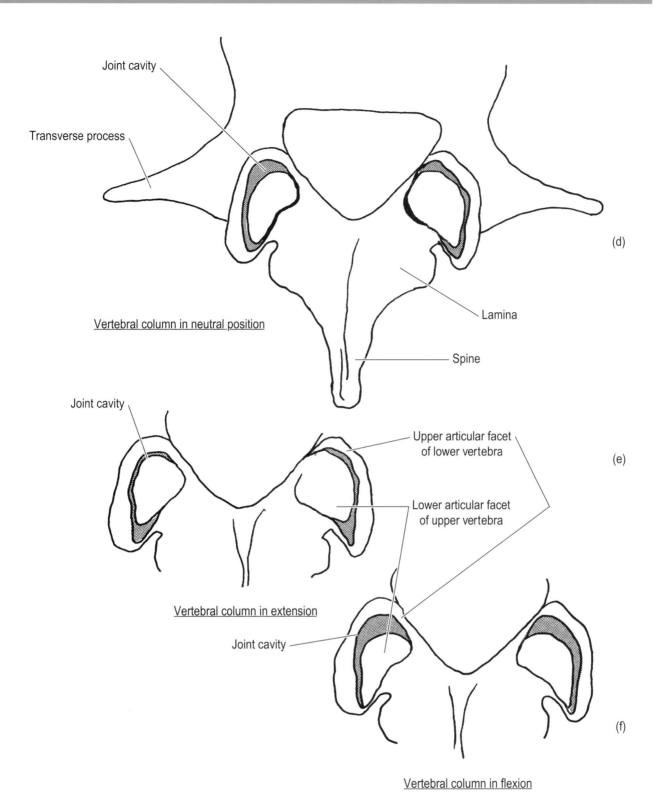

Fig. 6.2 (d)–(f)
Zygapophyseal joints of lumbar section of vertebral column (viewed from above)

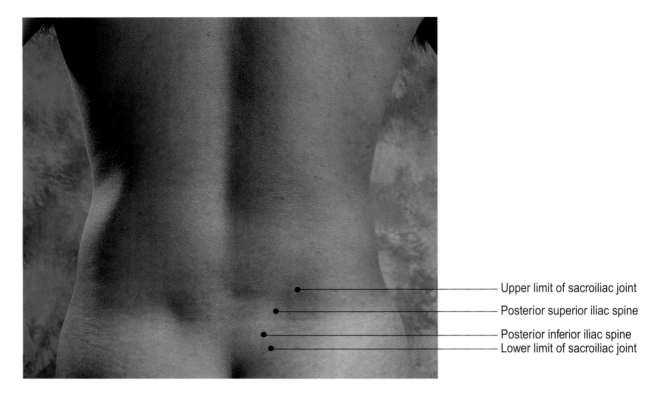

Upper limit of sacroiliac joint

Posterior superior iliac spine

Posterior inferior iliac spine
Lower limit of sacroiliac joint

Fig. 6.3 (a)
Sacroiliac joint (posterior aspect)

The pelvis [Figs 6.3 and 6.4]

Posteriorly, the sacrum articulates on either side with the ilium (innominate) bone at the sacroiliac joints (also discussed in Chapter 3). Anteriorly, the two pubic bodies articulate with each other at the pubic symphysis. The former is a very stable plane synovial joint supported by powerful interosseous and accessory ligaments. The latter is also stable, but is a secondary cartilaginous joint containing a modified disc of fibrocartilage. The sacroiliac joints allow a small degree of rotation of the sacrum, with respect to the innominate bones, about an axis through its interosseous ligament. Movement is more noticeable in young females, particularly during pregnancy and childbirth, reducing considerably after the third decade. In males, movement is negligible and virtually nil after the second decade.

The pubic symphysis allows a slight rocking and twisting to occur, which accompanies any movements which may occur at the sacroiliac joints.

The sacroiliac joint

Palpation

With the subject lying prone and the abdomen resting on a pillow, identify the posterior superior iliac spine. The sacroiliac joint lies 1 cm lateral and 1 cm anterior to this spine, on an oblique line extending above and below a further 2 cm. The line of the joint can also be marked by an oblique line passing downwards and medially, at an angle of approximately 25°, from a point 5 cm lateral to the spine of the fifth lumbar vertebra to a point just lateral to the posterior inferior iliac spine (Fig. 6.3b). It is impossible to palpate this joint.

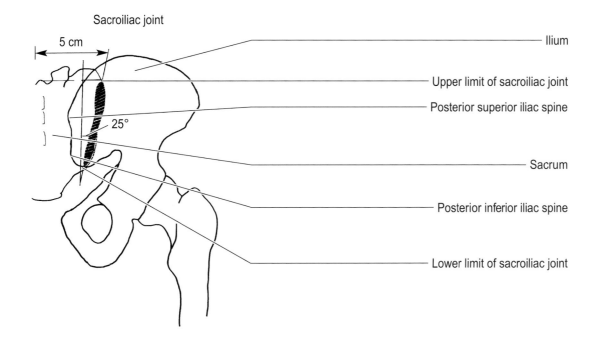

Fig. 6.3 (b)
Sacroiliac joint (posterior aspect)

Accessory movements

Little movement occurs at the sacroiliac joint, there being more in the young female and less in the middle-aged and elderly male (see above).

Rocking the sacrum around a frontal axis can be achieved in the prone subject by placing the heel of one hand over the apex and the heel of the other over the base of the sacrum. Alternate pressure applied to the apex and base produces a slight rocking movement of the sacrum between the two innominate bones. This movement can be increased locally on one side if one hand is placed on the apex of the sacrum and the other on the posterior aspect of the crest of the ilium. The opposite movement can be produced by placing one hand on the base of the sacrum and the other on the ischial tuberosity. The pressure applied to

these two areas must be downwards and towards each other, in the same direction as the movement of each component. It is a difficult movement to obtain, and some skill and practice is necessary before it can be achieved.

The posterior aspect of the joint can normally be gapped or at least stressed by using the leverage of the femur. With the subject supine, flex the opposite knee and hip and roll the limb and pelvis towards you. When the pelvis is rotated approximately 45°, a downward and medial pressure toward the opposite hip joint can be applied to the femoral condyles. This technique is used in the examination and treatment of sacroiliac problems and is covered in greater detail in the manipulation literature.

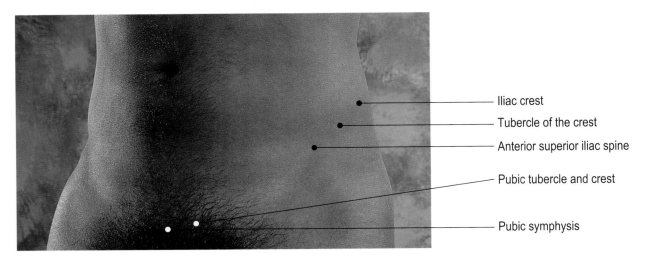

Iliac crest

Tubercle of the crest

Anterior superior iliac spine

Pubic tubercle and crest

Pubic symphysis

Fig. 6.4 (a)
The pelvis (anterior view)

The pubic symphysis

This joint is situated centrally at the lower aspect of the abdomen between the two pubic bones and just above the external genitalia. Locate the pubic tubercles on the upper border of the body of the pubis, either side of the midline. Between the two is a depressed line which can be traced downwards for about 2.5 cm. This indicates the anterior marking of the pubic symphysis, being the medial surfaces of the pubic bones separated only by the intervening interarticular disc.

Accessory movements

The slight twisting and gapping that occurs at this joint is due to stresses on the pelvis and sacrum which occur during movements at the sacroiliac and hip joint. With the subject lying supine, a slight gliding movement can be produced between the two bones by applying pressure to the anterior surface of the pubic body on one side only.

With the subject lying on the side, a downward compression force applied to the upper part of the ilium increases compression at the pubic symphysis, while also stressing the posterior sacroiliac ligament. With the subject supine, the two ilia can be stressed laterally by a downward and lateral pressure being applied to the two iliac crests. This produces a distraction force to the pubic symphysis and, in addition, an anterior gapping and stress on the anterior ligament of the sacroiliac joint

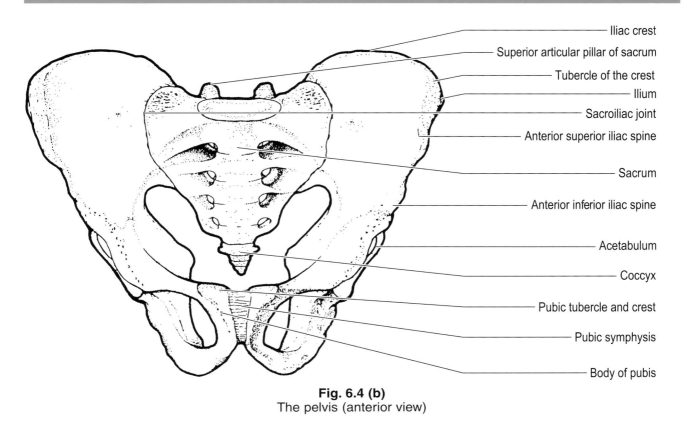

- Iliac crest
- Superior articular pillar of sacrum
- Tubercle of the crest
- Ilium
- Sacroiliac joint
- Anterior superior iliac spine
- Sacrum
- Anterior inferior iliac spine
- Acetabulum
- Coccyx
- Pubic tubercle and crest
- Pubic symphysis
- Body of pubis

Fig. 6.4 (b)
The pelvis (anterior view)

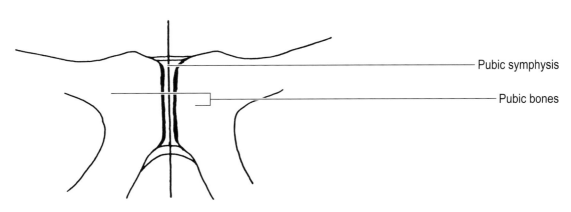

- Pubic symphysis
- Pubic bones

Fig. 6.4 (c)
The pelvis (anterior view)

SELF ASSESSMENT

Page 340

1. Describe the bony boundaries of the thoracic outlet.

2. Give the names and positions of the bones which comprise the pelvic inlet.

3. Which bones form the posterior boundary of the abdomen?

4. The costal angle is formed by which costal cartilage?

5. What forms the lowest extremity of the thoracic outlet?

6. On a level with what part of which vertebra does the tip of the 12th rib lie?

7. Name any other structure which lies on this level.

Page 341

8. Describe the steps involved in locating the anterior superior iliac spine.

9. What bony feature lies on the lateral lip of the crest of the ilium 5 cm posterior to the anterior superior spine?

10. Which bony features are palpable 5 cm above the genitalia?

11. What structure lies centrally at this point?

12. Describe the attachments of both ends of the inguinal ligament.

Page 342

13. How many lumbar vertebrae are found in the vertebral column?

14. Of these vertebrae, which is the largest and which is the smallest?

15. Which lumbar vertebra presents the largest transverse processes?

16. On a typical lumbar vertebra, in which direction do the upper articular processes face?

17. Generally, in which direction do the inferior articular facets face?

18. Identify any exceptions.

Please complete the labels below.

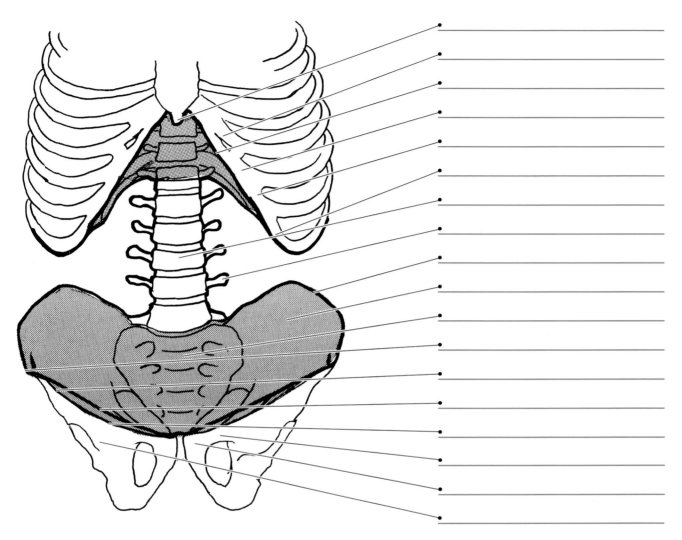

Fig. 6.1 (a) The bones surrounding the abdomen (anterior aspect)

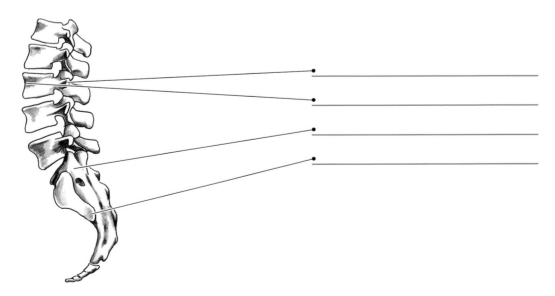

Fig. 6.1 (b) The bones surrounding the abdomen (lateral aspect, viewed from left)

19. Viewed from above, what shape is the neural canal in the lumbar spine?

20. What shape are the lumbar spines posteriorly?

21. Explain why there is a small hollow immediately above the central part of the sacrum.

22. When the spine is flexed, explain why the small gaps between the spines normally disappear.

23. What structure can be palpated 5 cm lateral to the spines?

24. Which muscles make the identification of bony features difficult in this region?

25. Which vertebrae are normally fused to form the sacrum?

26. Describe the shape and position of the sacrum.

27. In which area is there visible evidence of the sacrum being composed of five vertebrae?

28. What bony features lie down the middle of the sacrum's posterior surface?

29. What structure can be palpated on either side of the sacrum?

30. Which bones comprise the lateral mass of the sacrum?

31. With what structure does the lateral mass of the sacrum articulate?

Page 343

32. Between which two bones does the sacrum lie?

33. Which part of the sacrum projects backwards?

34. Name the bone which lies at the lower end of the sacrum.

35. From which bones is this structure formed?

36. Describe the method by which this bone can be palpated.

Please complete the labels below.

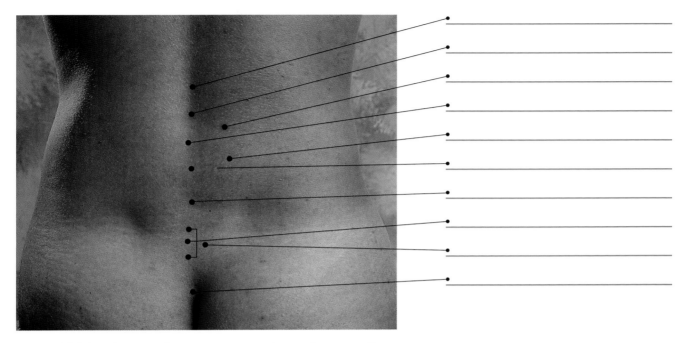

Fig. 6.1 (c) Lumbar vertebrae and sacrum (posterior aspect)

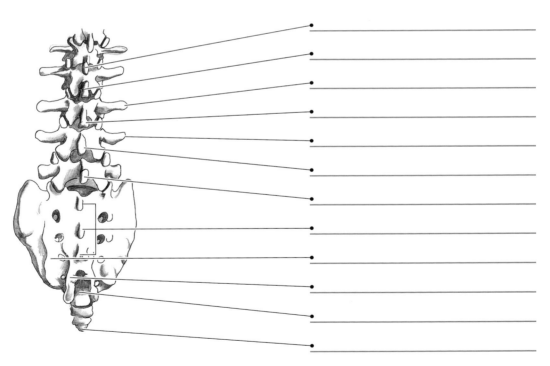

Fig. 6.1 (d) Lumbar vertebrae and sacrum (posterior aspect)

Page 344

37. Where does the zygapophyseal joint lie in relation to the spine of each lumbar vertebra?

Page 345

38. What is the only true accessory movement of the lumbar spine?

39. In which positions are these movements difficult to perform?

40. Why are they difficult to perform in these positions?

41. What methods of traction are available for the lumbar spine?

42. Describe one method of giving traction to the lumbar spine.

Page 348

43. Give the type and class of the sacroiliac joint.

44. What type of joint is the pubic symphysis?

45. Which movements may be possible in the sacroiliac joint?

46. Describe the movements which may be possible at the pubic symphysis.

47. List the surface markings of the sacroiliac joint.

Page 349

48. In which sex is the sacroiliac joint most mobile?

49. Is the joint more mobile in the young or the old?

50. Describe how an accessory movement may be performed at the sacroiliac joint.

Page 350

51. List the surface markings of the pubic symphysis.

52. Describe the method by which the pubic symphysis can be palpated.

53. What movement occurs naturally at this joint?

54. Describe the method by which a possible accessory movement may be produced at the pubic symphysis.

Please complete the labels below.

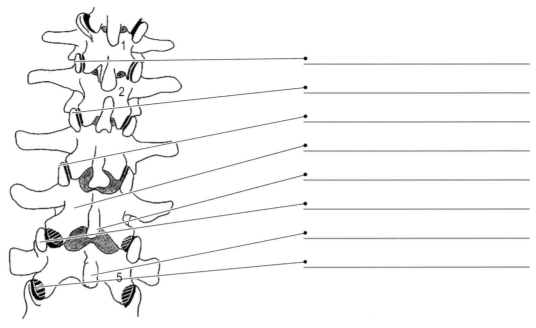

Fig. 6.2 (b) Zygapophyseal joints of lumbar spine (posterior view)

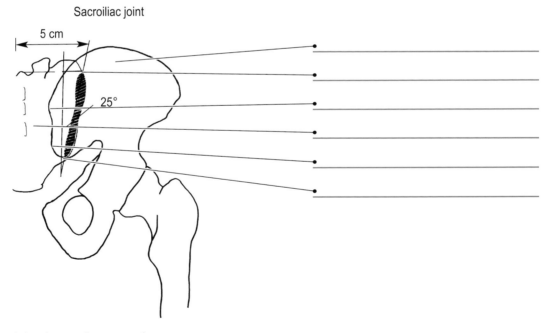

Fig. 6.3 (b) Sacroiliac joint (posterior aspect)

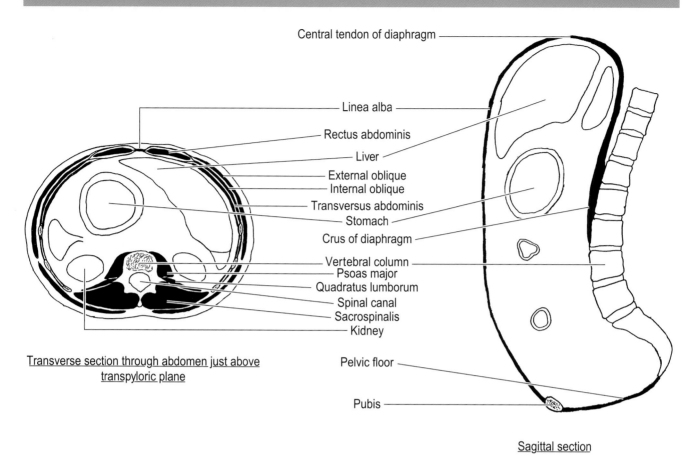

Central tendon of diaphragm

Linea alba

Rectus abdominis

Liver

External oblique

Internal oblique

Transversus abdominis

Stomach

Crus of diaphragm

Vertebral column

Psoas major

Quadratus lumborum

Spinal canal

Sacrospinalis

Kidney

Transverse section through abdomen just above
transpyloric plane

Pelvic floor

Pubis

Sagittal section

Fig. 6.5 (a), (b)
The abdomen

MUSCLES

The abdominal muscles form a continuous wall around the abdominal viscera. The cavity so formed is enclosed by the diaphragm above; the vertebral column and psoas major posteroinferiorly; quadratus lumborum posterolaterally; the internal and external oblique abdominal muscles anterolaterally, supported on their deep surface by transversus abdominis; rectus abdominis anteriorly; and inferiorly by the muscles which form the pelvic floor, i.e. levator ani and coccygeus. Some of these muscles may be palpable when they are contracting, although they may not always appear distinct (Fig. 6.5).

Palpation

Identification of structures and muscles in this area is dependent, to a certain extent, on the physique of the subject. Subcutaneous fat in the superficial fascia covering the abdomen can hinder accurate identification.

With the subject lying supine, place both hands on the central area of the abdomen, one above and one below the umbilicus. If the subject now raises the head, a column of muscle can be palpated running down either side of the central depressed line (the linea alba) (Fig. 6.5a–d). These two columns of muscle are the left and right sections of the rectus abdominus muscle. Each muscle is narrow inferiorly and can be traced from the pubic tubercle and crest below to its broader superior attachment to the fifth, sixth and seventh ribs. The upper attachment is V-shaped, as the attachment to the fifth rib laterally is higher than that to the seventh costal centrally. The lateral border of each muscle is convex. The muscle is interrupted

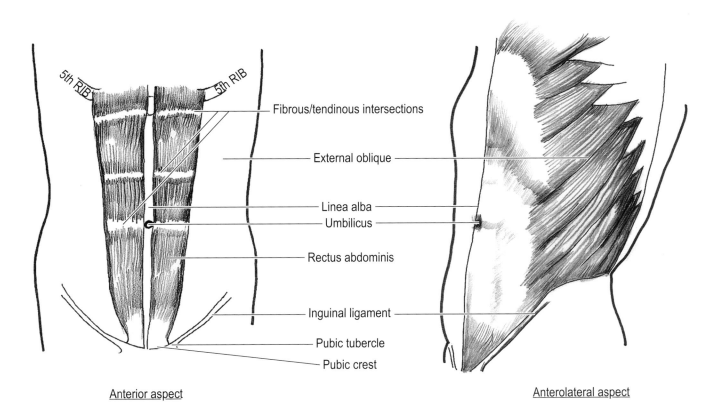

5th RIB

5th RIB

Fibrous/tendinous intersections

External oblique

Linea alba

Umbilicus

Rectus abdominis

Inguinal ligament

Pubic tubercle

Pubic crest

Anterior aspect

Anterolateral aspect

Fig. 6.5 (c), (d)
Muscles of the abdomen

by three transverse depressed **fibrous inter-sections**, which are at the level of the xiphoid, the umbilicus and midway between the two. These appear as transverse grooves across the muscles.

Both the external and internal oblique muscles contract during flexion of the trunk, but each can be identified more easily if its action is resisted. To facilitate palpation of the right external oblique, resistance must be applied to oppose upper trunk rotation to the left. This can be achieved with the subject supine, by standing to the left side and applying resistance to the right shoulder, preventing the head and shoulder being lifted and turned to the left. Contraction of the muscle tightens the aponeurosis just above its attachment to the right iliac crest.

The internal oblique lies deep to the external oblique so that, during the same actions as outlined above (rotation to the left), the left internal oblique also contracts, palpable between the left iliac crest and the umbilicus.

Quadratus lumborum can be palpated either side of the vertebral column, between the twelfth rib above and the posterior part of the iliac crest below. It mostly lies deep to latissimus dorsi, but its anterior border can be palpated just posterior to the mid-axillary line. If the subject is lying prone and raises the head and shoulders, the muscle becomes easier to palpate.

In this region sacrospinalis (erector spinae) lies close to the spinous processes of the lumbar vertebrae, forming two firm columns of muscle passing from the posterior part of the iliac crest and sacrum below, to the angle of the ribs and transverse processes of the thoracic vertebrae. They become visible and palpable lateral to the lumbar spines when the subject raises the head and shoulders in a prone position.

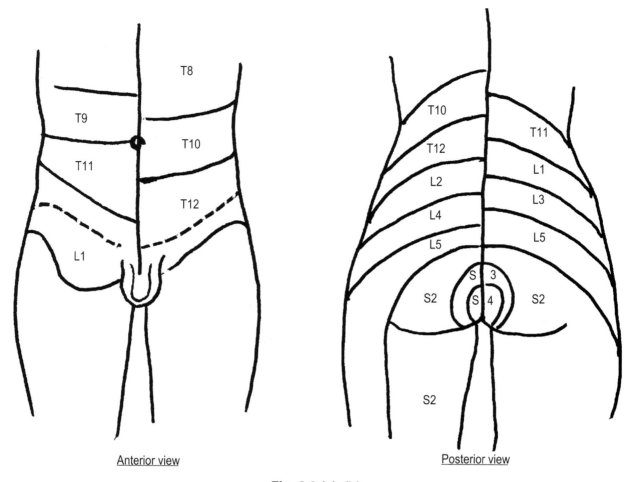

Anterior view   Posterior view

Fig. 6.6 (a), (b)
The cutaneous nerve supply

NERVES [Fig. 6.6a,b]

The nerve supply to the abdomen and lower limbs is derived from the thoracic 8–12, all five lumbar, all five sacral and the coccygeal nerve roots. The arrangement of these nerves is extremely complex (see *Anatomy and Human Movement*, Palastanga, Field and Soames 1998) and is dealt with here in outline only.

The thoracic nerves

Nerve roots T8–11 behave in a similar manner to intercostal nerves, supplying muscles in intercostal spaces and anteriorly contributing to the supply to the abdominal muscles. Their cutaneous branches follow the same general direction, supplying a band of skin running downwards and forwards.

The lumbar plexus

This is formed by part of T12 and L1–4. It supplies muscles of the lower abdomen, pelvis and front and inner side of the thigh. Its cutaneous supply is to the lower back and running downwards and forwards to the lower abdomen and the front and inner side of thigh and the inner side of the leg and foot.

The sacral plexus

Deriving its fibres from the ventral rami of L4, 5 and S1, 2, 3, 4, it supplies the muscles of the gluteal region, hamstrings, leg and foot. Its cutaneous supply is the gluteal region, back of the thigh, anterior, lateral and posterior aspects of the leg and plantar and dorsal aspects of the foot.

The coccygeal plexus supplies an area of skin around the anus.

The larger nerves of this region are situated deeply within the abdomen. Those of the lumbar plexus are formed within psoas major, while those of the sacral plexus mainly lie in front of the sacrum. All nerves that reach the surface of the abdominal and lumbar areas are too small to palpate. Nevertheless, these cutaneous nerves often influence their areas of distribution, with palpable signs such as changes in temperature and sweating. It is therefore important to study the plan of cutaneous distribution over the abdomen and lumbar area. There is, similar to the costal area, an overlap of root supply, each nerve covering an area of skin above and below.

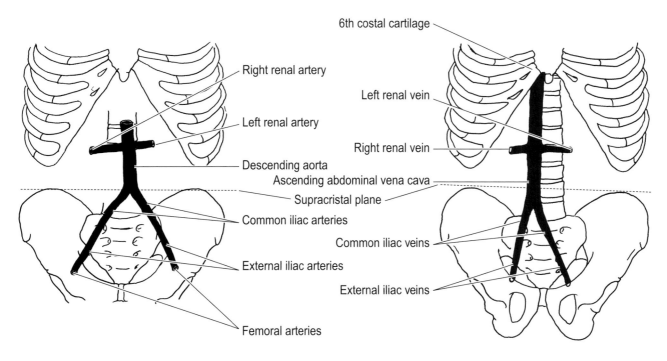

Fig. 6.6 (c)
Abdominal aorta and common iliac arteries

Fig. 6.6 (d)
Ascending abdominal vena cava and common iliac veins

ARTERIES [Fig. 6.6c]

All the larger arteries of the abdomen are also situated deeply within the abdominal cavity and are difficult or impossible to find. The pulsations of the abdominal aorta can be palpated in the supine subject if the fingers are pressed deeply to the left of the umbilicus, thereby compressing the abdominal aorta against the lumbar vertebral bodies. This technique is unpleasant for the subject, but can be improved by encouraging relaxation of the abdominal muscles. The abdominal aorta can be marked by a line drawn vertically from a point on the midline 2.5 cm above the transpyloric plane (see Fig. 6.7b) to a point just to the left of the midline 2.5 cm below the supracristal plane (Fig. 6.6c). Here it divides into the common iliac arteries which diverge from each other at an angle of approximately 37° to bifurcate again one vertebra below (lower border of the fifth lumbar vertebra) into the internal and external iliac arteries. The external iliac artery can be marked as it passes to the mid point of the inguinal ligament to be continued below the ligament as the femoral artery.

VEINS [Fig. 6.6d]

Again, all the large veins of the abdomen are deep within the cavity and impossible to palpate. It is, however, quite important to know where the abdominal portion of the inferior vena cava commences and leaves the abdominal cavity. It commences at the junction of the two common iliac veins at the level of the fourth lumbar vertebra and progresses upwards and slightly to the right, first accompanied on its left by the abdominal aorta. It leaves the abdominal cavity by passing behind the liver and through the diaphragm at the level of T8 (Fig. 6.6d).

The vena cava can be marked by a line 2.5 cm broad, commencing at a point just to the right of the midline 2.5 cm below the supracristal plane (lower body of the fourth lumbar vertebra), to a point just above the sixth costal cartilage on the right, where it passes through the vena caval opening in the tendinous portion of the diaphragm (Fig. 6.6d).

SELF ASSESSMENT

Page 358

1. List the muscles which surround the abdominal cavity.

2. Which muscle forms the upper boundary?

3. The floor of the pelvis is composed of which muscles? (fr)

4. State the general location of each of the above muscles.

5. What factors may hinder palpation of the abdominal muscles?

6. Name the fibrous line which runs down the front of the abdomen between the columns of muscle.

7. Which muscle forms the columns on either side of this line?

8. To what structures does this muscle attach above?

9. Describe its inferior attachment.

Page 359

10. In which area may fibrous intersections be palpated?

11. Which abdominal oblique muscles are brought into action when resistance is offered to upper trunk rotation to the left?

12. In which area may the quadratus lumborum be palpated?

13. Give the upper attachment of quadratus lumborum.(fr).

14. Where is it attached distally? (fr)

15. Which muscle lies superficial to the upper part of quadratus lumborum?

16. Describe the method whereby quadratus lumborum may be put into action.

17. Which muscle forms the two columns on either side of the spines of the lumbar vertebral column?

18. Describe the method whereby these muscular columns may be put into action.

Please complete the labels below.

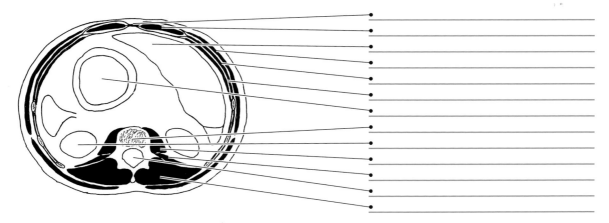

Fig. 6.5 (a) The abdomen

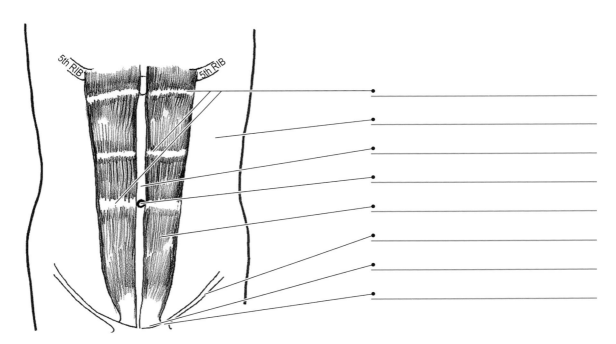

Fig. 6.5 (c) Muscles of the abdomen

SELF ASSESSMENT

Page 360

19. Which nerve roots are involved in supplying the abdomen and lower limbs?

20. Describe the route and distribution of a lower thoracic nerve.

21. Which nerve roots combine to form the lumbar plexus?

22. Outline the muscular supply of the lumbar plexus.

23. From which ventral rami does the sacral plexus derive its fibres?

24. List the muscles supplied from the sacral plexus.

25. Outline the cutaneous areas supplied by the sacral plexus.

26. Which nerve roots combine to form the coccygeal plexus?

27. Outline the cutaneous area supplied by the coccygeal plexus.

28. In which muscle is the lumbar plexus formed?

Page 361

29. Describe a method whereby the abdominal aorta may be palpated.

30. List the surface markings of the abdominal aorta.

31. Into which two arteries does the abdominal aorta divide?

32. Name the two arteries into which these two arteries bifurcate.

33. Specify the surface marking where the femoral artery emerges from the pelvis.

34. Why are the veins of the abdomen difficult to palpate?

35. At which vertebral level does this take place?

36. What accompanies the inferior vena cava as it passes through the abdomen?

37. Through which structures does it pass as it leaves the abdomen?

38. At which vertebral level does the inferior vena cava leave the abdomen?

39. Give the surface markings of the abdominal vena cava.

Please complete the labels below.

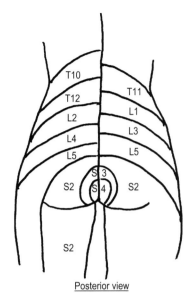

- _____
- _____
- _____
- _____
- _____
- _____
- _____
- _____
- _____
- _____

Fig. 6.6 (b) The cutaneous nerve supply

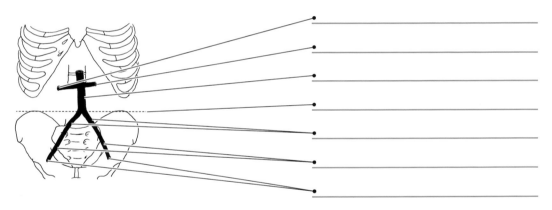

Fig. 6.6 (c) Abdominal aorta and common iliac arteries

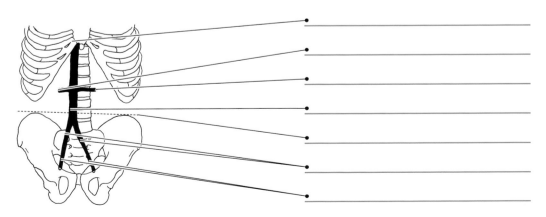

Fig. 6.6 (d) Ascending abdominal vena cava and common iliac veins

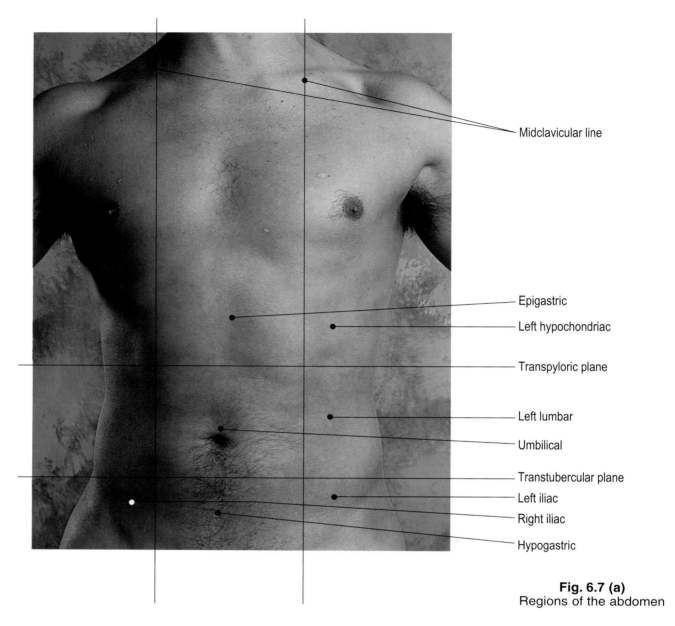

Midclavicular line

Epigastric

Left hypochondriac

Transpyloric plane

Left lumbar

Umbilical

Transtubercular plane

Left iliac

Right iliac

Hypogastric

Fig. 6.7 (a)
Regions of the abdomen

STRUCTURES WITHIN THE ABDOMINAL CAVITY

For convenient location of viscera, the abdomen may be divided into nine regions by two vertical and two horizontal lines (Fig. 6.7a, b). Other methods of dividing the abdomen into regions also exist but will not be covered here (Keogh and Ebbs 1984). The two vertical lines pass superiorly from the mid-inguinal point, which is halfway between the anterior superior iliac spine and the pubic tubercle, to the mid point of the clavicle. They are usually referred to as the midclavicular lines. The upper horizontal line is drawn level with the tip of the ninth costal cartilage: it crosses the tip of the twelfth rib and the spine of the first lumbar vertebra. This is known as the transpyloric plane, as it also passes through the pylorus of the stomach. The lower horizontal line is drawn across the abdomen between the tubercle of the crest of each ilium and is known as the transtubercular

plane (Fig. 6.7a,b). It crosses the vertebral column level with the upper portion of the body of L5, and may serve as a useful landmark when identification of lumbar vertebrae is necessary.

The three regions above the transpyloric plane are the right and left hypochondriac, with the epigastric centrally. The three regions between the transpyloric and transtubercular planes are the right and left lumbar, with the umbilical centrally, while the three lower regions are the right and left iliac, with the hypogastric centrally.

Organs in the abdominal cavity are normally quite movable, with some changing their shape and size according to their contents. This makes surface marking difficult and often unreliable. It is, however, important to be able to mark the areas in which the particular organ lies and note any fixed sites where markings are constant.

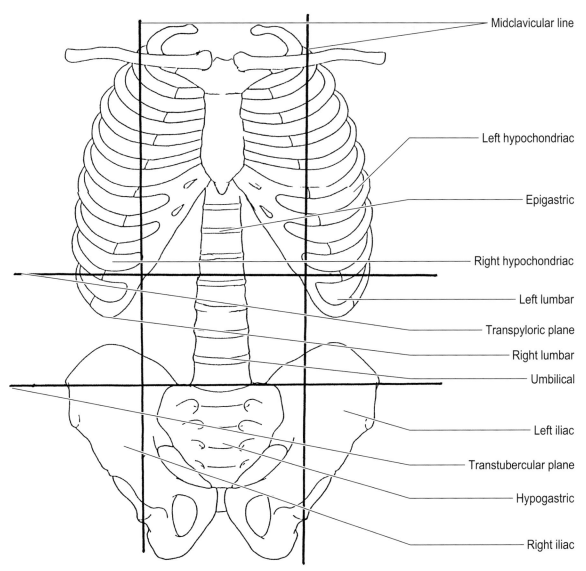

Midclavicular line

Left hypochondriac

Epigastric

Right hypochondriac

Left lumbar

Transpyloric plane

Right lumbar

Umbilical

Left iliac

Transtubercular plane

Hypogastric

Right iliac

Fig. 6.7 (b)
Regions of the abdomen

General locations

The liver lies mainly in the right hypochondriac and epigastric areas.

The spleen is located mainly in the left hypochondriac and extends posteriorly into the epigastric area.

The pancreas lies on the transpyloric plane between the epigastric and umbilical areas. The gall bladder again lies on the transpyloric plane where it crosses the right midclavicular line.

The stomach varies considerably in size but is normally in the left hypochondriac and umbilical areas.

The duodenum is partly in the umbilical and partly in the epigastric areas, the transpyloric plane passing through its second part.

The small intestine lies mainly in the hypogastric area.

The caecum and appendix lie in the right iliac region.

The large intestine passes through the right iliac and lumbar, umbilical, left lumbar and iliac areas and passes down through the hypogastric area.

The kidneys lie partly in the epigastric and partly in the umbilical areas.

The bladder lies behind the two pubic bones and pubic symphysis.

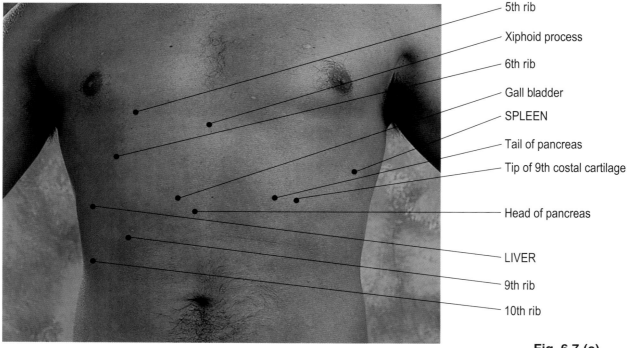

5th rib
Xiphoid process
6th rib
Gall bladder
SPLEEN
Tail of pancreas
Tip of 9th costal cartilage
Head of pancreas
LIVER
9th rib
10th rib

Fig. 6.7 (c)
The liver and spleen (anterior aspect)

The liver [Fig. 6.7c and d]

The liver is a large wedge-shaped organ situated mainly in the right hypochondriac and epigastric region of the abdomen just below the diaphragm. Its upper surface is moulded by the under surface of the diaphragm. The right side is thicker, narrowing as it passes towards the left. Posteriorly it is grooved by the inferior vena cava.

Surface markings

The position of the liver is fairly constant in healthy subjects. The upper boundary can be marked by a line drawn horizontally at the level of the xiphisternal joint, extending some 7 cm to the left of the midline and all the way round the right side of the thoracic cage. Its lower border is an oblique line beginning 7 cm to the left of the midline, crossing the left costal margin at the eighth costal cartilage, reaching the right costal margin at the ninth costal cartilage and continuing around the costal margin.

The spleen [Fig. 6.7c and d]

The spleen [*splen* (L) = spleen] is a reservoir for blood. It is soft and highly vascular and is just deep to the lower left ribs below the diaphragm and behind the stomach. In addition to the storage of blood, it is part of the reticuloendothelial system. It contains phagocytes which engulf micro-organisms, foreign particles and damaged cells. It is involved with the manufacture of white blood cells and in the infant it will also produce red blood cells.

The spleen lies under cover of the ribs, although it is an abdominal organ. This is due to the domes of the diaphragm rising into the thorax from its costal attachments.

The spleen lies posteriorly on the left side deep to the ninth, tenth and eleventh ribs, extending as far forwards as the mid-axillary line. It is approximately 10 cm long, 7 cm deep and 3–4 cm thick. Although it occasionally projects just below the costal margin, the spleen cannot usually be palpated unless it is enlarged to approximately three times its normal size. It is often ruptured in severe accidents where the chest is crushed and may well be overlooked. This will lead to large amounts of blood escaping into the abdominal cavity. The spleen can be removed without affecting the human body too seriously.

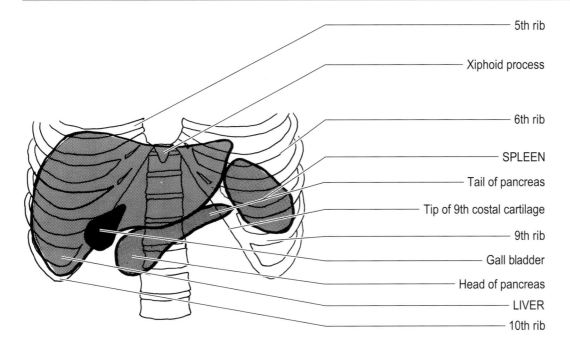

5th rib

Xiphoid process

6th rib

SPLEEN

Tail of pancreas

Tip of 9th costal cartilage

9th rib

Gall bladder

Head of pancreas

LIVER

10th rib

Fig. 6.7 (d)
The liver and spleen (anterior
aspect)

The pancreas [Fig. 6.7c and d]

The pancreas [*pan* (Gk) = all, *keras* (Gk) = flesh]
is a strangely shaped gland resembling a large
tadpole, having a head to the right with a body
and tail which narrows as it passes to the left.
It is approximately 10 cm long and 4 cm broad at
its head. It is situated anterior to the vertebral
column, level with the body of the first lumbar
vertebra. The head is surrounded by the four
sections of the duodenum, the pylorus of the
stomach lying anterior to the body. The pancreatic
duct passes from the head to the right, emptying
into the second part of the duodenum at a point
on the transpyloric plane 2 cm to the right of the
median line (Fig. 6.7c, d). Behind the body lie the
superior mesenteric and splenic veins; just below,
they form the portal vein. The head is related
posteriorly with the inferior vena cava and the
right crus of the diaphragm and the body lies just
in front of the abdominal aorta. The tail is related
to the spleen at its far left and with the stomach
anteriorly. The pancreas is not palpable in the
normal subject.

The gall bladder [Fig. 6.7c and d]

The gall bladder is a small reservoir, approximately
3 cm in diameter, with a short tail passing posteriorly. It is situated below the centre of the anterior
border of the liver, projecting a little below the
right costal margin deep to the costal angle level
with the ninth costal cartilage (Fig. 6.7c, d). In the
normal subject it is difficult to palpate. It dis-
charges bile through the bile duct into the second
part of the duodenum, which aids in the breakdown of fatty foods during digestion. Sometimes
stones are formed in the gall bladder and are
passed down the tortuous and sometimes narrowing tubes of the cystic and bile ducts. The blockage
of these tubes causes acute pain and often irritates
other structures in this area. If this is a recurring
problem, the gall bladder can be removed
(cholecystectomy).

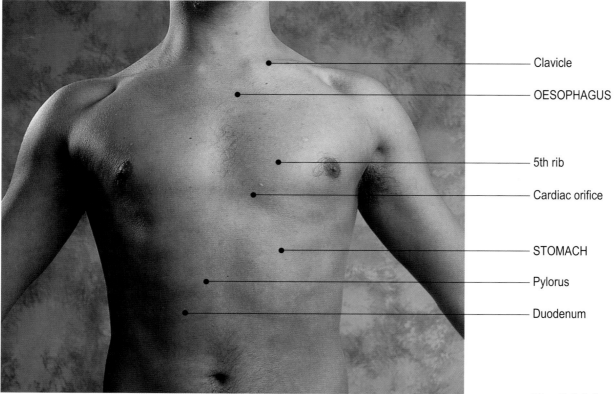

Clavicle

OESOPHAGUS

5th rib

Cardiac orifice

STOMACH

Pylorus

Duodenum

Fig. 6.8 (a)
The oesophagus, stomach and
duodenum

The stomach [Fig. 6.8]

The stomach [*stomachos* (Gk); the Greeks used this word for the gullet and the oesophagus, they later used '*gaster*' to denote the lower end] is a mobile, muscular, highly vascular container in the digestive system situated deep to the lower left rib cage, below the diaphragm, to the left of the liver and in front of the spleen. It receives food from the oesophagus [*oiso* (Gk) = I carry, *phagein* (Gk) = food] through its cardiac orifice into its upper part (the fundus) and after passing through the body of the stomach the partially digested food is passed on through the pylorus and pyloric orifice into the first part of the duodenum. It varies enormously in shape and size according to its contents. It is basically J-shaped, with its upper section being thicker and more expanded, while its lower end becomes narrower as it passes medially and slightly upwards, continuing as the first part of the duodenum.

A full stomach can be palpated as it extends below the rib cage on the left side and can be felt contracting and moving during the early part of digestion. An empty stomach is hidden beneath the rib cage.

Surface markings

Although the central section of the stomach varies in shape and size, its two openings – the cardiac and pyloric orifices – remain comparatively fixed. The former can be marked by a short oblique line, approximately 2 cm long, along the seventh costal cartilage 2.5 cm to the left of the midline, being level with the tip of the xiphoid process. The latter lies on the transpyloric plane 1.5 cm to the right of the midline. The fundus, or upper part of the stomach, may rise up as far as the fifth intercostal space 7 cm left of the midline or as far down as the tenth costal cartilage.

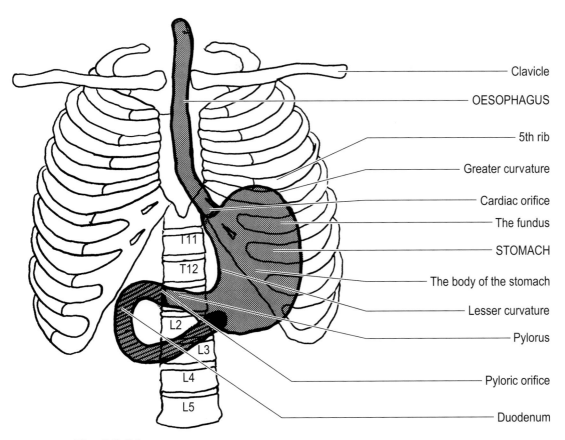

Fig. 6.8 (b)
The oesophagus, stomach and
duodenum

The lesser curvature of the stomach can be represented by a curved line, concave to the right, joining the cardiac and pyloric openings, while the greater curvature is represented by a line, convex to the left, joining the upper limit of the stomach at the fifth intercostal space to approximately the tenth costal cartilage (Fig. 6.8a, b).

The duodenum [Fig. 6.8]

The duodenum [*duoden arius* (L) = continuing twelve; Herophilus in 344 BC measured the duodenum as twelve finger breadths] is the continuation of the digestive tract beyond the pylorus of the stomach. It is approximately 25 cm long, passing initially upwards, backwards and to the right for 5 cm as far as the costal margin (first part), and then downwards to the left for 7.5 cm, to reach the level of the tenth costal cartilage (second part), across the front of the body of L3, passing upwards and to the left for approximately 10 cm (third part), and finally ascending for 2.5 cm (fourth part) to become continuous with the jejunum at the duodenojejunal flexure at the level of L2, 2 cm left of the mid line. The common bile duct and pancreatic duct drain into the duodenum midway along its second part.

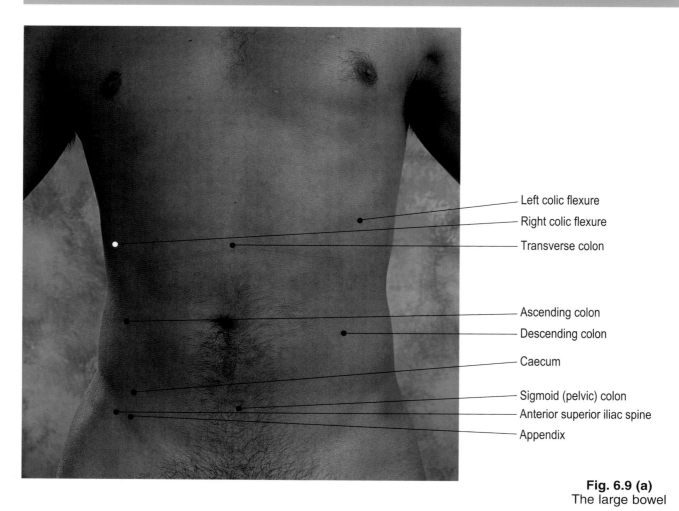

Left colic flexure
Right colic flexure
Transverse colon

Ascending colon
Descending colon

Caecum

Sigmoid (pelvic) colon
Anterior superior iliac spine
Appendix

Fig. 6.9 (a)
The large bowel

The small intestine

The small intestine is described in two parts, the first being termed the jejunum and the second, the ileum. The jejunum begins as a continuation of the duodenum (Fig. 6.8a, b) at the level of L2, 2 cm to the left of the midline and continues as the ileum which ends at its junction with the caecum (Fig. 6.9a, b) at the junction of the right mid-clavicular line with the transtubercular plane (drawn through the tubercles of the crest of the ilium). Each end is fixed in its position; the central portion, which may be up to 8 m long, is continually mobile. It is, however, contained within the confines of the large bowel.

The caecum [Fig. 6.9a and b]

The caecum [*caecus* (L) = blind; Galen confused the caecum with the appendix] is the first section of the large intestine and receives the contents of the small intestine. It fills the right iliac region of the abdomen, lying above the lateral half of the right inguinal ligament, with the appendix lying in the mid-clavicular line, 1.5 cm medial to the anterior superior iliac spine. The caecum and appendix are not palpable, but pressure applied to this region can be extremely painful, particularly if the appendix is inflamed.

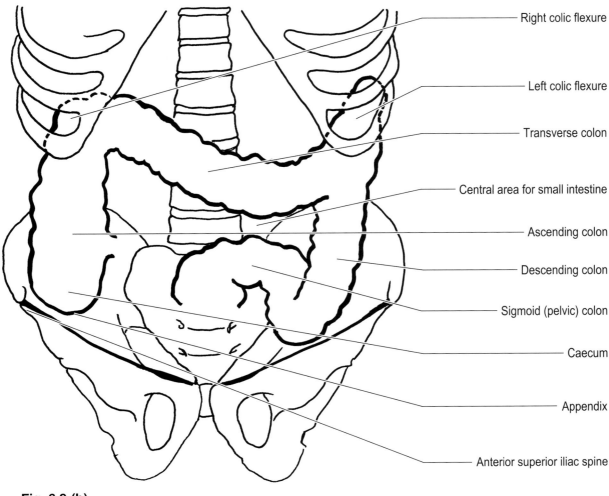

- Right colic flexure
- Left colic flexure
- Transverse colon
- Central area for small intestine
- Ascending colon
- Descending colon
- Sigmoid (pelvic) colon
- Caecum
- Appendix
- Anterior superior iliac spine

Fig. 6.9 (b)
The large bowel

The large intestine (large bowel)
[Fig. 6.9a and b]

For descriptive purposes, the large intestine is normally divided into four sections: ascending, transverse, descending and sigmoid (pelvic). It can be represented by a band, approximately 5 cm wide, but varies considerably according to its contents. The ascending colon commences in the right iliac region at the caecum and ascends through the right lumbar region, deep to the costal margin, to the level of the transpyloric plane, where it arches backwards and to the left, forming the right colic (hepatic) [*hepar* (Gk) = liver] flexure. The transverse colon passes from the colic flexure, across the umbilical region below the liver towards the spleen, where it turns downwards, forming the left colic (splenic) flexure just above the transpyloric plane. The descending colon passes through the left lumbar and iliac regions, turning backwards at the inguinal ligament to become the sigmoid [*sigma* (Gk) = letter C, *-oeides* (Gk) = shape, form] colon. This latter section passes backwards and downwards in an S-shaped curve to pass vertically downwards in front of the sacrum becoming the rectum. This is continuous with the anal canal and reaches the surface at the anus.

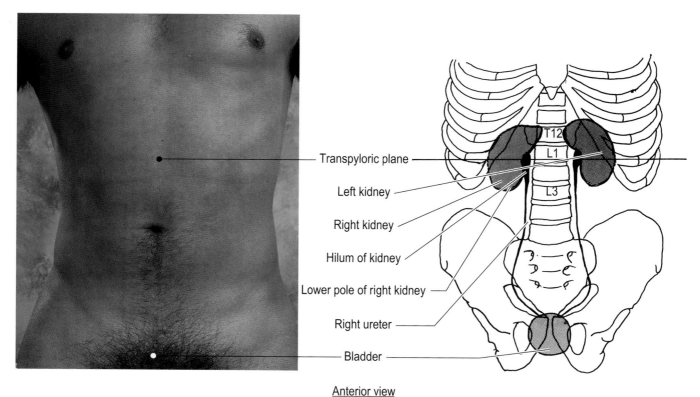

Transpyloric plane

Left kidney

Right kidney

Hilum of kidney

Lower pole of right kidney

Right ureter

Bladder

Anterior view

Fig. 6.10 (a), (b)
The kidneys, ureters and bladder

The kidneys [Fig. 6.10]

The kidneys are situated on the posterior abdominal wall anterior to quadratus lumborum behind the peritoneum. Each kidney lies obliquely with its anterior surface facing slightly laterally. The anterior relations of the right kidney are the right suprarenal gland and liver superiorly, the duodenum and right colic flexure inferomedially. The left kidney has the left suprarenal gland above, the tail of the pancreas and splenic vessels, the stomach and left colic flexure anteriorly, with the spleen postero-superiorly. Each kidney is related posteriorly to quadratus lumborum, the diaphragm, and the medial and lateral arcuate ligaments. The right kidney lies mainly in front of the twelfth rib, while the left lies anterior to the eleventh rib. Each kidney is approximately 11 cm in length, 6 cm broad and 3 cm thick. The hilum lies level with the spine of the first lumbar vertebra (the transpyloric plane), the right normally slightly lower than the left.

Surface markings

Each kidney can be located between two horizontal and two vertical lines, forming a rectangle either side of the vertebral column. The upper and lower limits of both kidneys lie between horizontal lines through the upper margin of T12 above and the L3 vertebra below. It may be easier to locate these lines if the following procedure is adopted: draw a horizontal line through the lower edge of the spine of L1; draw a second line 5.5 cm above this (i.e. level with the upper border of T12) and a third line 5.5 cm below (i.e. level with L3).

Because the two kidneys lie obliquely, the two vertical lines enclosing them are closer together than the width of the organ. Draw two vertical lines, one 3 cm and one 6.5 cm, lateral to the lumbar spines; these represent the medial and lateral margins of the kidneys.

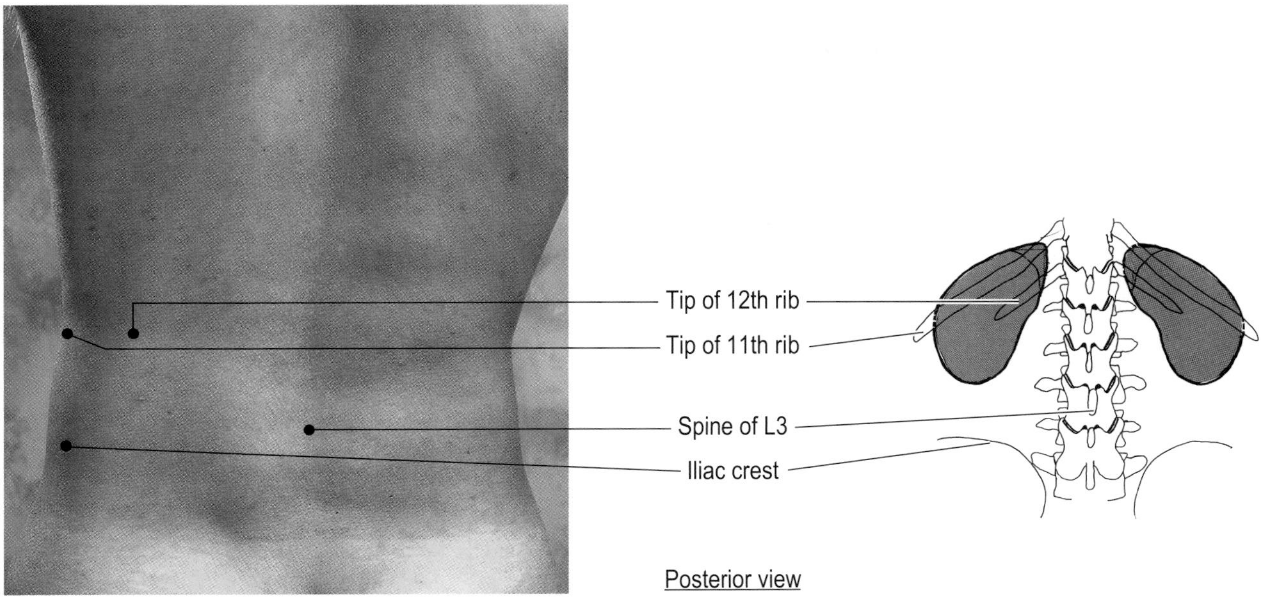

Tip of 12th rib
Tip of 11th rib
Spine of L3
Iliac crest

Posterior view

Fig. 6.10 (c), (d)
The kidneys

Palpation

The kidneys are well protected, lying anterior to the lower ribs and strong back muscles, below the diaphragm. The vertebral column, with the attachments of the crura of the diaphragm, lies between the two kidneys and the psoas major and minor lie behind them. The kidneys are protected in front by the large and small bowel and the powerful abdominal muscles. They are thus virtually impossible to palpate. However, the lower pole of the right kidney can be palpated with difficulty using deep pressure through a relaxed abdominal wall at a point just lateral to the vertical mid-clavicular line and just below the level of the tenth rib.

The bladder [Fig. 6.10a and b]

The bladder is a thin-walled muscular reservoir which varies in size according to the volume of fluid it contains. It is estimated that it is able to hold about 250 mL of urine before having to be emptied, but this estimate appears to be a little on the low side practically. Its volume obviously grows according to the frequency it is filled with large quantities of fluid.

The bladder is situated directly behind the two pubic bones and pubic symphysis, with its upper border reaching to the crest on either side. When full, however, it rises above the pubic rami by up to 5 cm.

The empty bladder is not palpable in the normal subject, but when full it can be felt as a soft swelling just above the pubic symphysis.

SELF ASSESSMENT

Page 366

1. For convenience of identification, the abdomen is normally divided into nine areas by four lines. Describe this process.

   _____

2. Name the vertical lines.

   _____

3. Through which structures does the upper horizontal line pass?

   _____

4. What name is given to this line?

   _____

5. Name the structures through which the inferior horizontal line passes.

   _____

6. By what name is this line known?

   _____

7. Give the locations of the vertical lines.

   _____

8. Name and locate each of these areas.

   _____

Page 367

9. With reference to the above lines and areas, describe the location of:

   a. the liver,

   _____

   b. spleen,

   _____

   c. pancreas,

   _____

   d. gall bladder,

   _____

   e. stomach,

   _____

   f. duodenum,

   _____

   g. small intestine,

   _____

   h. caecum,

   _____

   i. appendix,

   _____

   j. large intestine,

   _____

   k. kidneys,

   _____

   l. bladder.

   _____

Please complete the labels below.

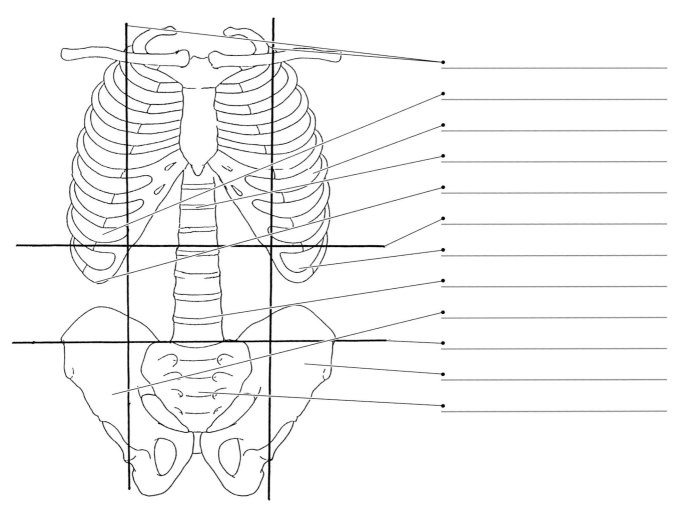

Fig. 6.7 (b) Regions of the abdomen

Page 368

10. Describe the general shape of the liver.

11. Describe the position of the liver in relation to other organs and structures.

12. By what structure is the liver grooved below?

13. List the surface markings of the liver.

14. Describe the shape of the spleen.

15. Identify the surface markings of the spleen.

16. Describe the position of the spleen in relation to other organs and structures.

17. List the functions performed by the spleen. (fr)

18. Describe the difference in these functions between the adult and the infant. (fr)

Page 369

19. Describe the shape of the pancreas.

20. Give the position of the pancreas in relation to other structures.

21. Explain the function of the pancreatic duct.

22. Name the structure to which it attaches.

23. List the surface markings of the pancreatic duct.

24. Which two veins unite to form the portal vein?

25. Describe the shape of the gall bladder.

26. Give its position in relation to other organs and structures.

27. List the surface markings of the gall bladder.

Please complete the labels below.

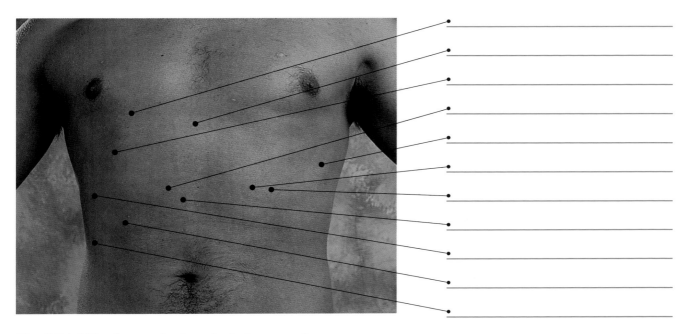

Fig. 6.7 (c) The liver and spleen (anterior aspect)

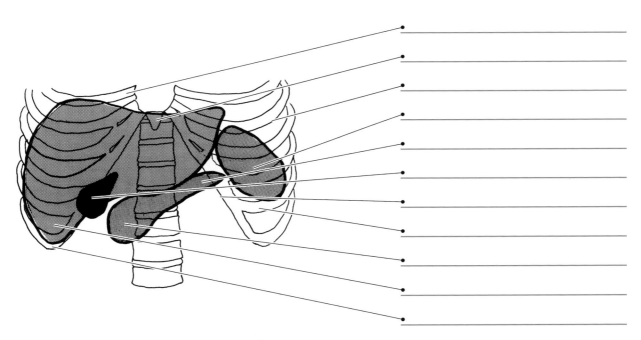

Fig. 6.7 (d) The liver and spleen (anterior aspect)

Page 370

28. Describe the general position of the stomach when empty.

_____

29. Explain how this position differs when the stomach is full.

_____

30. List the three regions of the stomach.

_____

31. Name the tubes and orifice through which food enters the stomach.

_____

32. Into which tube and through which orifice does the stomach empty?

_____

33. List the surface markings of the two orifices of the stomach.

_____

Page 371

34. Identify the length and direction of the four parts of the duodenum.

_____

35. With what structure does the fourth part of the duodenum become continuous?

_____

36. Identify the surface marking at which this occurs.

_____

37. What drains into the duodemum midway along its second part?

_____

38. What is the derivation and meaning of the word duodemum?

_____

39. Which gland is surrounded by the four parts of the duodenum?

_____

Page 372

40. By which names are the first and second part of the small intestine known?

_____

41. Approximately, how long is the small intestine?

_____

42. Identify the surface markings where the small intestine meets the caecum.

_____

43. Describe the location of the caecum.

_____

44. What is the derivation and meaning of the word caecum?

_____

45. Identify the surface markings of the appendix.

_____

Please complete the labels below.

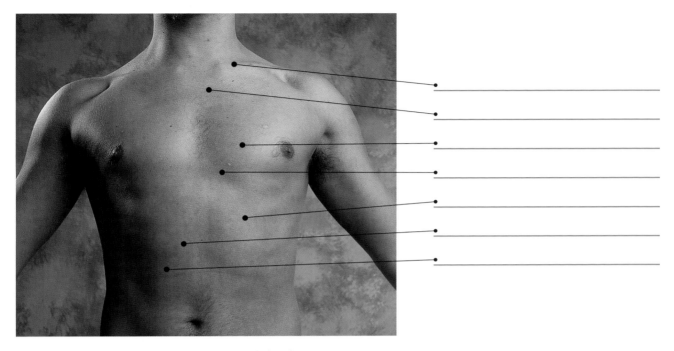

Fig. 6.8 (a) The oesophagus, stomach and duodenum

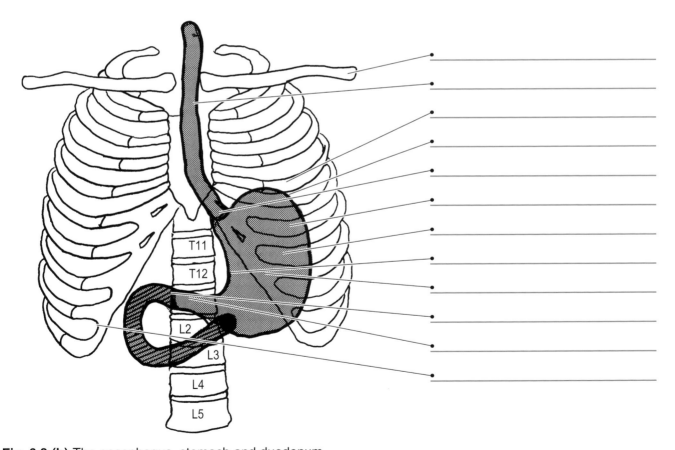

Fig. 6.8 (b) The oesophagus, stomach and duodenum

Page 373

46. List the four sections of the large intestine.

47. Describe the general position of each section.

48. What are the hepatic and splenic flexures?

49. Into what tube does the final part of the large intestine empty?

Page 374

50. What structures lie immediately in front and behind the kidneys?

51. List the other structures which lie close to the left kidney.

52. What other structures lie close to the right kidney?

53. Which ribs lie posterior to the kidneys?

54. In centimetres, what is the approximate size of each kidney?

55. At which vertebral level does the hilum of the kidney lie?

56. List the surface markings of both kidneys.

57. Explain why the two vertical lines of the surface markings are slightly closer together than the breadth of the actual kidneys.

58. Name the tubes through which urine is passed to the bladder. (fr)

59. How and where can the lower pole of the right kidney possibly be palpated?

Page 375

60. In which region of the body is the bladder situated?

61. Describe its structure.

62. How much urine is it estimated that the bladder can contain before having to be emptied?

63. Give the surface markings of the bladder.

64. Is it possible to palpate the bladder?

Please complete the labels below.

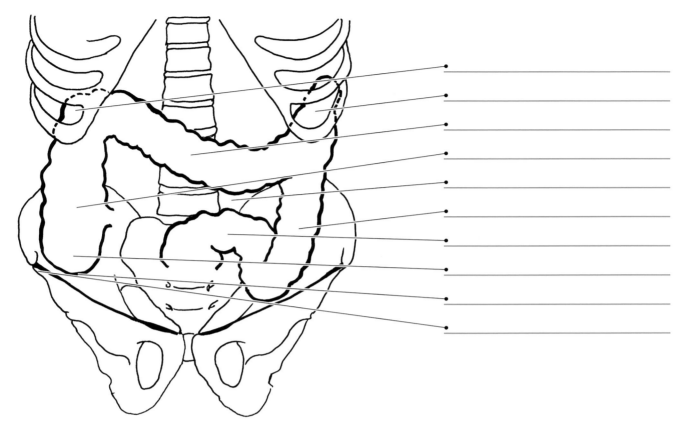

Fig. 6.9 (b) The large bowel

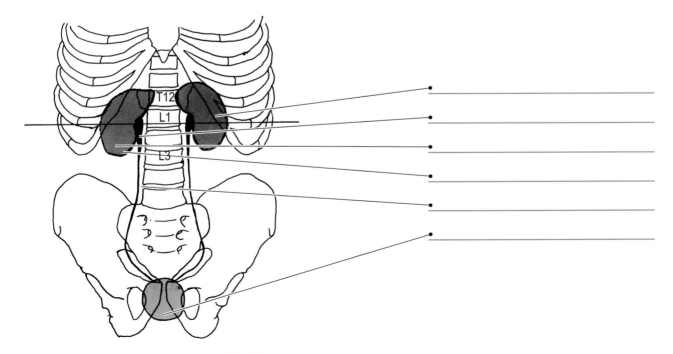

Fig. 6.10 (b) The kidneys, ureters and bladder

7
Conclusion

Although the major part of this book is devoted to encouraging readers to acquire anatomical knowledge through familiarization with the surface markings of underlying tissues, its principle aim is to promote the development of manual skills to improve clinical practice. If the suggested manoeuvres have been carried out, a thorough knowledge of the surface markings will have been gained together with an increased awareness of the sense of touch and the consequent improvement of palpation techniques. This knowledge will be invaluable to all practitioners during their subsequent clinical practice.

These palpation skills will, of course, be developed further with regular practice in which exploration of the basic techniques can take place. Regular evaluation and modification of all techniques will be crucial if improvement in performance is to be achieved. Indeed, the benefits of continually upgrading palpation skills extend far beyond the clinical setting. The activities of many skilled craftspeople provide excellent examples of highly developed manual skills. It may be useful to consider the following examples in which observation of the activities of craftspeople confirms their awareness of the importance of tactile input and the high level of skill in manual dexterity:

• the care with which a carpenter approaches the task of preparing and working on a piece of wood
• the attention to detail demonstrated by a dressmaker when selecting appropriate material prior to creating a particular garment
• the respect of a potter for a piece of clay
• the fine dexterity of the gardener's fingers when pricking out seedlings
• the careful smoothing and moulding carried out by a tailor when fitting a suit
• the care with which a hairdresser handles the hair of a client.

It is evident from the above examples that these craftspeople have great reverence for the materials with which they work. In the case of the hairdresser, the recipient gains something from the interaction which is far more subtle and psychologically significant than the experience of physical contact would initially suggest.

This is also true within the clinical context. Observation of the care and sensitivity with which a physiotherapist handles a painful limb confirms the intrinsic value of acquiring expertise in manual techniques. Most recipients acknowledge the importance of, and pleasure associated with, this physical contact and many recognize and express appreciation of its psychological benefits. The value of such non-verbal communication can never be underestimated. The gripping of a hand, an arm around the shoulder or a touch on the elbow can all be comforting to a person who is under some stress. All convey empathy and understanding and sometimes represent the only means by which such feelings can be effectively conveyed to the recipient.

As stated in Chapter 1, the art of palpation involves a combination of the appropriate use of touch, the application of methodical investigatory techniques, accurate interpretation of sensory feedback (based upon sound general knowledge), the ability to draw on previous experience, to reflect, critically, upon findings and arrive at a reasoned conclusion. The acquisition of this skill provides the therapist with valuable supplementary information to that which can be obtained through observation and verbal questioning and is crucial to arriving at a meaningful clinical diagnosis. Not until the practitioner becomes skilled at being able to 'read' the patient, however, can this art be regarded as having been fully developed. In order to help those with whom professionals have the privilege to come into contact, clinicians need to strive towards making conscious those processes which, in so many practitioners, often remain unconscious. By developing the sense of touch through the practise of palpation skills, we come closer to attaining this ideal.

The objective of this book is to inspire readers to improve their clinical practice by developing an expertise in palpation skills. All too often, evidence suggests that these skills remain underused and under-valued by professionals involved in the care and treatment of patients, not forgetting animals. Our experience confirms that the benefits of pursuing this form of study far outweigh the perceived drawbacks in terms of time and effort. Communication through touch has the potential to reveal information that may otherwise remain undiscovered: its power should never be underestimated and its status in relation to therapeutic practice should never be undermined.

References and further reading

Bayne R, Nicolson P, Horton I (eds) 1998 Counselling and Communication Skills for Medical and Health Practitioners. BPS Books, Leicestershire

Chairman R (ed) 2000 Complementary Therapies for Physical Therapists. Butterworth Heinemann, Oxford

Chaitow L 2003 Palpation and Assessment Skills: Assessment and Diagnosis Through Touch (2nd edn.), Churchill Livingstone, Edinburgh

Christensen N, Jones M, Edwards I 2004 Clinical reasoning in the diagnosis and management of spinal pain In: Boyling J, Jull G (eds) Grieve's Modern Manual Therapy: The Vertebral Column (3rd edn.) Churchill Livingstone, Edinburgh, pp 391–403

Dennis M, Jones C, Holey E 1995 Complementary Medicine In: Everett T, Dennis M, Ricketts E (eds) Physiotherapy in Mental Health: a Practical Approach. Butterworth-Heinemann, Oxford, pp 252–280

Evans D 2000 The reliability of assessment parameters: accuracy and palpation techniques. In: Boyling J, Palastanga N (eds) Grieve's Modern Manual Therapy: the Vertebral Column, 2nd edn. Churchill Livingstone, Edinburgh, pp 539–546

Evrett T 1997 Psychological treatment in physiotherapy practice. In French S (ed) Physiotherapy: a Psychosocial Approach, 2nd edn. Butterworth-Heinemann, Oxford pp 421–432

Field E J, Harrison R J 1974 Anatomical Terms: Their Origin and Derivation. W Heffer, Cambridge

Grieve G 1986 Modern Manual Therapy of the Vertebral Column. Churchill Livingstone, Edinburgh

Guyton A C 1991 Medical Physiology, 6th edn. WB Saunders, Philadephia, pp 605–606

Hengeveld E, Banks K (eds) 2005 Maitland's Peripheral Manipulation, 4th edn. Elsevier, Edinburgh

Hinkle C 1997 Fundamentals of Anatomy and Movement: a Workbook and Guide. Mosby, St. Louis

Keogh B, Ebbs S 1984 Normal Surface Anatomy. Heinemann, London

Krieger D 1986 The Therapeutic Touch: How to use Your Hands to Help or Heal, Prentice Hall, New York

Krieger D 1993 Accepting Your Power to Heal: the Personal Practice of Therapeutic Touch. Bear, Vermont

Krieger D 1997 Therapeutic Touch: Inner Workbook. Bear, New Mexico

Krieger D 2002 Therapeutic Touch as Transpersonal Healing. Lantern Books, New York

Macrae J 1987 Therapeutic Touch: A Practical Guide, Alfred A Knoff, New York

MacWhanell 1992 Communication in physiotherapy. In: French S (ed.) Physiotherapy: a Psychosocial Approach. Butterworth-Heinemann, Oxford

Magee D 1997 Orthopedic Physical Assessment, 3rd edn. WB Saunders, Philadelphia

Maitland A D 1991 Peripheral Manipulation, 3rd edn. Butterworth-Heinemann, Oxford

Mason A 1985 Something to do with touch. Physiotherapy, 71:167–169

Montague A 1978 Touching: the Human Significance of Skin, 2nd edn. Harper and Row, New York

Nathan B 1999 Touch and Emotion in Manual Therapy. Churchill Livingstone, Edinburgh

Owen Hutchinson J 2004 Health, health education and physiotherapy practice. In: French S, Sim J (eds) Physiotherapy: a Psychosocial Approach, 3rd edn. Elsevier, Edinburgh, pp 25–43

Owen Hutchinson J, Atkinson K, Orpwood J 1998 Breaking Down Barriers: Access to Further and Higher Education for Visually Impaired Students. Stanley Thornes, Gloucestershire

Palastanga N, Field D, Soames R 2004 Anatomy and Human Movement: Structure and Function, 4th edn. Elsevier, Edinburgh

Phillips N 2004 Motor learning. In: Trew M, Everett T (eds) Human Movement: an Introductory Text, 4th edn. Churchill Livingstone, Edinburgh, pp 129–141

Poon K 1995 Touch and handling. In: Everett T, Dennis M, Ricketts E (eds) Physiotherapy in Mental Health: a Practical Approach. Butterworth-Heinemann, Oxford, pp 91–101

Porter S 2002 The Anatomy Workbook. Butterworth Heinemann, Oxford

Ramsden E (ed) 1999 The Person as Patient: Psychological Perspectives for the Health Care Professional. WB Saunders, London

Sayre-Adams J, Wright S 2001 Therapeutic Touch. Churchill Livingstone, Edinburgh

Standing S (ed) 2004 Gray's Anatomy: the Anatomical Basis of Clinical Practice, 39th edn. Churchill Livingstone, Edinburgh

Stevenson C, Grieves M, Stein-Parbury 2004 Patient and Person: Empowering Interpersonal Relationships in Nursing. Elsevier, Oxford

Sunderland S 1978 Nerves and Nerve Injuries, 2nd edn. Churchill Livingstone, Edinburgh, p 355

Index